CHEST RADIOLOGY

Patterns and Differential Diagnoses

Seventh Edition

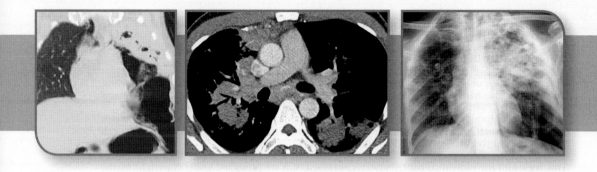

CHEST RADIOLOGY
Patterns and Differential Diagnoses

James C. Reed, MD

Professor of Radiology
University of Louisville
Louisville, Kentucky

ELSEVIER

ELSEVIER

1600 John F. Kennedy Blvd.
Ste 1800
Philadelphia, PA 19103-2899

Notices

Knowledge and best practice in this field are constantly changing. As new research and experience broaden our understanding, changes in research methods, professional practices, or medical treatment may become necessary.

Practitioners and researchers must always rely on their own experience and knowledge in evaluating and using any information, methods, compounds, or experiments described herein. In using such information or methods, they should be mindful of their own safety and the safety of others, including parties for whom they have a professional responsibility.

With respect to any drug or pharmaceutical products identified, readers are advised to check the most current information provided (i) on procedures featured or (ii) by the manufacturer of each product to be administered, to verify the recommended dose or formula, the method and duration of administration, and contraindications. It is the responsibility of practitioners, relying on their own experience and knowledge of their patients, to make diagnoses, to determine dosages and the best treatment for each individual patient, and to take all appropriate safety precautions.

To the fullest extent of the law, neither the Publisher nor the authors, contributors, or editors assume any liability for any injury and/or damage to persons or property as a matter of products liability, negligence, or otherwise or from any use or operation of any methods, products, instructions, or ideas contained in the material herein.

Previous editions copyrighted 2011, 2003, 1997, 1991, 1987, 1981 by Mosby, Inc., an affiliate of Elsevier Inc.

Library of Congress Cataloging-in-Publication Data
Names: Reed, James C. (James Croft), 1942- author.
Title: Chest radiology : patterns and differential diagnoses / James C. Reed.
Description: Seventh edition. | Philadelphia, PA : Elsevier, [2018] |
   Previous editions have subtitle: Plain film patterns and differential
   diagnoses. | Includes bibliographical references and index.
Identifiers: LCCN 2017043419 | ISBN 9780323498319 (hardcover : alk. paper)
Subjects: | MESH: Radiography, Thoracic | Diagnosis, Differential |
   Respiratory Tract Diseases--diagnostic imaging
Classification: LCC RC941 | NLM WF 975 | DDC 617.5/40757--dc23
LC record available at https://lccn.loc.gov/2017043419

Executive Content Strategist: Robin Carter
Senior Content Development Specialist: Rae Robertson
Publishing Services Manager: Catherine Albright Jackson
Senior Project Manager: Doug Turner
Designer: Maggie Reid

Printed in China

Last digit is the print number: 9   8   7   6   5   4   3   2   1

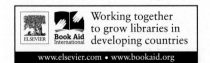

Working together
to grow libraries in
developing countries

www.elsevier.com • www.bookaid.org

Thank you to my wife, Sharon,
for the support and encouragement that have made it possible
for this text to reach a seventh edition.

This edition is dedicated to our grandchildren:
Samantha, Hailey, Zachary, James III, Morgan, Connor, Madeline, and Andrew

PREFACE

Chest radiology is sometimes considered to be the static part of a radiology practice, but chest radiology has shared the benefits of the imaging revolution. The chest x-ray contains a lot of information that is compressed into one or two images compared with several hundred images in a complete chest computed tomography (CT) examination with axial, coronal, and sagittal images. Chest CT provides a better understanding of chest disease and has become an important part of chest radiology. CT has added new descriptive patterns to our lexicon, including ground glass opacities, ground glass nodules, mosaic perfusion, and crazy paving. Special CT protocols such as high-resolution CT and CT angiography have given us the ability to make more specific diagnoses. The impact of magnetic resonance imaging and ultrasound are more limited because of the air in the lungs, but they also have important thoracic applications.

Continued medical progress and our collaborations with colleagues in medicine, surgery, and pathology have enhanced our understanding of chest diseases. By combining our new understanding of tumor biology with technical advancements, new imaging strategies such as low-dose CT screening for lung cancer have been developed.

Over the course of seven editions of this text there have been many changes in chest radiology, but a patient with chest symptoms still almost always has a chest x-ray as a first examination. Evaluation of the chest x-ray continues to require accurate perception of the abnormalities, recognition of the basic patterns, and development of a working differential diagnosis.

James C. Reed, MD

ACKNOWLEDGMENTS

A special thank you to Mr. Danny McGrath for assistance with production of the new digital illustrations and Ms. Lisa Floore for technical assistance and advice on manuscript preparation.

James C. Reed, MD

CONTENTS

PART 3 Hyperlucent Abnormalities

PART 1

Chest Wall, Pleura, and Mediastinum

1 | INTRODUCTION

The simplicity of performing a chest radiograph often leads to the mistaken impression that interpretation should also be a simple task. Despite the fact that the chest radiograph was one of the first radiologic procedures available to the physician, the problems of interpreting chest radiographs continue to be perplexing as well as challenging. The volume of literature on the subject indicates the magnitude of the problem and documents the many advances that have been made in this subspecialty of radiology. A casual review of the literature quickly reveals the frustrations a radiologist encounters in evaluating the numerous patterns of chest disease. There are as many efforts to define the patterns identified on chest radiographs as there are critics of the pattern approach. Because radiologists basically view the shadows of gross pathology, it is not surprising that the patterns are frequently nonspecific and that those who expect to find a one-to-one histologic correlation of the radiographic appearances with the microscopic diagnosis will be frustrated. It is much more important to develop an understanding of gross pathology to predict which patterns are likely in a given pulmonary disease. With this type of understanding of pulmonary diseases, we are better qualified to use nonspecific patterns in developing a differential diagnosis and planning the procedures required to make a definitive diagnosis.

Colonel William LeRoy Thompson of the Armed Forces Institute of Pathology first developed the concept of differential diagnosis based on radiologic findings. Later, Reeder and Felson amplified and popularized the approach in their book *Gamuts in Radiology* by providing an extensive list of the various patterns and the corresponding differential diagnoses.[467]

This manual illustrates the common patterns of chest disease to facilitate recognition. After recognition, the second step in evaluating a pattern is to develop an appropriate differential diagnosis. The complete differential diagnosis must include all of the major categories of disease (Chart 1.1) that might lead to the identified pattern. Next, the differential must be significantly narrowed by (1) careful analysis of the image for additional radiologic findings, (2) consideration of the evolving patterns of the disease by review of serial examinations, and (3) correlation of patterns with clinical and

---

Chart 1.1	**CATEGORIES OF DISEASES**

   I. Congenital/developmental
  II. Inflammatory
 III. Neoplastic
 IV. Traumatic
  V. Vascular
     A. Thromboembolic
     B. Cardiovascular
     C. Collagen-vascular
 VI. Iatrogenic
VII. Idiopathic

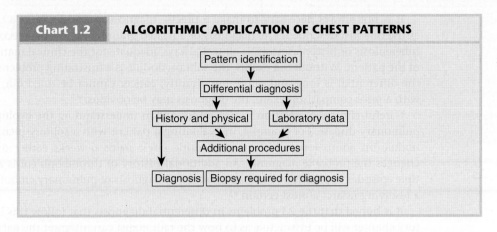

Chart 1.2   **ALGORITHMIC APPLICATION OF CHEST PATTERNS**

laboratory data (Chart 1.2). With this narrowed differential, we will be able to function as consultants, suggesting further procedures that may lead to a precise diagnosis. These procedures vary from simple radiographic examinations, such as those taken with the patient in oblique positions, to percutaneous biopsy under fluoroscopic, computed tomography (CT), or ultrasound guidance.

A radiologist should have a thorough understanding of the radiologic differential diagnosis to determine appropriate procedures for investigating diseases of the chest. It should be obvious that the first step in evaluating many abnormalities identified on the standard posterior-anterior (PA) and lateral chest radiograph is to confirm that the abnormality is real. A newcomer to radiology frequently forgets the value of simple techniques such as reviewing examinations taken in oblique positions, PA chest radiographs with nipple markers, fluoroscopy, full chest lordotic views, and, most important, old exams. These simple procedures should be used to confirm the presence of an abnormality before considering more complicated procedures such as radionuclide scanning, arteriography, CT scanning, magnetic resonance imaging (MRI), or biopsy. In fact, the latter procedures are special procedures that should be undertaken to answer specific questions.

After deciding that an observation is a true abnormality, one of the most important radiologic decisions to be made is to localize the abnormality. Localization to soft tissues, chest wall, pleura, diaphragm, mediastinum, hilum, peripheral vessels, or the lung parenchyma is absolutely necessary before a logical differential diagnosis can be developed. Once the suspected abnormality is localized to a specific anatomic site, it is necessary to classify or describe the pattern. Some of the patterns of parenchymal lung disease considered in this text are nodules, masses, diffuse opacities, cavities, calcifications, and atelectasis. If the pattern is nonspecific, a moderately long differential must be offered. As mentioned earlier, one of the objectives of this manual is to further refine pattern analysis and develop methods of improving diagnostic specificity. For example, in the analysis of parenchymal lung disease, assessment of the distribution—deciding whether the process is localized or diffuse, peripheral or central, in the upper vs. lower lobes, or alveolar vs. interstitial—is extremely helpful. In correlating these features, we are able to eliminate a number of possible diagnoses from initial consideration. Once the differential has been narrowed on the basis of identification of the disease pattern and distribution, examination of old exams is valuable. Unfortunately, a common mistake is oversight of the very dynamic changes in the patterns of chest disease. A typical case history may be as follows:

This is the first admission for this patient, and therefore the first chest radiograph examination. The knowledge that a solitary nodule was present on an exam taken 2 years earlier at another hospital, or even 5 or 10 years earlier at still other hospitals, could completely resolve the problem of how to manage the patient.

It is not always necessary to make a precise diagnosis, particularly in a case such as the one just described. The diagnosis of a healed granuloma, whether secondary to tuberculosis or histoplasmosis, is almost always adequate for the clinical management of the patient. Without old exams, the solitary nodule is a frustrating problem because the differential is long and, more importantly, cancer cannot be ruled out, whereas with a prior comparison exam, the diagnosis may be obvious.[469]

Careful clinical correlation is also important in understanding the evolution of a pulmonary disease. For example, in evaluating a patient with a solitary pleural-based nodule on admission, a history of pleuritic chest pains 6 weeks earlier drastically changes the probable diagnosis. An additional history of thrombophlebitis and multiple episodes of pleuritic chest pain makes the diagnosis of pulmonary embolism with a resolving infarct almost certain.[637]

It is hoped that the 23 problems in differential diagnosis that follow this introductory chapter will be instructive as to how the radiologist can interpret the pattern on a single chest radiograph, consider a moderately long differential diagnosis, narrow the differential diagnosis to a shortlist of most likely possibilities, and make recommendations for further procedures, leading to a definitive diagnosis.

2 | CHEST WALL LESIONS

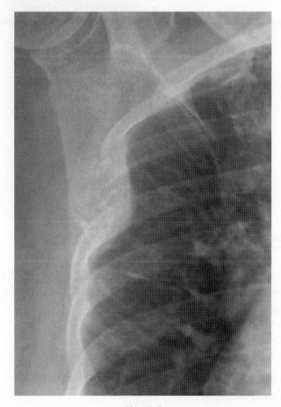

Fig. 2.1

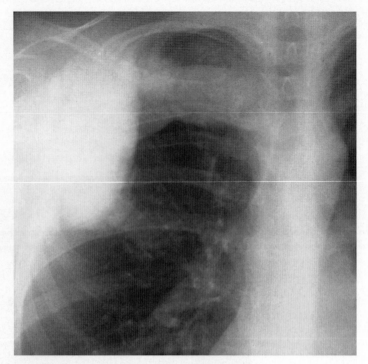

Fig. 2.2

QUESTIONS

1. The most likely diagnosis in the afebrile patient in Fig. 2.1 is:
   a. Neurofibroma.
   b. Lipoma.
   c. Multiple myeloma.
   d. Osteosarcoma.
   e. Chondrosarcoma.

2. The most likely diagnosis in Fig. 2.2 is:
   a. Ewing sarcoma.
   b. Osteosarcoma.
   c. Chondrosarcoma.
   d. Metastatic lung cancer.
   e. Plasmacytoma.

Mark the following questions **True** *or* **False:**

3. _____ Chest wall lesions may sometimes be distinguished from pulmonary nodules by identification of an incomplete border.

4. _____ Lipoma is a common chest wall lesion.

5. _____ Neurofibroma of an intercostal nerve will probably cause rib destruction.

6. _____ Rib detail views or computed tomography (CT) scans are rarely needed to identify the rib destruction of a primary bone tumor in the chest wall.

7. _____ Metastases and multiple myeloma are among the most common causes of a chest wall mass with associated rib destruction in an adult.

8. _____ Ewing tumor and neuroblastoma should be considered when a chest wall mass is observed in a child or young adult.

Chart 2.1	**PATTERN: CHEST WALL LESIONS**

I. Nipples,[387] supernumerary nipples[206]

II. Artifact

III. Skin lesions (e.g., moles, neurofibromas, extrathoracic musculature)[88]

IV. Mesenchymal tumors (muscle tumors, fibromas, lipomas,[137] liposarcoma,[63] desmoid tumor,[109] synovial sarcoma[191])

V. Neural tumors (schwannoma,[459] neurofibroma, ganglioneuroma, neuroblastoma[580])

VI. Hodgkin and non-Hodgkin lymphoma[438]

VII. Vascular tumors (angiosarcoma, glomus tumor, hemangioma, Kaposi sarcoma)[63,352,579,580]

VIII. Benign bone tumors (fibrous dysplasia, osteochondroma, giant cell tumor, aneurysmal bone cyst, fibroma, chondromyxoid fibroma)[579]

IX. Malignant bone tumors (metastases,[325] multiple myeloma, plasmacytoma [solitary myeloma])[580]

X. Ewing sarcoma, chondrosarcoma,[419] osteosarcoma,[191] fibrosarcoma, malignant undifferentiated pleomorphic sarcoma

XI. Hematoma

XII. Rib fractures

XIII. Infection (actinomycosis,[618] aspergillosis,[14] nocardiosis, blastomycosis, tuberculosis, empyema necessitans, osteomyelitis [rare])[210]

XIV. Thoracopulmonary small cell (Askin) tumor[157]

XV. Invasion by contiguous mass (lung cancer)[167,313]

XVI. Lymphangioma (cystic hygroma)

Discussion

Chest wall lesions (Chart 2.1) may arise from both extrathoracic and intrathoracic locations as well as normal and abnormal structures. Common extrathoracic causes of radiographically visible opacities include nipples, moles, and various cutaneous lesions (e.g., neurofibromas of von Recklinghausen disease).[155,535] Extrathoracic chest wall opacities are seen as soft-tissue opacities with an incomplete, sharp border (Fig. 2.3). The border is produced by the interface of the mass with air and is lost where the mass is continuous with the soft tissues of the chest wall. Cutaneous lesions should not have the tapered borders that are seen in Fig. 2.1. The tapered border indicates displacement of the pleura inward by the mass and has been described as an extrapleural sign.[151] Physical examination is also essential in the evaluation of cutaneous lesions. Nipple shadows may be easily identified when they are symmetric and when their borders are incomplete, but caution is warranted.[387] Repeat examination with small, lead nipple markers should be performed if there is any possibility of confusing a nipple shadow with a pulmonary nodule.

Intrathoracic chest wall lesions are radiologically visible because of their interface with aerated lung. Like the cutaneous lesions, their borders are incomplete where they are contiguous with the chest wall.[132] Thus the incomplete border is helpful in distinguishing chest wall lesions from pulmonary lesions (answer to question 3 is *True*), but not in distinguishing cutaneous from intrathoracic chest wall lesions. The tapered superior and inferior borders, however, are valuable signs for confirming an intrathoracic extrapulmonary location. Unfortunately, the tapered border may not be observed if the lesion is seen *en face*; in fact, the lesion may not be visible. Lateral and oblique cone-down views are frequently helpful in eliciting this sign.

Lipomas are common chest wall lesions[313] and may be seen as either subcutaneous or intrathoracic masses (Fig. 2.4, *A*). (Answer to question 4 is *True*.) They may even grow between the ribs, presenting as both intrathoracic and subcutaneous masses.

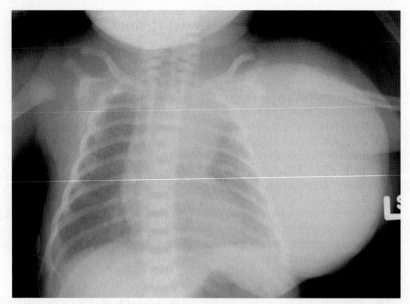

Fig. 2.3 This large, left mass has a sharp lateral border because it is outlined by air, but has no medial border illustrating the incomplete border sign. The mass is obviously outside of the rib cage and easily identified as a chest wall mass. Physical examination revealed this to be a soft, pliable mass in this neonate, making lymphangioma the most likely diagnosis.

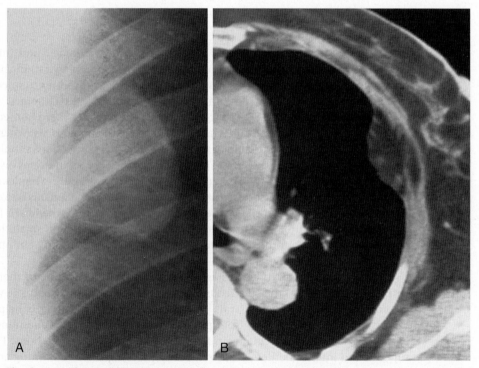

Fig. 2.4 **A,** Chest wall lipoma appears to be of tissue opacity, in contrast to aerated lung. Location of lipoma against the lateral chest wall and its incomplete border (sharp medial but absent lateral border) suggest that it is nonpulmonary. There is no rib destruction to confirm chest wall origin. Both chest wall and pleural masses should be considered in differential. **B,** Computed tomography scan of another patient with a chest wall lipoma shows a mass that is of greater opacity than the aerated lung but less opaque than the musculature of the chest wall. This intermediate fat attenuation mass is shown to extend through chest wall muscles. (Case courtesy of Thomas L. Pope, Jr., M.D.)

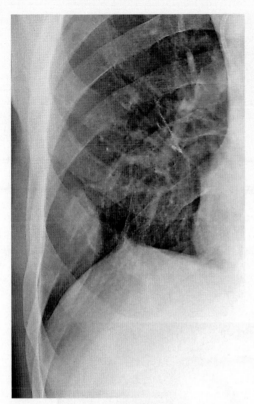

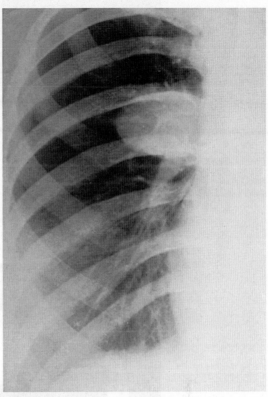

Fig. 2.5 This elongated tapered mass in the right costophrenic angle has invaded and destroyed a portion of the adjacent rib, which confirms chest wall involvement. These observations narrow the differential to metastasis vs. multiple myeloma or plasmacytoma. The patient's history of renal cell carcinoma confirms the diagnosis of metastasis.

Fig. 2.6 Schwannoma has not destroyed the rib but has eroded its inferior cortex. Note sclerotic border, which virtually ensures the benign nature of the lesion.

Physical examination reveals a soft, movable mass when there is a significant subcutaneous component. CT should show the extent of the mass and, more importantly, confirm that the lesion is of fat attenuation[137] (Fig. 2.4, *B*).

Rib destruction is a key observation in Fig. 2.5.[151] This finding excludes lipoma and other benign tumors, such as neurofibroma, from the diagnosis. Benign neural tumors, such as schwannoma and neurofibroma, may erode ribs inferiorly and even produce a sclerotic reaction (Fig. 2.6). Multiple chest wall masses in combination with rib deformities and inferior rib erosions should suggest neurofibromatosis (Figs. 2.7, *A-C*). Neural tumors should not destroy the rib, as shown in Fig. 2.6. (Answer to question 5 is *False*.) Rib destruction is not always obvious on a frontal examination and may be better visualized with rib detail views or CT scan. (Answer to question 6 is *False*.)

Metastases and small, round cell tumors are the most common tumors to produce the pattern of rib destruction seen in Figs. 2.1 and 2.5. The most common primary tumors to metastasize to the chest wall are lung, breast, and renal cell, but knowledge of a primary tumor is essential because any tumor that spreads by hematogenous dissemination may produce a chest wall lesion. Multiple myeloma, plasmacytoma (solitary myeloma), and Ewing tumors are primary round cell tumors that may arise in the bones of the chest wall. The differential diagnosis in the adult patient with a chest wall mass and bone destruction is most often metastasis vs. multiple myeloma. (Answer to question 7 is *True*.) In a child, however, the pattern is more suggestive of metastatic neuroblastoma or Ewing tumor. (Answer to question 8 is *True*.) Fig. 2.1 shows a typical

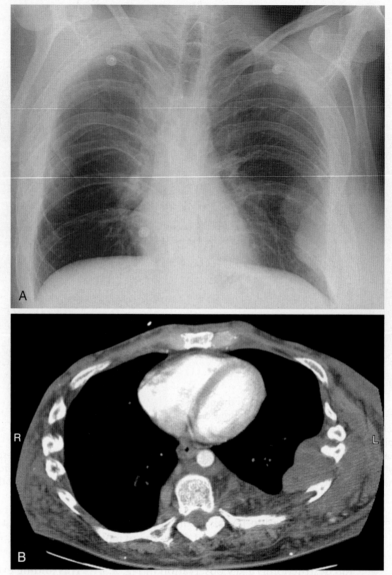

Fig. 2.7   A, This patient with neurofibromatosis has bilateral, elongated, tapered, smooth, peripheral masses, and multiple ribs are inferiorly eroded. **B,** Computed tomography confirms the peripheral masses with extension of the left lateral mass through the chest wall. The posterior extension of the mass was not suspected from the radiograph.

example of multiple myeloma (answer to question 1 is *c*), but there are a number of common variations. Myeloma (Figs. 2.8, *A-C*) may occur with complete loss of a rib, large expanded ribs, or only a small, ill-defined area of bone destruction. The patient may even present with a pathologic fracture of the involved rib. Occasionally, the soft-tissue mass may be rather large and the bone lesion minimal. Lymphoma is another tumor that may infrequently produce a peripheral soft-tissue mass with incomplete or tapered borders and extend through the chest wall.[438] This indicates an advanced stage of lymphoma and is not an expected abnormality at the time of presentation. The chest wall extension may not be seen on the chest radiograph, but it can be confirmed with a CT scan (Figs. 2.9, *A* and *B*). Extrathoracic subcutaneous metastases are more likely to be detected by physical exam than on the chest radiograph. Subcutaneous metastases are often best shown by CT (Fig. 2.10)

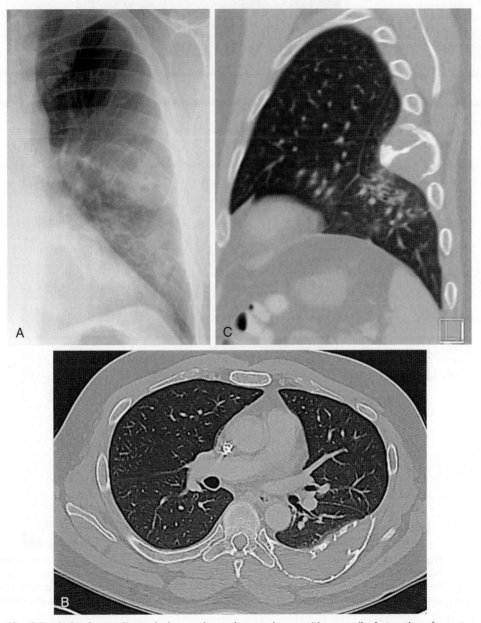

Fig. 2.8   A, PA chest radiograph shows a large elongated mass with expansile destruction of a posterior rib. **B,** Axial computed tomography confirms the large mass with expanded rib cortex. **C,** Sagittal reconstruction shows destruction of the anterior rib cortex and a large soft-tissue mass with tapered superior and inferior borders. These findings could result from metastasis, but this is another case of multiple myeloma.

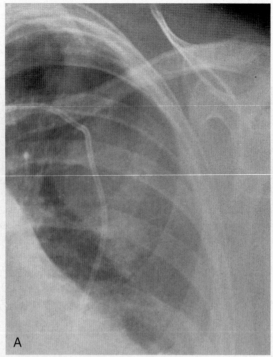

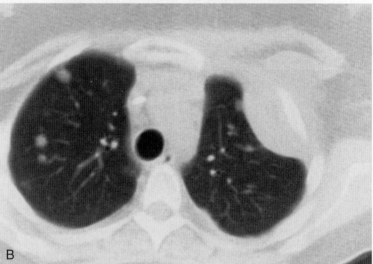

Fig. 2.9 **A,** Advanced Hodgkin lymphoma has caused this large soft-tissue mass. The incomplete borders indicate an extrapulmonary location, but the chest radiograph reveals no evidence of the chest wall extension. **B,** Computed tomography scan shows the peripheral soft-tissue opacity to have tapered borders and to extend through the chest wall. Multiple pulmonary nodules were also confirmed.

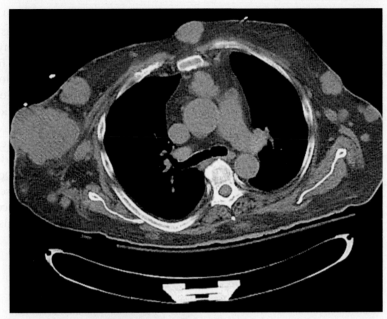

Fig. 2.10 Metastases to the subcutaneous soft tissues are not surrounded by air and are best diagnosed by physical exam and computed tomography. This patient with melanoma has an anterior mediastinal mass and multiple large subcutaneous metastases

Benign and malignant bone tumors may arise in the scapula, sternum, vertebra, and ribs. Some of the common benign rib lesions, such as benign cortical defect and fibrous dysplasia, do not produce soft-tissue masses, but hemangiomas and osteochondromas do produce soft-tissue opacities that project inward and should be considered in the differential diagnosis of intrathoracic chest wall masses. Hemangiomas may produce a significant extraosseous mass and resemble other chest wall masses, but they can best be identified by their typically reticular, or "basket weave," pattern of bone destruction. Osteochondromas may elevate the pleura and present as an intrathoracic chest wall mass. The typical pattern of the calcified matrix should confirm the diagnosis of osteochondroma (Fig. 2.11). Hereditary multiple exostoses are the result of an autosomal dominant disorder that frequently involves multiple flat bones. These patients may have deformity of the ribs and multiple osteochondromas. They are also at increased risk for the development of chondrosarcoma. Malignant transformation of osteochondromas in this group of patients has been reported to vary from 3% to 25%. Signs of malignancy include pain, swelling, soft-tissue mass, and growth (Figs. 2.12, *A-C*).

Osteosarcoma and chondrosarcoma may arise from the bones of the chest wall in patients without any known risk factors. Chondrosarcoma is the most common primary bone tumor of the scapula, sternum, and ribs. Ten percent of all chondrosarcomas are reported to arise in the thorax.[63,419] Chondrosarcoma might have been considered in the case seen in Fig. 2.2; however, the tumor matrix of chondrosarcoma is typically more spotted with calcified rings, arcs, dots, or bands as compared with the more homogenous matrix seen in this case. In answer to question 2, Ewing sarcoma, metastatic lung cancer, and plasmacytoma may all involve the chest wall, but should be eliminated by the blastic appearance. Osteosarcoma[280] typically produces a more homogeneous blastic matrix. (Answer to question 2 is *b*.) Blastic metastases from breast and prostate cancer (Figs. 2.13, *A* and *B*) to the ribs and vertebrae are much more common.

Inflammatory lesions of the chest wall may arise from puncture wounds, hematogenous seeding, or direct extension from intrathoracic infections. Septicemia by bacterial infections and even miliary spread of tuberculosis may cause osteomyelitis of the spine or ribs with chest wall involvement, but infectious chest wall masses most often arise from empyema or pneumonias with empyema. Actinomycosis is one of the more aggressive granulomatous infections, and it may produce a parenchymal opacity, pleural effusion, chest wall mass, rib destruction, and even cutaneous fistulas.[164,618] Occasionally, air-fluid levels are seen in the soft tissues. Other granulomatous infections that produce a similar appearance include aspergillosis,[14] nocardiosis, blastomycosis, and tuberculosis (Figs. 2.14, *A* and *B*). Patients with these infections usually have a febrile course, although it may be somewhat indolent.

Hematoma is usually suggested by a history of trauma and is frequently associated with rib fractures (Figs. 2.15, *A-C*). Care must be taken not to overlook an underlying lytic lesion that would indicate that the fracture is pathologic. Occasionally, old rib fractures may be mistaken for nodules because of their callus. These are best evaluated with coned views of the ribs. Rarely, chest wall desmoid tumor occurs as a late complication of trauma.[303] Desmoid tumors are locally invasive but histologically benign chest wall masses.[109]

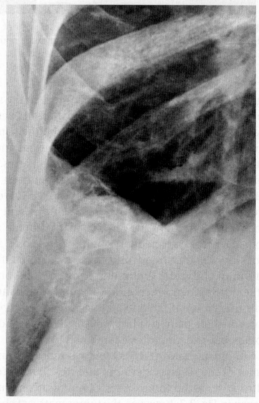

Fig. 2.11 This mass has protruded into the thorax, elevating the pleura, as evidenced by the tapered borders. The calcified matrix has a speckled, reticulated appearance that is typical of a cartilage matrix. In addition, there is a well-defined, calcified cortex. These features are diagnostic of an osteochondroma.

Primary lung abnormalities sometimes invade the pleura and chest wall with rib destruction and resemble primary chest wall abnormalities. This is observed with both infections and primary lung tumors. The apical lung cancer (Pancoast tumor) is best known for this presentation. When a lung cancer invades the pleura, it may spread along the pleura in a manner that produces a tapered border. However, close observation often reveals irregular or even spiculated borders, which should strongly suggest the pulmonary origin of the tumor (Fig. 2.16). CT is sometimes

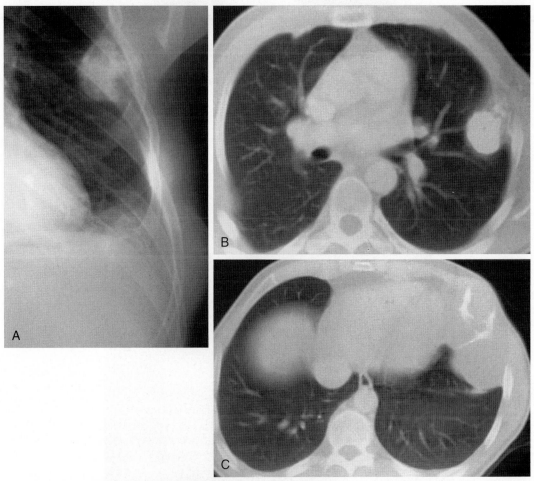

Fig. 2.12 A, Multiple osteochondromas produce calcified soft-tissue masses. These masses often cause considerable chest wall deformity with spreading of ribs. They may also cause intrathoracic and extrathoracic soft-tissue masses. This patient with hereditary multiple exostoses has two large masses. The smaller superior mass is an osteochondroma. The large inferior mass obliterates the costophrenic angle and extends into the extrathoracic soft tissues. Because of recent growth, a biopsy was performed confirming the diagnosis of chondrosarcoma. **B,** Computed tomography (CT) of the smaller superior osteochondroma shows a typical pattern of calcification. **C,** CT of the larger inferior chondrosarcoma shows a large soft-tissue mass with irregular bands of calcified matrix.

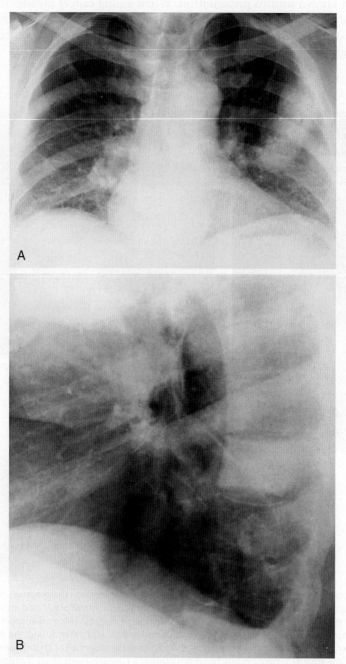

Fig. 2.13   A, Compare this case with the case seen in Fig. 2.2, *A.* This elongated opacity follows the left anterior third rib, indicating a chest wall origin. The opacity is lobulated and blastic. Blastic rib lesions are a common appearance of prostate metastases, but the lobulated, expansile chest wall mass is unusual. **B,** The blastic lesion in the lower thoracic vertebra confirms the presence of multiple blastic bone lesions. This is a common appearance of metastatic prostate cancer.

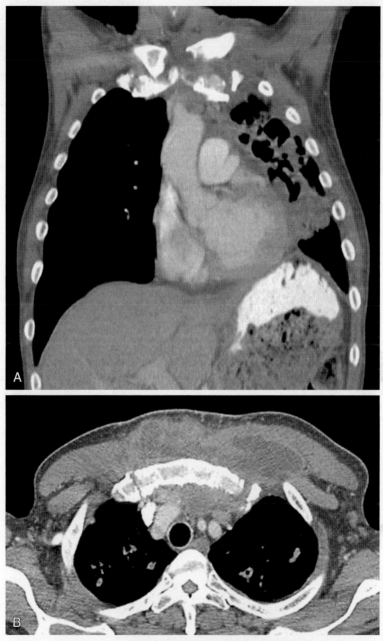

Fig. 2.14   A, This coronal computed tomography (CT) reveals multiple left upper lobe cavities that are highly suggestive of active tuberculosis (discussed in Chapter 24). **B,** The axial CT images reveal extensive anterior soft-tissue swelling with a central low attenuation fluid-filled structure. This is the result of extension of the infection through the chest wall causing tuberculous cellulitis and abscess.

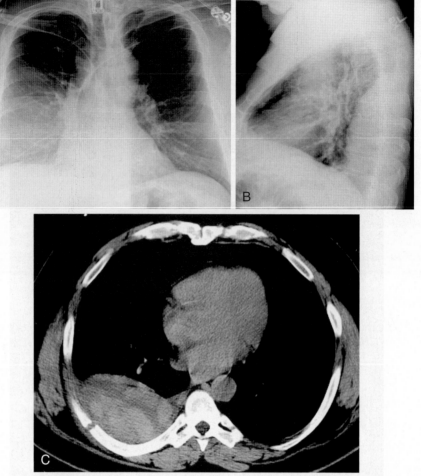

Fig. 2.15 **A,** This right-lower thoracic opacity has no detectable borders on the PA radiograph. **B,** The lateral review reveals a well-circumscribed, posterior, elongated, mass-like opacity. **C,** Computed tomography reveals mixed attenuation of the posterior opacity with an associated rib fracture. This confirms a chest wall hematoma.

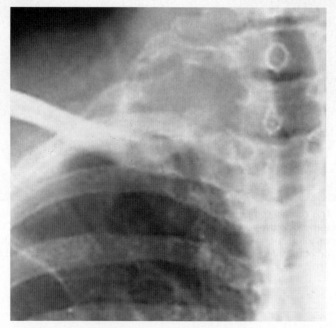

Fig. 2.16 Superior sulcus (Pancoast) tumors are primary lung cancers that often invade the pleura and chest wall. Notice the poorly defined inferior border of the mass that distinguishes it from a chest wall or pleural mass. The tumor has destroyed multiple ribs and vertebrae.

required to visualize the irregular interface with the lung and confirm the pulmonary origin of the tumor. Patients with apical lung cancer frequently present with shoulder and arm pain. This combination is described as *Pancoast syndrome*. When the tumor invades the paravertebral sympathetic chain, the patient may also have Horner syndrome,[17] which includes ipsilateral ptosis, miosis, anhidrosis, and enophthalmos.

Top 5 Diagnoses: Chest Wall Lesions

1. Metastases
2. Multiple myeloma
3. Neural tumors
4. Invasive lung cancer
5. Hematoma

Summary

The incomplete border sign, which may be seen as the result of both extrathoracic and intrathoracic chest wall masses, is suggestive of an extrapulmonary process.

Chest wall masses have smooth, tapered borders that are helpful in distinguishing them from pulmonary lesions. These are best seen with tangential views.

Benign chest wall tumors such as lipoma, schwannoma, and neurofibroma should not destroy ribs but may erode the inferior surface of a rib.

Chest wall tumors that destroy ribs are most commonly metastases or multiple myeloma in adults and Ewing tumor or neuroblastoma in children.

Rib destruction may be subtle, requiring coned views, CTs, and even radionuclide bone scans for visualization.

Actinomycosis, aspergillosis, nocardiosis, tuberculosis, and blastomycosis may all produce chest wall lesions with rib destruction. The history and physical findings should alert the radiologist to these possibilities.

A CT scan is often required to confirm chest wall involvement by metastases, myeloma, lymphoma, and even benign masses.

Lung, breast, and renal cell tumors are the most common primary tumors to metastasize to the chest wall.

ANSWER GUIDE

Legends for introductory figures

Fig. 2.1 The tapered border of this mass indicates an intrathoracic extrapulmonary location. The expansile lytic destruction of the adjacent rib confirms the chest wall origin of the mass. The patient has a known diagnosis of multiple myeloma.

Fig. 2.2 This large, right-upper, lateral thoracic mass has tapered superior and inferior borders with the additional finding of an opacity that follows the posterior aspect of the right third and fourth ribs. The widening of the interspace between the second and third ribs is the result of the mass. There is also lateral destruction of the third rib. The opacity is greater than that of the surrounding ribs, indicating a blastic bone reaction that is the result of calcified tumor matrix. This is a rare case of osteosarcoma arising from the chest wall. Prostate and breast cancers are common primary tumors and are common causes of blastic bone metastases that may involve the thoracic skeleton.

ANSWERS

1. c   2. b   3. T   4. T   5. F   6. F   7. T   8. T

3 | PLEURAL AND SUBPLEURAL OPACITIES

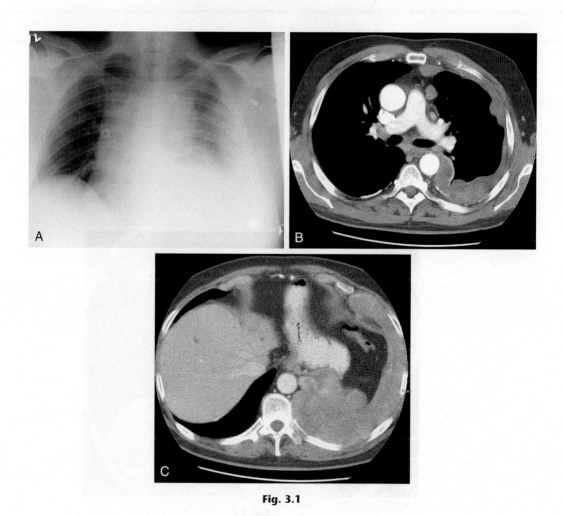

Fig. 3.1

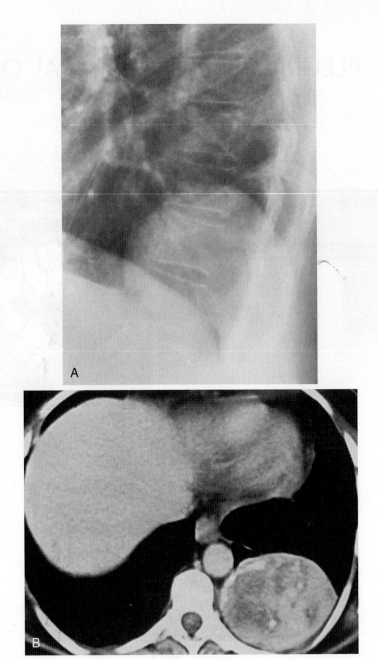

Fig. 3.2

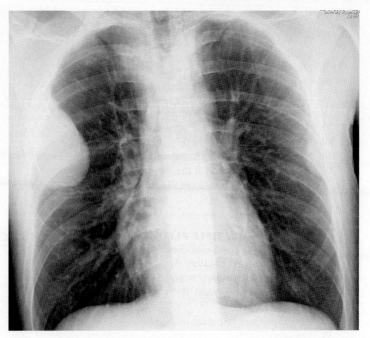

Fig. 3.3

QUESTIONS

1. Referring to Fig. 3.1, *A-C*, which of the following is the most likely diagnosis?
   a. Metastatic melanoma.
   b. Metastatic breast carcinoma.
   c. Invasive thymoma.
   d. Mesothelioma.
   e. Metastatic ovarian carcinoma.

2. Referring to Fig. 3.2, *A* and *B*, the most likely diagnosis for this case is:
   a. Rounded atelectasis.
   b. Localized fibrous tumor of the pleura.
   c. Multiple myeloma.
   d. Infarct.
   e. Mesothelial cyst.

3. Referring to Fig. 3.3, which of the following is the most likely diagnosis?
   a. Mesothelioma.
   b. Neurofibromatosis.
   c. Localized fibrous tumor of the pleura.
   d. Multiple myeloma.
   e. Invasive thymoma.

Mark the following questions **True** *or* **False:**

4. _____ A shaggy, irregular border favors a subpleural, parenchymal lung lesion over a pleural lesion.

5. _____ Mesothelioma frequently causes bone destruction.

6. _____ Pleural lesions may be confused with mediastinal masses.

Chart 3.1	SOLITARY PLEURAL OPACITY

I. Loculated pleural effusion
II. Metastasis[131]
III. Mesothelioma[47] (rare)
IV. Lipoma[153,160,183,195,466]
V. Organized empyema[519,625]
VI. Hematoma
VII. Mesothelial cyst
VIII. Neural tumor (schwannoma, neurofibroma)[459]
IX. Solitary fibrous tumor of the pleura[116,483]

Chart 3.2	MULTIPLE PLEURAL OPACITIES (EACH >2 CM)

I. Loculated pleural effusion[318]
II. Metastases (particularly from adenocarcinomas)
III. Invasive thymoma (rare)[318,600]
IV. Mesothelioma[256,500,588]
V. Pleural plaques (asbestos related)[480]
VI. Splenosis[270,493]
VII. Neural tumors

Chart 3.3	SUBPLEURAL PARENCHYMAL LUNG OPACITIES

I. Infarct[218]
II. Granuloma (tuberculosis, fungus)
III. Inflammatory pseudotumor
IV. Metastasis
V. Rheumatoid nodule
VI. Primary carcinoma of the lung including Pancoast tumor[17,193]
VII. Lymphoma
VIII. Round atelectasis[35,375]

Discussion

SOLITARY PLEURAL OPACITY

The radiologic evaluation of a solitary pleural opacity (Chart 3.1) is complicated by the paucity of reliable signs for accurate localization.[519,588] The opacity should be in a peripheral extrapulmonary location, which may be confirmed by identifying the incomplete border sign (see Fig. 2.4, A and B). The peripheral position is easily recognized when the mass is against the lateral chest wall, but the correct location may be more difficult to identify when the mass is either anterior or posterior (Fig. 3.4, A). The lateral view (see Fig. 3.2, A), or even a computed tomography (CT) scan[124] (see Fig. 3.2, B, and Fig. 3.4, B), may be needed to confirm the peripheral location. A peripheral mass requires consideration of three locations: (1) chest wall, (2) pleura, and (3) subpleural area of the lung. Smooth, incomplete tapered borders with obtuse pleural angles localize a mass to either the chest wall or pleura, whereas shaggy borders and acute pleural angles confirm the diagnosis of a subpleural peripheral lung opacity (Fig. 3.5, A-C).

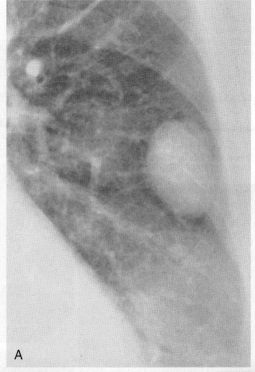

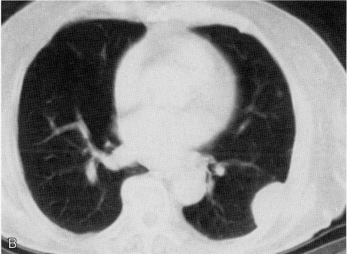

Fig. 3.4   A, This solitary metastasis from a malignant fibrous histiocytoma presents as a sharply circumscribed peripheral mass. Its pleural location may be suspected because of the less definite lateral borders, but this cannot be confirmed on the posteroanterior chest radiograph. **B,** Computed tomography scan shows the mass to have a broad pleural attachment with obtuse pleural angles, confirming its pleural origin.

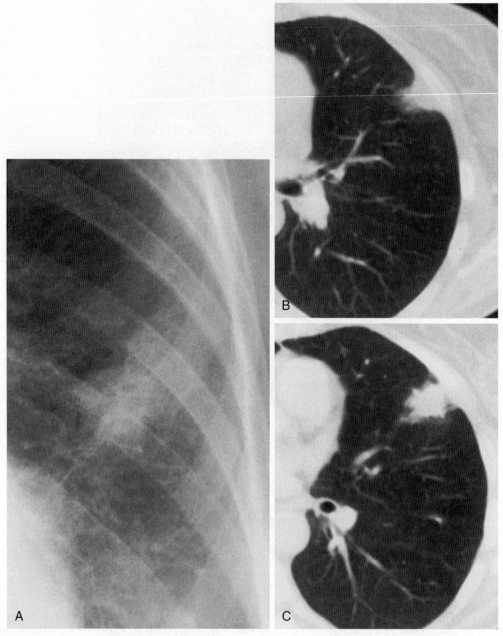

Fig. 3.5   A, Posterior-anterior chest radiograph shows a poorly defined opacity in the periphery of the left upper lobe. **B,** Computed tomography (CT) section of the upper portion of the opacity shows a tapered border, suggesting either a pleural mass or pleural extension of a lung mass. **C,** A lower CT section shows irregular margins, confirming a subpleural origin of a pulmonary mass. Biopsy confirmed primary lung cancer.

One pitfall is that a peripheral lung mass, such as a metastasis, may have smooth borders. Some metastatic tumors and even lymphoma can also disseminate to both the lung and pleura. The foregoing signs for localizing peripheral masses are sometimes indeterminate on the chest radiograph, but they are also applicable in CT scan interpretation. In fact, CT is often required for the precise localization of abnormalities seen on the chest radiograph.

Some pleural tumors lack the broad-based pleural signs described previously because they have a small area of attachment to either pleural surface and appear more round. The case shown in Fig. 3.2, *A* and *B*, was described at surgery as a pedunculated pleural mass. Berne and Heitzman[43] have reported that pedunculated pleural tumors may be fluoroscopically observed to change shape or move with respiration. This motion may also be recorded on inspiration and expiration views. Documentation of free movement in the pleural space distinguishes the chest wall from pleural masses.

Medial pleural opacities are probably the most confusing. A mass in this position is often more suggestive of a mediastinal mass. Because pleural masses and mediastinal masses are seen as a result of their interface with the lung, both have a sharp incomplete border that is frequently tapered; therefore, diagnosis of a medially located mesothelioma can be made only by biopsy. Similarly, mesothelioma arising from an interlobar fissure is difficult to identify correctly as a pleural mass. This is best accomplished by identification of the fissures on the lateral view or with a CT scan.

Pleural tumors, cysts, and loculated effusions all appear homogeneous on chest radiographs, but should be distinguished with ultrasound, CT, or magnetic resonance imaging (MRI) scanning. Pleural tumors may be regarded as solid, but they are not always entirely homogeneous. The large mass shown in Fig. 3.2, *A* and *B*, is shown by CT to be heterogeneous, with soft-tissue opacity, a calcification, and areas of low attenuation caused by necrosis. It does not have uniform low attenuation, which is expected with a mesothelial cyst.

Localized fibrous tumor of the pleura (see Fig. 3.2, *A* and *B*; answer to question 2 is *b*) probably arises from submesothelial mesenchymal cells rather than mesothelial cells and is usually benign, although 37% of such tumors have been reported to be malignant.[124,483] Localized fibrous tumor of the pleura should present as a well-circumscribed peripheral mass and should not invade the chest wall or lung. The chest radiographs in this case are not adequate for exclusion of a chest wall mass, but the CT scan shows the mass to be separate from the chest wall and thus makes multiple myeloma an unlikely choice. The CT appearance of this heterogeneous mass further excludes mesothelial cyst. Both pulmonary infarcts and rounded atelectasis are pulmonary processes that typically have a subpleural location. They usually have poorly defined borders, and the CT scan should confirm their pulmonary origin.[375]

A solitary pleural metastasis is impossible to differentiate on the basis of its radiologic features from the mass seen in this case. The similarity of a solitary metastasis is illustrated in Fig. 3.4, *A* and *B*. Metastatic disease is the most common cause of a pleural mass, with lung and breast cancer accounting for 60% of cases.

MULTIPLE PLEURAL OPACITIES

Multiple pleural opacities (Chart 3.2) are usually the result of loculated effusion, pleural masses, or a combination of the two. The radiologic appearance is that of multiple, separate, sharply circumscribed, smooth, tapered opacities (Fig. 3.6) or of diffuse pleural thickening with lobulated inner borders. Loculated pleural effusion is probably the most common cause of this appearance. The causes of loculated effusion include empyema (Fig. 3.7, *A*), hemorrhage, and neoplasms. Lateral decubitus views are of little value in recognizing the condition because some free fluid may coexist with either loculated collections of fluid or solid masses. Sequential radiographs showing a change

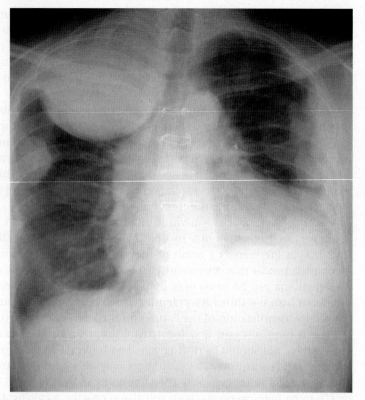

Fig. 3.6 Multiple bilateral pleural masses are the result of the contiguous spread of invasive thymoma. Observe the sharply defined interface with the lung and the incomplete borders. The large right apical mass has obtuse pleural angles. These features confirm an extrapulmonary origin. The prior sternotomy was for resection of the primary mediastinal tumor.

over a short period should suggest the presence of loculated fluid collections (Fig. 3.8, *A* and *B*). Ultrasound and CT scans (see Fig. 3.7, *B*) may be useful for confirming the presence of loculated fluid collections and for thoracentesis or drainage procedures. A history of recent pneumonia is evidence that favors a loculated empyema.[220,519]

Metastases are the most common cause of multiple pleural nodules or masses. Adenocarcinomas are especially known for their tendency to produce pleural metastases. Knowledge of either a primary lung tumor or an extrathoracic primary tumor, such as breast cancer or melanoma, should strongly suggest the diagnosis. The radiologic combination of bilateral lobulated pleural thickening and a known primary cancer should virtually ensure the diagnosis (Fig. 3.9, *A* and *B*).

Invasive thymoma[600] spreads contiguously and may invade the pleura, spreading around the lung with the radiologic appearance of multiple pleural masses (see Fig. 3.6). It should be suspected when associated with an anterior mediastinal mass or a history of resected thymoma.

Multiple myeloma often presents with extrapulmonary masses (see Chapter 2) and may mimic multiple pleural masses. It is not likely to result in the appearance of diffuse nodular pleural thickening, as seen with either pleural metastases or mesothelioma. Bone destruction is a reliable feature of multiple myeloma (see Fig. 2.1).

Neurofibromatosis may present with multiple tapered masses that require consideration of chest wall vs. pleural masses.[168] These masses often arise from the intercostal nerves and are expected to erode or scallop their associated ribs, but they may not

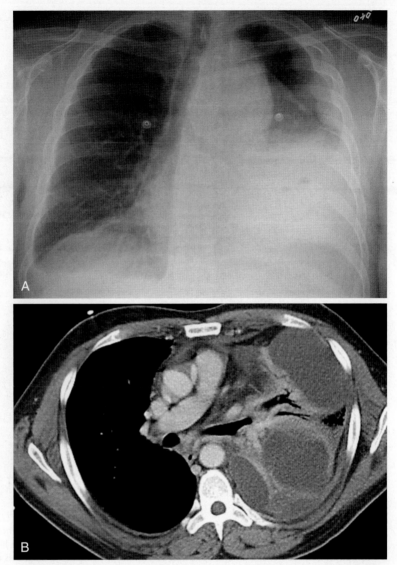

Fig. 3.7 A, This large mass-like opacity fills the left lower chest, obscuring the left heart border and costophrenic angle. **B,** Axial computed tomography reveals a large loculated fluid collection with thick walls resulting from empyema.

always show this feature. Without the rib erosion, their appearance is more suggestive of pleural masses (see Fig. 3.3). The chest radiograph in this case shows bilateral smooth, tapered peripheral masses, with no evidence of rib erosion. Localized fibrous tumor of the pleura presents as a solitary pleural mass, and mesothelioma causes multiple unilateral pleural masses. Multiple myeloma is unlikely in the absence of rib destruction, and invasive thymoma usually presents with an anterior mediastinal mass that may invade the pleura.

Mesothelioma is an important cause of lobulated or nodular pleural thickening (Fig. 3.1, *A-C,* and Fig. 3.10).[124,131,239] Mesothelioma spreads around the pleura and is virtually always unilateral. (Answer to question 1 is *d.*) Radiologic distinction of mesothelioma from pleural metastases[124] is often impossible in patients with

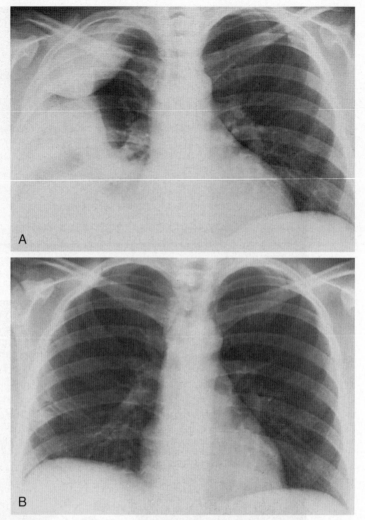

Fig. 3.8   A, This diffuse, mass-like, pleural thickening was the result of hemothorax in a hemophiliac. **B,** Follow-up posterior-anterior chest radiograph after 2 weeks from the case illustrated in **A** reveals complete resolution of the pleural opacities, confirming the suspected diagnosis of pleural effusion.

unilateral pleural masses, but bilateral pleural masses are strong evidence for pleural metastases. Either may have an associated bloody pleural effusion. Even the histologic distinction of these two lesions may be difficult, requiring special stains. CT studies have shown mesotheliomas to be more extensive than suspected from chest radiographs, with extension into the lung, chest wall, and mediastinum.[13] Invasion of lung or bone is considered evidence of advanced disease but is not common. (Answer to question 6 is *False*.)

The association of asbestos exposure with both primary carcinoma of the lung and mesothelioma is well known.[47,239,376] Because the incidence of primary lung and pleural tumors is increased by asbestos exposure, a history of exposure is of no value in making the distinction of pleural metastases from a primary lung cancer vs. mesothelioma. Another curious feature of the relationship between asbestos exposure and these tumors is that patients who develop the neoplasms usually do not have the typical pulmonary findings of asbestosis (see Chapters 18 and 19).

Asbestos-related pleural plaques may be flat or nodular. They are easily overlooked or mistaken for artifacts in the early stages of the disease.[184,480] The plaques usually

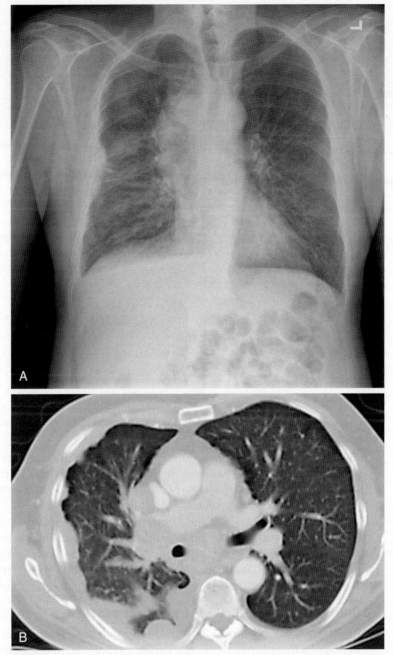

Fig. 3.9   A, This patient has a large right hilar opacity, with nodular thickening of the lateral pleura. **B,** Axial computed tomography reveals nodular pleural masses that resemble mesothelioma, but the hilar mass extends into the mediastinum and is confirmed to be metastatic small cell lung cancer that has spread around the pleura, resembling the appearance expected with diffuse mesothelioma.

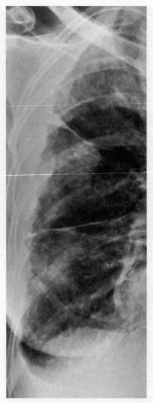

Fig. 3.10 Diffuse nodular pleural thickening, with thickening of interlobar fissures, was unilateral in this case. Unilateral nodular pleural thickening is the most common appearance of mesothelioma.

cause areas of flat pleural thickening, but occasionally they produce a nodular appearance. They do not spread around the lung and rarely extend to the apex. Although they may be confused with the early stages of mesothelioma, they should not be confused with advanced cases, such as that illustrated in Fig. 3.1.

Splenosis[270,493] occurs after the autotransplantation of splenic tissue into the pleural space following combined splenic and diaphragmatic injuries. The presence of multiple masses in the left pleural space requires questioning the patient for a history of prior severe upper abdominal or lower thoracic trauma. This is particularly important when the patient has undergone splenectomy and repair of a ruptured diaphragm.

SUBPLEURAL PARENCHYMAL LUNG OPACITIES

Another problem to be considered in the evaluation of a peripheral opacity is the distinction of a true pleural abnormality from a subpleural lung lesion (Chart 3.3). Sometimes, peripheral lung opacities are so sharply defined that they completely mimic a true pleural opacity. Additional signs that suggest the true nature of the opacity are (1) ill-defined or shaggy borders, (2) associated linear opacities, (3) heterogeneous texture with small areas of lucency or air bronchograms, and (4) acute pleural angles. These clues to a pulmonary origin of the opacity may be enhanced by CT scanning, which reveals the texture of a suspected mass and its interface with the surrounding lung.[193] This provides a sensitive means for detecting local invasion of lung parenchyma and even confirming a pulmonary origin (see Fig. 3.5, *A-C*). CT has the added advantage of being more sensitive for the detection of very small lesions. This is most important when evaluating patients with a known primary neoplasm. (Answer to question 5 is *True*.)

Neoplasms, including metastases and primary lung cancer, often develop in a peripheral subpleural location. The frequency with which metastases occur in this setting was not appreciated prior to the use of CT scanning for staging metastatic disease. Metastatic nodules are typically well-circumscribed opacities. Some have acute pleural angles and can be labeled intrapulmonary, whereas others have more obtuse angles, indicating pleural involvement (see Fig. 3.4, *A* and *B*). Because they are incompletely surrounded by air and are often small, the chest radiograph is not sensitive for the detection of small subpleural metastases.

Primary carcinoma of the lung, including superior sulcus tumors,[415] often presents as a peripheral subpleural nodule. These masses grow by contiguous invasion and are distinguished radiologically from pleural masses by their irregular, poorly defined margins or irregular borders (see Fig. 3.5, *A-C*). Because they are locally very invasive, they often spread through the pleura into the chest wall. The chest radiograph finding of bone destruction indicates advanced disease (see Fig. 2.16). In the absence of bone involvement on the radiograph, CT and MRI scans are used for detecting extension into the soft tissues of the chest wall, particularly in confirming brachial plexus invasion. The superiority of CT over chest radiograph for staging these tumors is well documented, but the axial display of CT does not show the pleural fat planes optimally. Coronal CT or MRI scans may provide the optimal means for detecting penetration of the mass through the apical pleura. The cell types of apical lung cancer include adenocarcinoma, invasive mucinous adenocarcinoma, and squamous cell carcinoma. These tumors are accessible to needle aspiration biopsy, which yields a diagnosis in a high percentage of cases. Scar carcinoma is another variant of lung cancer that often occurs in the apices. This variant includes all lung cancers that arise around a preexistent scar. Scar carcinoma may be suggested by serial radiographs that reveal an old calcified scar from a previous granulomatous infection and an associated growing soft-tissue opacity. Lymphoma may also cause an irregular apical mass that resembles a superior sulcus or Pancoast tumor. It is usually associated with evidence of lymphadenopathy or with a history of previously treated nodal disease.

Organizing pulmonary processes, including organizing pneumonia, inflammatory pseudotumor, granulomas, infarcts, and rounded atelectasis, must also be considered in the differential diagnosis of subpleural pulmonary opacities. Granulomas are often peripheral and may resemble either metastases or primary lung tumors. Likewise, infarcts may organize into well-circumscribed, subpleural opacities that are radiologically indistinguishable from granulomas, metastases, or lung cancers, but they more typically form pleural-based triangular opacities. This characteristic triangular or wedge-shaped opacity may be more confidently identified by CT. A history of prior pleuritic chest plain or thrombophlebitis should provide further confirmatory evidence of an infarct.

Rounded atelectasis or folded lung is another benign cause of peripheral lung opacities that resemble lung cancer.[60,64] These opacities are associated with pleural thickening and may be caused by retracting pleural fibrosis. They are usually spherical, with irregular borders, typically extend to the pleura with an acute angle, and are usually posterior. Air bronchograms may be observed at the periphery. This phenomenon is usually seen in patients with a history of asbestos exposure and must be distinguished from mesothelioma and lung cancer. CT may be diagnostic in revealing the associated pleural thickening and characteristic retraction of pulmonary vessels and bronchi into a curved shape following the contour of the mass of scarred collapsed lung[64,122,375] (Fig. 3.11). Confirmation of stability with an old radiograph is essential because lung cancer may appear to be nearly identical, sometimes requiring biopsy.

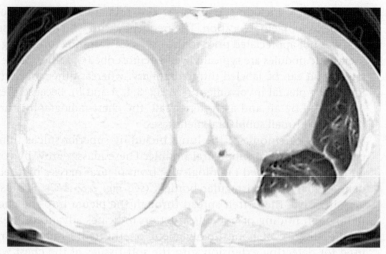

Fig. 3.11 Rounded atelectasis causes a peripheral, mass-like opacity, often with associated pleural thickening. Volume loss leads to retraction of surrounding pulmonary vessels with a characteristic computed tomography appearance of vessels curving around the round opacities.

Top 5 Diagnoses: Pleural and Subpleural Opacities

1. Metastases
2. Loculated pleural effusion
3. Mesothelioma
4. Neural tumor
5. Hematoma

Summary

Pleural opacities may be confused with either chest wall lesions or subpleural parenchymal lung lesions.

Identification of bone destruction or extension of the mass through the ribs is the most reliable chest radiograph feature for confirming a chest wall lesion.

A solitary pleural opacity may be caused by a loculated fluid collection or a solid mass such as a metastasis, mesothelioma, or lipoma.

Localized fibrous tumor of the pleura has no association with asbestos exposure, but may require biopsy to exclude a solitary malignant mass.

Multiple pleural opacities result from loculated effusion, mesothelioma, and metastases. Primary tumors that frequently metastasize to the pleura include lung, breast, gastrointestinal tract, and melanoma.

Splenosis is a rare cause of multiple pleural masses that should be suspected on the basis of a history of prior splenic injury and thoracoabdominal surgery.

Ill-defined or shaggy borders, associated linear opacities, and a heterogeneous appearance with air bronchograms should be reliable findings for the identification of a subpleural parenchymal lung process that may have secondarily involved the pleura. These findings should suggest tuberculosis, fungal infection, organizing infarct, or even primary lung tumor.

Rounded atelectasis is associated with pleural scarring, occurs in patients with a history of asbestos exposure, and must be distinguished from primary lung cancer or mesothelioma.

ANSWER GUIDE

Legends for introductory figures

Fig. 3.1 **A,** The peripheral and medial opacities of the left hemithorax obscure the diaphragm and could result from extensive peripheral masses with pleural effusion. **B,** Axial computed tomography (CT) through the midthorax reveals nodular pleural masses with posterior plaques of pleural calcification. **C,** Axial CT through the lower thorax reveals a large pleural mass rather than the pleural effusion that was suspected from the chest radiograph. The combination of unilateral pleural masses with calcified pleural plaques makes the diagnosis of asbestos-related mesothelioma almost certain.

Fig. 3.2 **A,** This localized fibrous tumor of the pleura is seen as a sharply circumscribed mass in the left posterior pleural space. Other differential considerations include loculated pleural fluid and a solitary metastasis. **B,** Computed tomography (CT) scan from the same case confirms that the opacity is a heterogeneous mass with soft tissue, a calcification, and low-attenuation areas of necrosis. The mass is bounded posteriorly by the pleural fat and does not involve the chest wall. The CT findings rule out the options of a mesothelial cyst, myeloma, infarct, and rounded atelectasis.

Fig. 3.3 Bilateral, peripheral, tapered masses require consideration of chest wall vs. pleural masses. The presence of rib involvement would confirm a chest wall origin, but in this case, the masses have not destroyed or eroded the ribs. Therefore, both pleural and chest wall masses must be considered. Because a number of tumors may metastasize to the ribs or pleura, metastases cannot be excluded by the chest radiograph findings. Diffuse mesothelioma is expected to be unilateral and therefore is not a likely diagnosis. These are noninvasive masses that resemble multiple pleural masses, but this is neurofibromatosis, with neurofibromas arising from the intercostal nerves that are actually chest wall tumors. This case further illustrates the difficulty of distinguishing chest wall masses from pleural masses.

ANSWERS

1. d   2. b   3. b   4. T   5. F   6. T

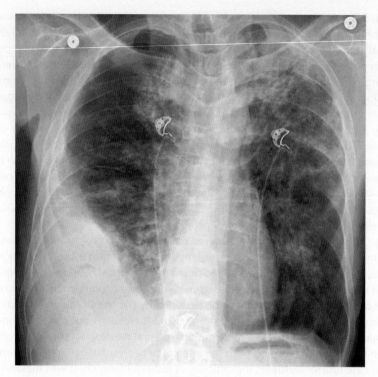

Fig. 4.1

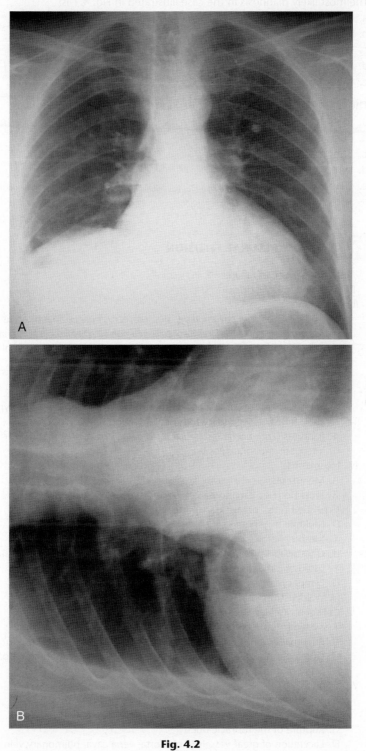

Fig. 4.2

QUESTIONS

1. The most likely diagnosis in the case illustrated in Fig. 4.1 is:
   a. Necrotizing pneumonia with empyema.
   b. Tuberculosis.
   c. Lung cancer.
   d. Mesothelioma.
   e. Metastases.

2. The most likely diagnosis in the case illustrated in Fig. 4.2, *A* and *B,* is:
   a. Right lower-lobe pneumonia.
   b. Pulmonary embolism.
   c. Subphrenic abscess.
   d. Lymphoma.
   e. Diaphragmatic hernia.

Chart 4.1	PLEURAL EFFUSION

   I. Congestive heart failure[6,390]
   II. Thromboembolic disease[660]
   III. Infection
      A. Bacteria (*Klebsiella pneumoniae, Staphylococcus aureus, Streptococcus pyogenes, Nocardia asteroides,*[29] *Streptococcus pneumoniae [Diplococcus],*[578] anaerobic organisms,[324] anthrax,[125,648] actinomycosis,[164] other necrotizing bacterial infections)
      B. Tuberculosis
      C. Viral (uncommon)
      D. Mycoplasma (uncommon)
      E. Fungus (blastomycosis, coccidioidomycosis,[431] histoplasmosis, cryptococcosis[504] [effusion secondary to fungal infection is rare])
      F. Parasites (*Entamoeba histolytica,*[639] *Echinococcus, Paragonimus,*[260,262] malaria)
      G. Infectious mononucleosis
   IV. Neoplasms
      A. Metastases
      B. Bronchogenic carcinoma
      C. Distant (e.g., breast, gastrointestinal, pancreatic)
      D. Multiple myeloma
      E. Mesothelioma
      F. Chest wall—primary bone cancer (e.g., Ewing sarcoma, chondrosarcoma, osteosarcoma, fibrosarcoma)
      G. Lymphoma[620]
      H. Waldenström macroglobulinemia
   V. Collagen vascular disease (autoimmune)
      A. Systemic lupus erythematosus[632]
      B. Rheumatoid arthritis[59,532]
      C. Granulomatosis with polyangitis[4] (formerly Wegener granulomatosis)
      D. Scleroderma (rare)[19]
   VI. Trauma
      A. Chest wall trauma
      B. Rupture of the esophagus
      C. Rupture of the thoracic duct
      D. Laceration of great vessels (e.g., aorta, vena cava, pulmonary veins)
   VII. Abdominal diseases
      A. Pancreatitis
      B. Pancreatic neoplasms

Chart 4.1	PLEURAL EFFUSION—cont'd

    C. Pancreatic pseudocyst
    D. Pancreatic abscess
    E. Subphrenic abscess
    F. Abdominal or retroperitoneal surgery (e.g., renal surgery, splenectomy)
    G. Urinary tract obstruction with extension of retroperitoneal urine[31]
    H. Ovarian tumors (e.g., Meigs syndrome)
    I. Cirrhosis of the liver
    J. Peritoneal dialysis
    K. Renal disease
    L. Renal failure
    M. Acute glomerulonephritis
    N. Nephrotic syndrome
    O. Whipple disease
VIII. Diffuse pulmonary diseases
    A. Lymphangioleiomyomatosis[424] (LAM)
    B. Asbestosis (rare)
    C. Usual interstitial pneumonitis (rare)
    D. Sarcoidosis (reported to be 4% of cases)[635]
  IX. Drug reactions
    A. Nitrofurantoin
    B. Methysergide
    C. Busulfan
    D. Procainamide
    E. Hydralazine
    F. Isoniazid (INH)
    G. Phenytoin sodium (Dilantin)
    H. Propylthiouracil
    I. Procarbazine
  X. Other
    A. Postmyocardial infarction syndrome (Dressler syndrome) and postpericardiotomy syndrome
    B. Coagulation defect
    C. Radiation therapy (very rare)[628]
    D. Idiopathic
    E. Pleural fistulas (bronchial, gastric, esophageal, subarachnoid)[220,638]
    F. Empyema from retropharyngeal and neck abscess
    G. Empyema in postpneumonectomy space[231]

Chart 4.2	PLEURAL EFFUSION WITH LARGE CARDIAC SILHOUETTE

  I. Congestive heart failure
  II. Pulmonary embolism with right-sided heart enlargement
  III. Myocarditis or pericarditis with pleuritis
    A. Viral infection
    B. Tuberculosis
    C. Rheumatic fever
  IV. Tumor: metastasis, mesothelioma
  V. Collagen vascular disease
    A. Systemic lupus erythematosus[632] (pleural and pericardial effusion)
    B. Rheumatoid arthritis[532]
  VI. Postpericardiotomy syndrome

Chart 4.3	**PLEURAL EFFUSION WITH SUBSEGMENTAL, SEGMENTAL, OR LOBAR OPACITIES**

  I. Postoperative (thoracic and abdominal surgery)
 II. Pulmonary embolism
III. Pneumonia with parapneumonic effusion or empyema
 IV. Abdominal mass
  V. Ascites
 VI. Rib fractures
VII. Tuberculosis
VIII. Neoplasms
    A. Bronchogenic carcinoma
    B. Lymphoma

Chart 4.4	**PLEURAL EFFUSION WITH HILAR ENLARGEMENT**

  I. Tumor
    A. Lung cancer
    B. Lymphoma
    C. Metastases
 II. Tuberculosis
III. Fungal infections
    A. Histoplasmosis
    B. Coccidioidomycosis
 IV. Anthrax[125,648]
  V. Sarcoidosis
 VI. Pulmonary embolism
VII. Congestive heart failure

Discussion

Pleural effusions may produce blunting of a costophrenic angle (see Fig 4.1), apparent elevation of the diaphragm (see Fig 4.2, *A*), peripheral homogeneous opacity with a line that parallels the lateral chest wall (Fig 4.3), opacity in interlobar fissures (Fig 4.4, *A-D*),[465] or complete opacification of an entire hemithorax, with a shift of the mediastinum (Fig 4.5). Detection and confirmation are often the first steps in the evaluation of a suspected pleural effusion. Small effusions with opacification of the costophrenic angle may be confirmed by a lateral decubitus examination, with the side of the suspected effusion down. The decubitus examination may show a change in position of the opacity and confirm free-flowing effusion. No change in the opacity may be the result of loculated effusion, pleural scarring, or possibly a pleural mass. Prior chest radiographs indicating that the blunting is a new finding also provide a good indicator of pleural effusion. Loculated effusions are difficult to confirm with chest radiograph, but ultrasound, computed tomography (CT), and even magnetic resonance imaging (MRI) may be used to verify a localized collection of pleural fluid. The differential diagnosis of pleural effusion entails consideration of a long list of entities (Chart 4.1),[465] but the radiologist should not be discouraged.[478] Pleural effusion is sometimes associated with additional radiologic findings that may be very specific, but clinical and laboratory correlation are almost always required to make a specific diagnosis.

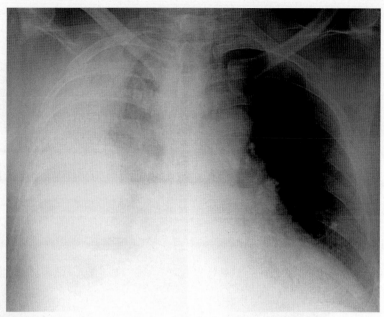

Fig. 4.3   A large homogeneous opacity in the right lateral chest has a sharp line separating it from the partially aerated lung. This is the result of a large pleural effusion caused by metastatic disease.

PLEURAL EFFUSION WITH LARGE CARDIAC SILHOUETTE

Congestive heart failure is one of the most common causes of pleural effusion, and it usually presents with a specific combination of cardiac and vascular findings. These cardiovascular changes include cardiomegaly, prominence of upper-lobe vessels, constriction of lower-lobe vessels, and prominent hilar vessels. In addition, there may be signs of interstitial edema, including fine reticular opacities, interlobular septal thickening (Kerley lines), perihilar haze, and peribronchial thickening. There may even be evidence of alveolar edema, with acinar nodules, confluent, ill-defined opacities with a perihilar distribution, and air bronchograms. The combination of cardiomegaly, pulmonary vascular changes, interstitial or alveolar edema, and pleural effusion is almost certainly diagnostic of congestive heart failure.

The pleural effusions resulting from congestive heart failure may be bilateral or unilateral. Unilateral effusions are usually on the right. Unilateral left pleural effusion in congestive failure is considered a great rarity and has even been cited as a reason to consider other diagnoses. It actually occurs in 10% to 15% of patients who develop pleural effusions secondary to congestive heart failure. Recurrent effusions caused by congestive heart failure tend to duplicate the appearance of the effusion seen in the previous episode of failure.

The combination of enlargement of the heart, pleural effusion in the absence of pulmonary vascular congestion, and signs of pulmonary interstitial or alveolar edema may be consistent with congestive heart failure. The presence of pleural effusion and cardiac enlargement alone is less specific; therefore, these require more careful review of serial examinations and correlation with clinical data to narrow the differential diagnosis (Chart 4.2). Because interstitial and alveolar edema may resolve rapidly in response to diuretics, these signs of congestive heart failure may disappear, leaving residual pleural effusion and cardiomegaly. Serial chest radiographs frequently confirm this possibility.

Chronic renal failure is another cause of pulmonary edema with associated pleural effusions that is usually confirmed by correlation with the clinical history. When renal

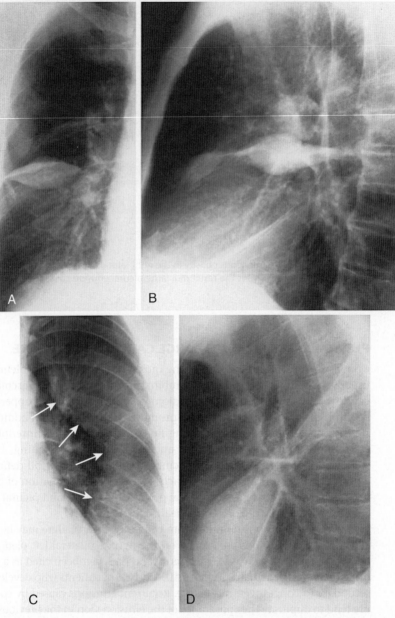

Fig. 4.4   A, Posterior-anterior (PA) chest radiograph demonstrates elliptic opacity in the horizontal fissure. **B,** Lateral view confirms that the opacity is in the horizontal fissure. This is the characteristic appearance of loculated fluid in the horizontal fissure. These collections may be rounder and are often called *pleural pseudotumors.* They may be transient and are sometimes described as vanishing tumors, especially when they are the result of congestive heart failure. **C,** PA view from another case demonstrates the appearance of fluid in the left oblique fissure. This is less mass-like, with the fluid spreading out in the fissure. The medial inferior border *(arrows)* is well circumscribed, with an arch that appears to outline the superior segment of the lower lobe. **D,** Lateral view of the case seen in **C** shows thickening of the entire length of the horizontal fissure.

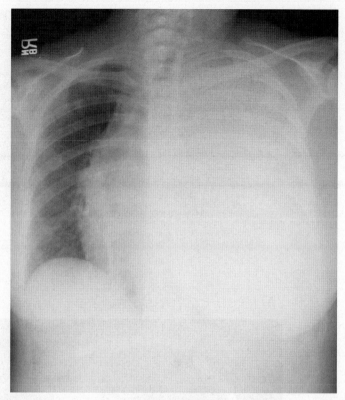

Fig. 4.5 This posterior-anterior chest radiograph shows complete opacification of the left hemithorax. Also note the shift of the trachea, mediastinum, and heart to the right. This is a large pleural effusion, with complete atelectasis of the left lung. This appearance does not reveal the cause of the effusion but is an important observation because it often indicates the need for urgent drainage.

failure is the cause of pleural effusions, the associated congestive heart failure is secondary to fluid overload.

Pulmonary embolism as a cause of pleural effusions is a more difficult diagnosis to confirm.[82] Right-sided heart enlargement and pleural effusions may be suggestive of embolism. A patient with congestive heart failure may have right-sided heart enlargement and pleural effusion and is also at increased risk for developing a pulmonary embolism. When the effusion is atypical (e.g., predominantly left sided) or if it increases after the pulmonary edema has begun to clear, the possibility of embolism should be considered. Any combination of additional clinical information indicating the development of chest pain, hemoptysis, sudden shortness of breath, pleural friction rub, decreased arterial P_{O_2}, or thrombophlebitis should be considered evidence for pulmonary embolism and thus would indicate more definitive evaluation.[396]

The combination of cardiac silhouette enlargement caused by pericardial effusion with associated pleural effusions may be seen in patients with metastatic or inflammatory disease. A history of a current or recurrent malignant neoplasm should suggest metastatic pleural and pericardial effusions. A febrile illness with clinical findings of pericarditis or myocarditis are helpful in suggesting inflammatory diseases, in particular viral and tuberculous infections or even poststreptococcal infection (e.g., rheumatic fever).

Pleural and pericardial effusions are the most common radiologic manifestations of systemic lupus erythematosus (Fig 4.6, *A* and *B*).[632] This diagnosis is rarely suggested by the radiologist. In the absence of other radiologic or clinical features of the common causes of pleural effusion with cardiac enlargement, this diagnosis may be considered.

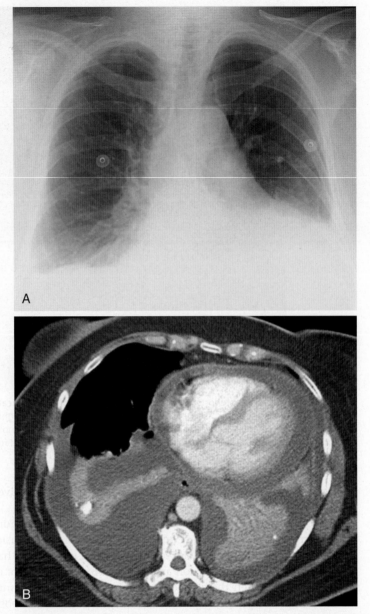

Fig. 4.6   A, The blunting of both costophrenic angles with apparent elevation of the left diaphragm provides the clue to suspect bilateral pleural effusions that are greater on the left. The heart is partially obscured on the left but appears to be enlarged. **B,** Computed tomography confirms bilateral pleural effusions and reveals that the apparent cardiac enlargement is the result of pericardial effusion. This patient had a known diagnosis of lupus erythematosus. Effusions are the most common manifestation of lupus in the chest.

The pericardial effusion may be confirmed with ultrasound as an alternative to CT. Correlation with clinical and laboratory data is required to confirm the diagnosis.

PLEURAL EFFUSION WITH MULTIPLE MASSES

Metastatic tumors and mesothelioma may both cause pleural masses and effusion. The case in Fig. 4.7, *A,* shows a large, left pleural effusion with multiple pleural masses. A CT scan from the same case (see Fig 4.7, *B*) reveals a large inferior chest wall mass that was obscured by the pleural effusion. This combination is not likely to result from empyema, tuberculosis, actinomycosis, or multiple myeloma. In this case, an

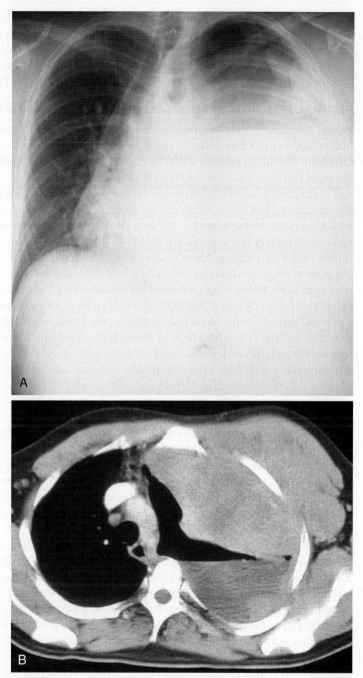

Fig. 4.7 A, The opacity of the left hemithorax with shift of the mediastinum to the right is the result of a large hydropneumothorax with an air-fluid level. The pneumothorax would suggest a bronchopleural fistula, but is iatrogenic secondary to thoracentesis. The additional finding of superior lobulated lateral masses is the result of pleural metastases. This combination of pleural effusion with pleural masses is difficult to evaluate on the chest radiograph, except for the pneumothorax. The combination of pleural effusion with pleural masses often requires computed tomography (CT) for confirmation. In this case, the masses were obscured by the pleural effusion prior to the thoracentesis and are visible because of the iatrogenic pneumothorax. **B,** The CT reveals a large inferior mass that has extended through the chest wall. This is a Ewing sarcoma that has spread to the pleura, with malignant effusion and multiple pleural masses.

iatrogenic pneumothorax accounts for the air-fluid level. The pleural masses were obscured by the large effusion prior to the thoracentesis. The combination of pleural effusion with pleural masses is most often confirmed with CT and is strongly suggestive of metastases. When there has been a history of asbestos exposure, mesothelioma becomes a likely explanation for unilateral pleural masses with pleural effusion.

PLEURAL EFFUSION WITH SEGMENTAL AND LOBAR OPACITIES

Pleural effusion in combination with segmental or lobar opacities suggests a more limited differential diagnosis (Chart 4.3). This combination is common and requires especially careful correlation with the clinical data. The postoperative patient requires the most careful consideration because subsegmental atelectasis is extremely common and is frequently secondary to a combination of thoracic splinting and small airway mucous plugs, but the coexistence of pleural effusions requires a separate explanation. Obviously, a thoracotomy explains effusion, and sympathetic effusion related to abdominal surgery is a well-known entity. In the previously noted clinical settings, the timing of the developing effusion should be considered. Late development or increasing pleural effusion could be secondary to postpericardiotomy syndrome or pulmonary embolism. Pulmonary embolism should be strongly suspected when a patient on bed rest develops dyspnea, hemoptysis, chest pain, or thrombophlebitis.

Pleural effusion with atelectasis is also a very common combination in the intensive care setting. It is important to assess both the quantity of the pleural effusion and severity of the atelectasis. Very large pleural effusions are a cause of compressive atelectasis and may even completely collapse a lung, with a contralateral shift of the mediastinum (see Fig 4.5). In contrast, small pleural effusions are often missed or underestimated on the supine portable radiograph. CT scans of patients from the intensive care unit often reveal unexpected or larger than expected pleural fluid collections. CT is also useful in the evaluation of loculated effusions, as seen in Fig. 4.8, *A* and *B*. Pleural effusions and atelectasis are also common in the coronary care setting. Pleural effusion is a common expected finding in patients who have congestive heart failure, but these sedentary patients are also at risk for pulmonary embolism and, rarely, may develop a postmyocardial infarction or Dressler syndrome. In the latter group, atelectasis may result from bronchial obstruction by mucous plugs or compression of the left, lower-lobe bronchus by the enlarged heart.

The outpatient who presents with pleural effusion and segmental or lobar opacities with minimal symptoms or a more chronic history of slowly developing dyspnea, cough, blood-tinged sputum, or weight loss over a period of months is likely to have a primary lung neoplasm. Endobronchial masses may cause atelectasis or obstructive pneumonia. The presence of pleural effusion in a patient with a primary lung cancer is an indication for thoracentesis to prove that the effusion is malignant. Patients with lymphoma may also have this combination of findings, but are much less likely to have pleural effusion and pulmonary opacities at the time of initial diagnosis than are patients with primary lung cancer. Pleural effusions and pulmonary opacities are seen in the late stages of lymphoma and must be distinguished from opportunistic infections. Tuberculosis is the granulomatous disease that is most likely to present with pulmonary opacities and pleural effusion (see Fig 4.1). Pleural effusions may occur in both primary and postprimary tuberculosis. (Answer to question 1 is *b*.)

PLEURAL EFFUSION WITH HILAR ENLARGEMENT

The combination of hilar enlargement, especially a hilar mass or adenopathy with pleural effusion, may be even more specific (Chart 4.4). A unilateral hilar mass in a middle-aged smoker is highly suggestive of primary lung cancer. These patients may even present with pleural effusion, hilar mass, and atelectasis. Pleural effusion and hilar mass may also result from lymphoma, metastases from distant primary tumors,

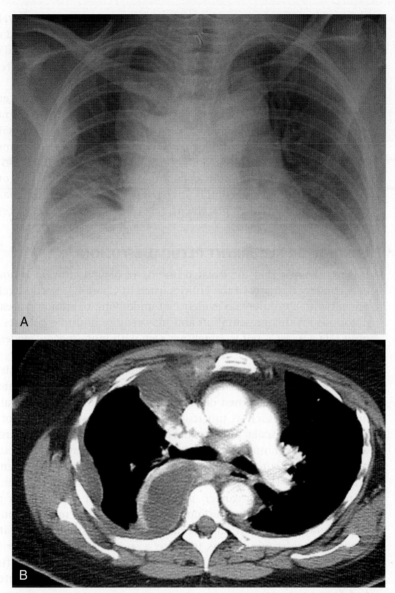

Fig. 4.8   A, A patient with a clinical and laboratory diagnosis of pneumonia has developed right localized medial and lateral pleural opacities. **B,** Computed tomography confirms multiple loculated pleural fluid collections consistent with empyema.

and granulomatous infections, including tuberculosis and less likely fungal infections such as histoplasmosis or coccidioidomycosis. There are a number of diagnostic procedures that may confirm the diagnosis, including the following: thoracentesis with culture and cytologic studies of fluid; bronchoscopy with cultures and biopsy; or CT-guided, fine-needle aspiration biopsy of the hilar mass.

Enlargement of the proximal pulmonary vessels with the appearance of hilar enlargement in combination with pleural effusion may occur in patients with congestive heart failure. However, this is rarely seen with pulmonary artery hypertension secondary to pulmonary embolism.

PARAPNEUMONIC EFFUSIONS AND EMPYEMA

Parapneumonic effusions and empyema develop in response to pneumonias. Parapneumonic effusions have a low white blood cell (WBC) count and low protein content, are sterile, and resolve completely in response to antibiotic therapy. In contrast, empyemas have an elevated WBC count and high protein content, and organisms may be cultured from the fluid. Thoracentesis specimens should be cultured for bacteria, fungi, and tuberculosis. Empyema is an active pleural infection that often requires pleural drainage to prevent chronic pleural scarring.[220,458]

The radiologic appearance of parapneumonic effusions and empyemas may be indistinguishable. Empyemas should be suspected when there is a rapid accumulation of a large quantity of pleural fluid or when the fluid is loculated. CT is often required for the precise localization of loculated empyemas (see Fig 4.8, *A* and *B*).

Empyemas are usually secondary to pneumonias, but may also be caused by the extension of an infection from a pharyngeal abscess, mediastinitis, or abdominal infection. Empyemas are also complications of penetrating chest trauma, pulmonary resections, thoracostomy tube placement, sclerosis of malignant effusions, and esophageal perforation.

CHRONIC OR RECURRENT PLEURAL EFFUSION

It is well known that the isolated finding of pleural effusion is nonspecific and may be secondary to many of the entities listed in Chart 4.1. Even infectious diseases may present with absolutely no evidence of underlying pulmonary disease. Tuberculosis is notorious for this presentation and may require multiple cultures for accurate diagnosis (Fig 4.9, *A-C*), but is sometimes seen with more specific evidence of tuberculosis (see Fig 4.1).

Rheumatoid disease of the pleura is another very elusive diagnosis unless the patient has obvious joint abnormalities. In the absence of joint abnormalities, the rheumatoid effusion may be diagnosed only after an extensive laboratory evaluation to exclude infectious causes such as tuberculosis and with positive results of serologic studies. Other collagen vascular diseases that cause chronic or recurrent effusions include lupus erythematosus, granulomatosis with polyangitis, and systemic sclerosis.

Malignant pleural effusions[358] should be suspected in patients with a known primary tumor (Fig 4.10), but effusion may also be the presenting abnormality in patients with lung cancer, mesothelioma, and even distant primaries such as ovarian carcinoma. The radiologic combination of multiple pulmonary nodules and pleural effusion virtually confirms the diagnosis of metastatic disease. Sometimes, unique combinations indicate a specific primary tumor. Because patients with malignant effusions are also at risk for opportunistic infections and are often treated with toxic drugs, malignant effusions must be differentiated from empyema and drug reactions.

ABDOMINAL DISEASES

Abdominal diseases must be considered in the evaluation of pleural effusion. A minimal radiologic examination of a patient with abdominal disease should include radiographs of the abdomen, with the patient in the supine and upright positions, as well as posterior-anterior (PA) and lateral chest radiographs. Fig. 4.2, *A* and *B*, illustrates a case of pleural effusion secondary to abdominal disease. In addition to the apparent elevation of the right hemidiaphragm and blunting of the right costophrenic angle, air is seen over the right-upper quadrant of the abdomen. A localized extraluminal collection of air is good evidence of a subphrenic abscess. (Answer to question 2 is *c*.) A cross-table lateral view or a lateral decubitus view (see Fig 4.2, *B*) will reveal an air-fluid level in the right-upper quadrant. The lateral decubitus view has the advantage of being easier to interpret and confirms the presence of the associated pleural effusion. A subphrenic abscess, which has definite radiographic findings such as in the present case, does require further confirmation, but a subphrenic abscess, which does not have air under the diaphragm, cannot be

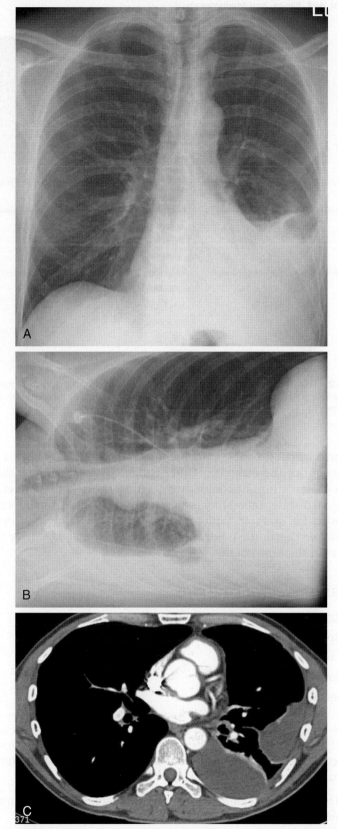

Fig. 4.9   A, Opacification of the lower-left thorax obscures the diaphragm and costophrenic angle. Effusions may layer between the diaphragm and base of the lung, resembling an elevated diaphragm. **B,** Left lateral decubitus view confirms pleural effusion with free-flowing fluid that changes position and separates the lung from the chest wall. **C,** Computed tomography (CT) reveals that the effusion is a complex effusion, with loculated fluid collections. Based on the CT scan, this was diagnosed as an empyema; 2 weeks after thoracentesis, the cultures were positive for tuberculosis.

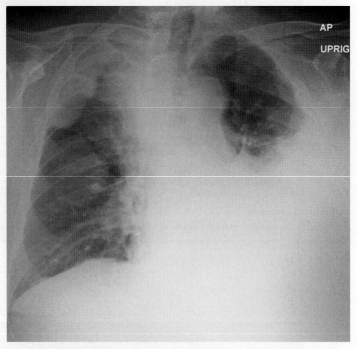

Fig. 4.10 This large left subpulmonic pleural effusion appears to spread around the lateral pleura. The right apical mass also appears to follow the pleura and makes the diagnosis of metastases almost certain. The history of renal cell carcinoma confirmed the diagnosis.

confirmed by chest or abdominal radiographic criteria. In such a case, ultrasound or CT confirms the diagnosis. Other patients with abdominal disease that might lead to pleural effusion require careful clinical correlation and evaluation of their abdominal disease. Laboratory evaluation of the pleural fluid is beneficial and often diagnostic; for example, patients with pancreatitis may have extremely elevated levels of amylase in the fluid, and patients with an amebic liver abscess may have parasites in their pleural fluid.[639]

Top 5 Diagnoses: Pleural Effusions

1. Congestive heart failure
2. Parapneumonic effusion
3. Metastases
4. Ascites
5. Tuberculosis

Summary

Free pleural fluid may be radiologically confirmed by lateral decubitus views or serial examinations that show a change in contour.

Loculated effusions are difficult to confirm by radiographic examination but may be confirmed by ultrasound or CT examination of pleural opacities.

The presence of pleural effusion must be carefully correlated with other radiologic findings, both on the chest radiograph and in other organ systems.

ANSWER GUIDE

Legends for introductory figures

Fig. 4.1 Blunting of the right costophrenic angle with opacity obscuring the right hemidiaphragm is a clue to suspected pleural effusion. The associated apical opacities strongly suggest that the effusion is the result of tuberculosis.

Fig. 4.2 **A,** This posterior-anterior chest radiograph demonstrates apparent elevation of the right hemidiaphragm. **B,** Lateral decubitus view confirms the presence of pleural fluid and reveals a large air-fluid level below the diaphragm. The latter finding confirms the diagnosis of subphrenic abscess.

ANSWERS

1. b   2. c

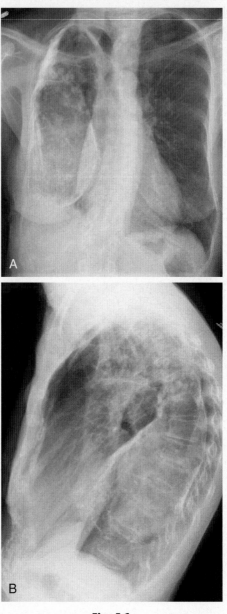

Fig. 5.1

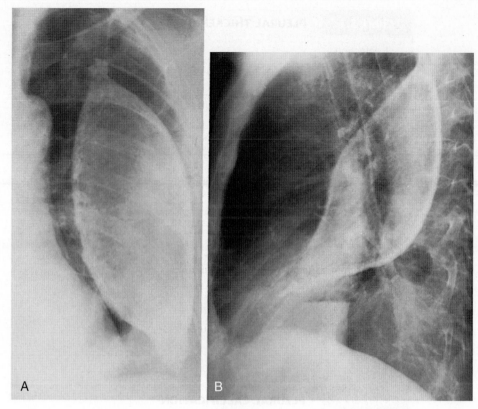

Fig. 5.2

QUESTIONS

1. What is the most likely diagnosis for the case illustrated in Fig. 5.1?
   a. Mesothelioma.
   b. Metastases.
   c. Empyema.
   d. Lung cancer.
   e. Lymphoma.

2. The large calcification in Fig. 5.2 is most probably caused by:
   a. Tuberculosis.
   b. Asbestosis.
   c. Mesothelioma.
   d. Empyema.
   e. Talcosis.

3. Which one of the following interstitial lung diseases is most likely to have associated plaques of pleural thickening?
   a. Rheumatoid lung.
   b. Scleroderma lung.
   c. Usual interstitial pneumonitis.
   d. Desquamative interstitial pneumonitis.
   e. Asbestosis.

Chart 5.1	**PLEURAL THICKENING**

I. Infection
   A. Empyema
   B. Tuberculosis[388]
   C. Aspergillosis (saprophytic form—i.e., fungus ball)[340]
II. Neoplasm
   A. Metastases
   B. Mesothelioma[376]
   C. Pancoast tumor[415]
   D. Leukemia[297]
III. Collagen vascular (rheumatoid arthritis[369])
IV. Trauma (healed hemothorax)
V. Inhalational diseases
   A. Asbestos related diseases[5,37,184,376,511-513]
   B. Talcosis[144]
VI. Other
   A. Organization of serous pleural effusion
   B. Sarcoidosis[635]
   C. Splenosis[270]
   D. Fat[160]
   E. Mimics (extrathoracic musculature)[88]

Chart 5.2	**PLEURAL CALCIFICATION**

I. Trauma (healed hemothorax)
II. Infection
   A. Chronic empyema[520]
   B. Tuberculosis[298]
III. Inhalation
   A. Asbestos-related plaques[179,513]
   B. Talcosis[144]

Discussion

Pleural thickening must be distinguished from pleural fluid (Chart 5.1). Like pleural effusion, pleural thickening is usually appreciated as a thick white line between the lucent lungs and ribs. Lateral decubitus views are frequently necessary for distinguishing free pleural effusion from pleural thickening, but loculated effusions are not as easily distinguished from pleural thickening. This may sometimes be accomplished by comparison with prior examinations. When the pleural thickening is of recent onset (days to weeks), pleural effusion is the most likely cause of the opacity, whereas if the process has been stable for months to years, it is most probably true pleural thickening. As with pleural masses, ultrasound or computed tomography (CT) may be essential for distinguishing loculated fluid collections from pleural thickening or nodules.

ORGANIZING EFFUSION

Organization of an infected pleural effusion (empyema) is one of the most common causes of pleural thickening. The detection of a small amount of associated pleural fluid may seem unimportant but is vital for diagnostic thoracentesis.[478] The fluid may appear to be nondiagnostic, but it provides material for culture and cytologic studies.

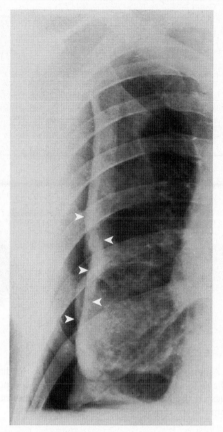

Fig. 5.3 This case of rheumatoid pleural thickening *(arrowheads)* illustrates involvement of visceral pleura. The distinction of visceral from parietal pleural thickening is possible only in the presence of pneumothorax. Recall that asbestosis is one of the few causes of pleural thickening that can appear to spare the visceral pleura.

An organizing fibrothorax is definitely less diagnostic because it usually consists of chronic inflammatory cells and fibrosis. It may be the end result of a variety of bacterial, fungal, and tuberculous pulmonary infections. In such cases, the radiologic finding of pleural thickening is nonspecific, and the radiologic diagnosis usually depends on associated pulmonary findings. Apical pulmonary cavities with associated pleural thickening are characteristic of prior granulomatous infection, such as tuberculosis or histoplasmosis.[388] A strongly reactive skin test may confirm the diagnosis. Additional complications should be suspected in patients with old cystic lesions or cavities who develop a new pleural opacity in the area of the old abnormalities. A new area of pleural thickening in the same vicinity is suggestive of new complications, which include reactivation of tuberculosis, scar cancer, or a new infection, such as aspergilloma, which develops in old cavities and may cause pleural thickening.[340] As with other causes of inflammatory pleural thickening, the histologic appearance of the pleural disease secondary to aspergilloma is nonspecific. The fungus is not usually identifiable in the pleural reaction.

The less specific appearance of extensive pleural thickening over the bases, with associated parenchymal scars, can best be diagnosed as chronic empyema when a definite history of previous pneumonia is obtained. Some noninfectious causes of pleural effusion, such as rheumatoid disease, occasionally fail to resolve, with the final result of a thick pleural reaction (Fig 5.3).[369] A history of known rheumatoid arthritis may suggest this diagnosis. In addition, positive results of serologic studies for rheumatoid factor may also suggest the diagnosis, particularly if there is a history of thoracic disease prior to the onset of joint disease.

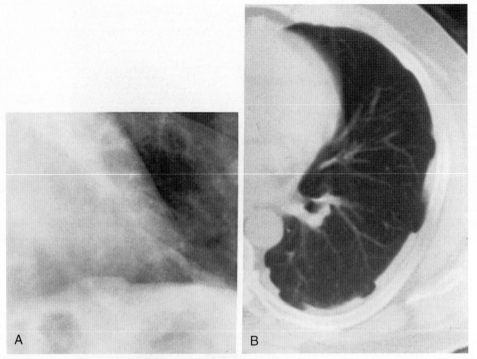

Fig. 5.4   A, Asbestos-related plaques typically involve the diaphragmatic pleura. Noncalcified plaques are often difficult to see on a chest radiograph. **B,** A computed tomography scan of the same case reveals plaques on the lateral and posterior pleura to be much more extensive than what has been suspected from the chest radiograph.

ASBESTOS-RELATED PLAQUES

Asbestos-related pleural plaques are a common cause of pleural thickening.[511-513] They are most likely seen along the lateral chest walls or on the diaphragmatic pleura (Fig 5.4, A and B), sparing the apices.[281] High-resolution CT (HRCT) has been advocated for distinguishing these plaques from other causes of pleural thickening.[179] Basilar interstitial disease is occasionally an associated finding that may also be more accurately assessed with HRCT.[5] The diagnosis of asbestosis requires a combination of basilar interstitial fibrosis with pleural plaques (answer to question 3 is *e*). The diagnosis requires a history of exposure to asbestos for confirmation.

A curious feature of the pleural thickening of asbestos exposure is the tendency for marked parietal pleural thickening and relative sparing of the visceral pleura. This is in contrast to other causes of pleural thickening, such as empyema, tuberculosis, and rheumatoid disease. The finding is rarely useful for the radiologist except for patients who at some time have had either spontaneous or iatrogenic pneumothorax.

NEOPLASM

As mentioned in the discussion of pleural masses (see Chapter 3), diffuse nodular pleural thickening raises the differential of (1) loculated effusion, (2) metastases, and (3) mesothelioma (Fig 5.5).[131] In such cases, the nodular character of the pleural reaction may not be appreciated prior to thoracentesis for the removal of an associated pleural effusion. Thoracentesis should be done in combination with a pleural biopsy, which frequently confirms the diagnosis.

Apical pleural capping is a common radiologic appearance[378,471,472] and must not be confused with normal structures, such as the subclavian artery, supraclavicular border, sternocleidomastoid muscle, or rib companion shadows. There is a tendency to attribute

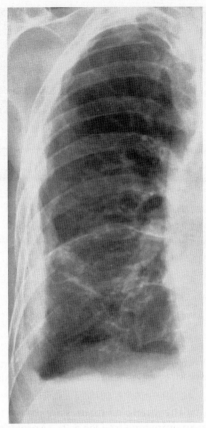

Fig. 5.5 This case of mesothelioma (like the one shown in Fig. 3.10) has produced diffuse, unilateral pleural thickening.

true pleural thickening to old tuberculosis, but it is often a fibrotic scar of obscure origin. It is possible to confuse tuberculous pleural thickening with a Pancoast tumor, but a convex inferior border should suggest a mass (Fig 5.6).[415] Coned views of the ribs or CT may show bone destruction, which indicates a neoplastic process, but the absence of bone destruction does not exclude a malignant neoplasm. Radionuclide bone scans are more sensitive than chest radiographs for early bone involvement by a Pancoast tumor. Comparison with old examinations that show the apical pleural cap to be stable over a period of years is essentially diagnostic of an old inflammatory process. When serial examinations demonstrate a change, it is strongly suggestive of tumor or active infection.

PLEURAL CALCIFICATION

The causes of pleural calcification (Chart 5.2) are limited to a small number of diagnoses, in contrast with the lack of specificity of both pleural effusion and pleural thickening.

Hemothorax is usually confirmed by a history of significant chest trauma. There may be associated healed rib fractures. Although pulmonary contusion may have accompanied the acute episodes, contusion usually resolves without any significant residual effect. Associated parenchymal scarring thus favors a diagnosis other than that of a previous hemothorax.

Chronic empyema is a more common cause of pleural calcification. Calcification was previously considered a sign of an old healed process, but CT studies have indicated that chronic empyema may calcify around the periphery while retaining collections of fluid for years.[520] Occasionally, calcified pleural thickening from empyema does assume unusual or bizarre configurations and may be very extensive. It must be

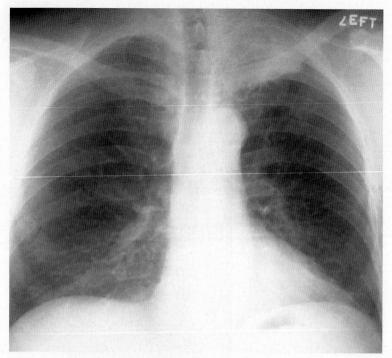

Fig. 5.6 Apical involvement of the pleura by tuberculosis may resemble apical lung cancer, but in this case the asymmetric left opacity is more mass-like and was caused by a superior sulcus or Pancoast tumor.

remembered that the interlobar fissures are part of the pleural space and may therefore be involved by an empyema (see Fig 5.2). (Answer to question 2 is *d.*) A careful history frequently dates these pleural reactions to a specific episode of pneumonia. Empyema may also be the result of penetrating injuries, such as bullet and stab wounds.

Tuberculosis is no longer a common cause of empyema, but because calcification indicates a long-standing process, tuberculosis is a likely cause of calcified empyema.[298] The pleural reaction is usually apical and asymmetric. Asymmetric pleural thickening and calcification, with apical scarring and cavities or cystic bronchiectasis, should strongly suggest tuberculosis (Fig 5.7, *A* and *B*).

Asbestos exposure is a common cause of pleural calcifications measuring less than 3 to 4 cm, but the pleural plaques may spread around the pleura. Pleural calcifications resulting from asbestos exposure usually affect the domes of the diaphragmatic pleura, but they may be extensive and bilateral (Fig 5.8, *A-C*). Anterior and posterior pleural plaques are not seen as sharp lines of pleural calcification on the posterior-anterior (PA) chest radiograph, but as less well-defined opacities that are termed *en face plaque.* These plaques are often mistaken for pulmonary opacities or may be recognized by their association with the more characteristic diaphragmatic or lateral pleural calcifications. Noncalcified plaques are the most common finding in patients with asbestos exposure, but they are more difficult to identify on chest radiograph and are less specific than the calcifications. CT scanning (Fig 5.9, *A* and *B*) has been shown to be the most sensitive means for detecting minimal pleural changes from asbestos exposure.[5,480,556] Pleural calcification is not seen in all cases of asbestos exposure, but can lead to one of the most specific appearances in chest radiology.

Talcosis is the result of exposure to a variety of talc mixtures.[144] Pure talc is not very fibrogenic, but mixtures of talc with silica or magnesium silicate are very fibrogenic. Both asbestos and tremolite talc contain magnesium silicate. The radiologic findings in this type of talcosis are the same as those in asbestosis.

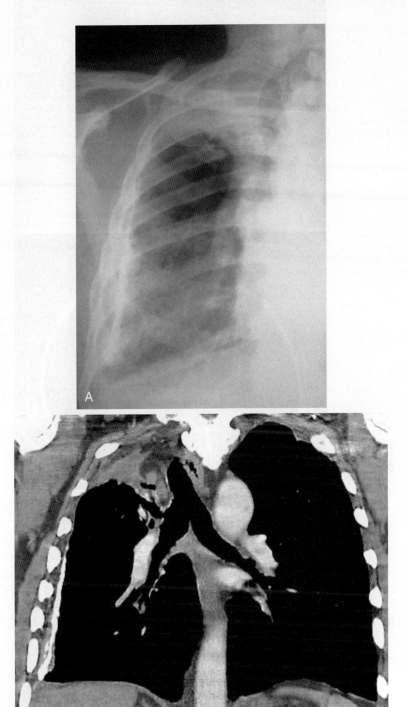

Fig. 5.7 **A,** The right apical opacity has an associated shift of the trachea to the right, which is the result of chronic scarring with lateral pleural thickening and calcification. **B,** Coronal computed tomography scan confirms the apical opacity with a shift of the trachea and the lateral pleural calcifications, which are the result of tuberculosis.

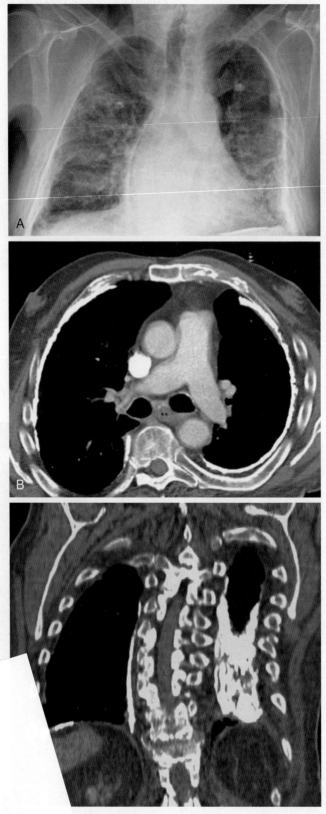

pleural calcifications that appear to encase the lungs are an unusually
-related plaques. In this case, the plaques involve the medial, lateral,
ura. The less well-defined opacities overlying the lungs are the result
are described as en face plaque. **B,** Computed tomography confirms
ions. **C,** A posterior section from the coronal reconstructions shows
ural calcification, but the posterior plaque on the left is even more
ification accounts for en face plaques on the chest radiograph.

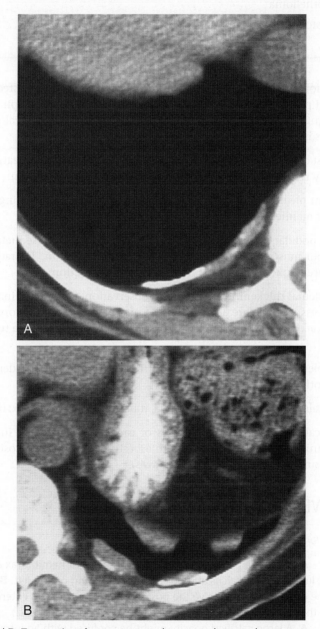

Fig. 5.9   A and **B,** Two sections from a computed tomography scan demonstrate calcified and non-calcified pleural plaques typical of asbestos exposure.

Top 5 Diagnoses: Pleural Thickening and Pleural Calcification

1. Empyema
2. Metastases
3. Tuberculosis
4. Mesothelioma
5. Asbestos-related plaques

Summary

Distinction of pleural thickening from effusion may be suggested by the configuration and position of the opacity on the upright chest radiograph (e.g., apical pleural thickening), but comparison with previous examinations, lateral decubitus views, or CT scans is frequently required.

The most common cause of chronic pleural thickening is organization of an empyema. This may result from a bacterial, tuberculous, or fungal infection.

Recurrent pleural effusion with development of pleural thickening is one of the more frequent manifestations of rheumatoid disease in the thorax.

Diffuse, nodular pleural thickening is consistent with diffuse metastases or mesothelioma, but must be distinguished from loculated effusion. Thoracentesis and pleural biopsy are frequently required for making the distinction.

Apical pleural thickening is a common observation. Serial examinations showing that the process is stable are adequate proof of a benign inflammatory process. A change suggests activity of the inflammatory process or the presence of a tumor (e.g., Pancoast tumor).

Apical pleural thickening with rib destruction should be considered neoplastic until proven otherwise.

Pleural calcification indicates empyema, tuberculosis, hemothorax, or asbestos exposure.

Pleural calcifications over the domes of each hemidiaphragm in combination with pleural thickening are consistent with asbestos exposure or talcosis. A history of such an exposure should confirm the diagnosis.

ANSWER GUIDE

Legends for introductory figures

Fig. 5.1   A, Extensive pleural calcification over the right hemithorax appears to encase the right lung, with no calcification or pleural thickening on the left. **B,** The lateral view shows the calcification to involve the posterior right thorax. This extensive pleural calcification is the result of chronic empyema. (Answer to question 1 is *c*.)

Fig. 5.2   A, A large calcified opacity might be confused with an intrapulmonary mass on the posteroanterior view. **B,** Lateral view localizes the abnormality to the oblique fissure and thus the pleural space. This pleural calcification resulted from an old empyema.

ANSWERS

1. c   2. c   3. e

6 | ELEVATED DIAPHRAGM

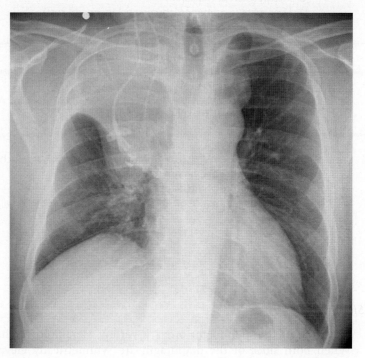

Fig. 6.1

QUESTIONS

1. Which one the following diagnoses is most likely in the case illustrated in Fig. 6.1?
   a. Hepatomegaly.
   b. Interposition of the colon.
   c. Right upper lobe atelectasis.
   d. Phrenic nerve paralysis.
   e. Right upper lobe pneumonia.

2. Which of the following is least likely to be associated with pleural effusion?
   a. Primary lung tumor.
   b. Interposition of colon.
   c. Subphrenic abscess.
   d. Echinococcal cyst.
   e. Metastasis.

3. Which of the following is not true of phrenic nerve paralysis?
   a. Results in complete loss of motion of the diaphragm at fluoroscopy.
   b. May be secondary to primary lung tumor in the apex.
   c. May be secondary to mediastinal malignant tumor.
   d. Occasionally is idiopathic.
   e. Results in paradoxic motion of the diaphragm.

Chart 6.1	**ELEVATED DIAPHRAGM**

I. Subpulmonic pleural effusion[32,53]
II. Abdominal disease
   A. Subphrenic abscess
   B. Distended stomach
   C. Interposition of the colon
   D. Liver mass (e.g., tumor, abscess, echinococcal cyst)
III. Decreased lung volume
   A. Atelectasis
   B. Postoperative lobectomy and pneumonectomy
   C. Hypoplastic lung
IV. Phrenic nerve paralysis
   A. Primary lung cancer
   B. Malignant mediastinal tumor
   C. Iatrogenic
   D. Idiopathic
V. Diaphragmatic hernia[336] (e.g., foramina of Morgagni and Bochdalek)
VI. Eventration of the diaphragm
VII. Traumatic rupture of the diaphragm
VIII. Diaphragmatic tumor (e.g., lipoma,[153] fibroma, mesothelioma, metastasis, lymphoma)

Discussion

Elevation of the diaphragm offers a variety of radiologic challenges (Chart 6.1). When both sides of the diaphragm are symmetrically elevated, the differential is significantly different from that with unilateral elevation. The most common cause of elevation of both sides of the diaphragm is failure of the patient to inspire deeply. This is frequently voluntary, but may be an indicator of a significant pathologic process. Obesity is probably the most common abnormality resulting in low lung volume. A similar appearance may be produced by a variety of abdominal conditions, including ascites and large abdominal masses. Bilateral atelectasis may also result in the elevation of both sides of the diaphragm, but is usually identifiable by increased opacity in the lung bases. Restrictive pulmonary diseases may likewise result in elevation of both sides of the diaphragm (see Cicatrizing Atelectasis in Chapter 13).

SUBPULMONIC PLEURAL EFFUSION

Subpulmonic pleural effusion is an important cause of apparent elevation of the diaphragm.[32,53] This is usually unilateral, but on occasion may be bilateral. The posteroanterior view may suggest this diagnosis when the diaphragm appears flat, with a lateral meniscus in the costophrenic angle (Fig. 6.2, *A*), or when the dome of the diaphragm is more lateral than normal, with an abrupt drop-off (Fig. 6.3, *A*). The lateral view may help confirm this impression by demonstrating a posterior meniscus (see Fig. 6.3, *B*). The diagnosis is often confirmed with a lateral decubitus view (see Fig. 6.2, *B*). Caution must be exercised in evaluating a subpulmonic pleural effusion because pleural effusions may be associated with other significant abnormalities, such as a subphrenic abscess, primary lung tumor, and liver masses (including abscesses and echinococcal cysts) that result in true elevation of the diaphragm.

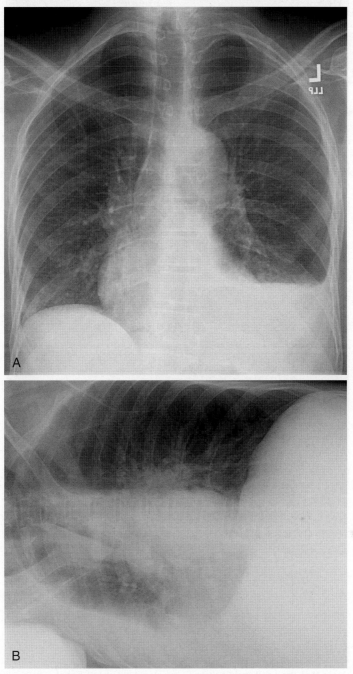

Fig. 6.2 A, The opacification of the left lower thorax is flat rather than domed, with a lateral meniscus. This is the result of a large fluid collection between the base of the lung and the diaphragm. **B,** Left lateral decubitus view confirms the presence of a large, free-flowing pleural effusion.

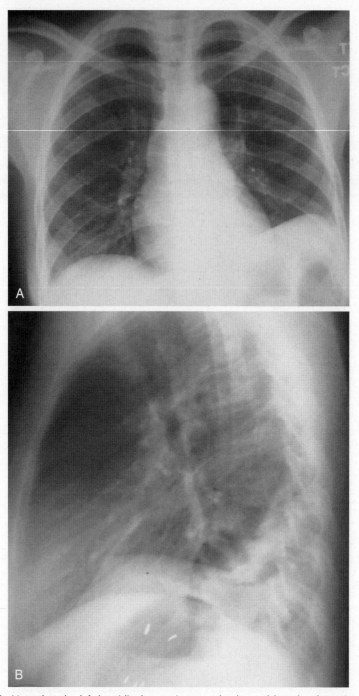

Fig. 6.3 **A,** Note that the left hemidiaphragm is not only elevated but the dome is more lateral than the normal right side due to a subpulmonic pleural effusion. **B,** Lateral view reveals a sharp right costophrenic angle but blunting of the left costophrenic angle. Only the posterior portion of the left hemidiaphragm appears elevated, and it appears to end at the major fissure. This unusual appearance is another clue to a subpulmonic pleural effusion, mimicking elevation of the left hemidiaphragm.

ALTERED PULMONARY VOLUME

Atelectasis is a common cause of diaphragmatic elevation and is recognizable by the associated pulmonary opacity. Elevation of the diaphragm is an expected complication of lower-lobe, lingula, or middle-lobe atelectasis, but is also seen in upper-lobe atelectasis (see Fig. 6.1). (Answer to question 1 is *c*.) Postoperative volume loss should be recognized easily in cases with rib defects, metallic sutures, and shift of the heart or mediastinum.

ABDOMINAL DISEASES

A subphrenic abscess is not a rare cause of unilateral elevation of the diaphragm following abdominal surgery. It is usually accompanied by pleural effusion. Chest radiographs alone may confirm the diagnosis when localized collections of air are demonstrated below the diaphragm (see Fig. 4.2, *A* and *B*). Ultrasound is the least invasive method for confirming the diagnosis, and it is virtually diagnostic when localized fluid collections are demonstrated below the diaphragm.

Distended abdominal viscera, such as the colon and stomach, may occasionally elevate one side of the diaphragm. Interposition of the colon is a completely benign condition in which the colon is interposed between the liver and right side of the diaphragm. It may result in elevation of the right side of the diaphragm, but is not an adequate explanation for pleural effusion. (Answer to question 2 is *b*.) Occasionally, large liver masses elevate the right diaphragm, and computed tomography (CT) with biopsy may be required to confirm the diagnosis.

PHRENIC NERVE PARALYSIS

Phrenic nerve paralysis is a common cause of elevation of one side of the diaphragm. It may be due to a variety of problems, including primary lung cancer, malignant mediastinal tumors, and surgery of the mediastinum. It may even be idiopathic. The combination of a lung or mediastinal mass and elevation of the diaphragm strongly suggests phrenic nerve paralysis. The condition can be confirmed by fluoroscopy, which will reveal paradoxic motion of the diaphragm—that is, as the patient inspires, the paralyzed side of the diaphragm appears to rise. This may be associated with slight flutter and is best demonstrated with the patient in the lateral position. (Answer to question 3 is *a*.) A sniff accentuates diaphragmatic motion and is therefore useful in eliciting paradoxic motion.

EVENTRATION OF THE DIAPHRAGM

Eventration of the diaphragm is similar to paralysis but represents an area of weakness and thinning of the diaphragm. With eventration, there may be motion of the diaphragm but a smaller excursion between inspiration and expiration. It should not entail a paradoxic movement of the diaphragm. In infancy, eventration may result in elevation of a large portion of the diaphragm. In these cases, the entire leaf of the diaphragm may consist of thin fibrous tissue. Older patients frequently have localized irregularities of the diaphragm that lead to a lobulated appearance but are of little pathologic significance.

TRAUMATIC RUPTURE OF THE DIAPHRAGM

Traumatic rupture of the diaphragm may result in apparent elevation of the diaphragm with intrathoracic herniation of an intraabdominal viscus. Left rupture with herniation of the stomach, small bowel, or colon often results in a lucent structure adjacent to the heart (Fig. 6.4). These structures are likely to contain air, fluid, or air-fluid levels in the left side of the chest rather than an elevation of the left hemidiaphragm. When there is a large amount of fluid in these structures, the radiologic appearance may be

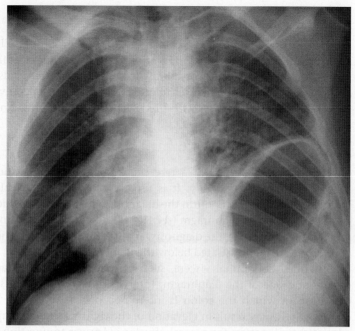

Fig. 6.4   This is a common appearance for traumatic rupture of the left hemidiaphragm. The elevated air-filled stomach following thoracoabdominal trauma should strongly suggest this diagnosis. Also, note the shift of the mediastinum to the right, indicating a space-occupying abnormality in the lower left thorax.

that of near-opacification of the left hemithorax. Right-sided injuries with herniation of the liver are often more difficult to recognize.[263] In this situation, the liver herniates into the right hemithorax and simulates elevation of the diaphragm (Fig. 6.5, *A* and *B*), which might be mistakenly attributed to paralysis, subphrenic pleural effusion, or atelectasis with elevation of the diaphragm. Diaphragmatic rupture is frequently associated with other signs of chest or abdominal trauma, including multiple fractures. Because of the severity of the injury, it may also be associated with pulmonary contusion and chest wall vascular injury, leading to pleural effusion. Although these signs of significant thoracic trauma should indicate the possibility of diaphragmatic injury, they may also obscure the direct signs that permit a confident diagnosis. Chest radiographs may provide the first clues to suspect the diagnosis, but CT with multiplanar imaging is more sensitive and specific for confirming the diagnosis (see Fig. 6.5, *C* and *D*).

DIAPHRAGMATIC TUMOR

Mesothelioma, fibroma, and lipoma may produce an apparent elevation of the diaphragm when the tumor assumes a massive size, but this is an infrequent occurrence. Serial radiographs may confirm growth of the mass, and CT should confirm the diagnosis.

Top 5 Diagnoses: Elevated Diaphragm

1. Eventration
2. Subpulmonic pleural effusion (apparent elevation of the diaphragm)
3. Atelectasis
4. Phrenic nerve paralysis
5. Diaphragmatic hernias (including traumatic hernias)

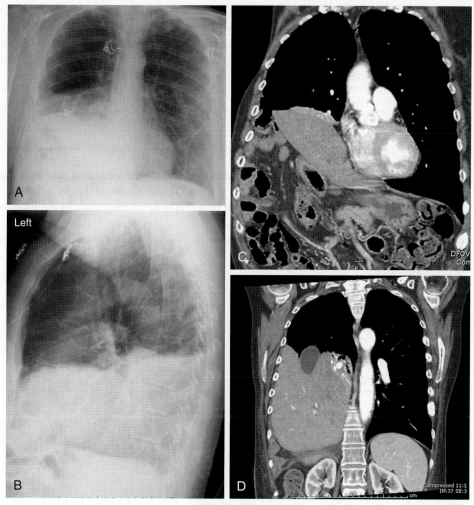

Fig. 6.5   A, The opacification of the right hemithorax could be the result of atelectasis of the right middle and lower lobes, a subpulmonic pleural effusion, or elevation of the diaphragm. **B,** Lateral chest radiograph shows a large opacity in the right lower thorax, which changes contour near the region of the oblique fissure and is suggestive of middle- and lower-lobe atelectasis. However, with the history of major abdominal trauma, a diaphragmatic injury should be considered. **C,** Coronal CT image through the anterior chest and abdomen reveals herniation of liver and bowel into the chest. **D,** Coronal CT scan through the posterior chest and abdomen confirms herniation of the liver, with the additional finding of inversion of the liver. Note the position of the gallbladder. This is a diaphragmatic rupture, with herniation and volvulus of the liver.

Summary

Subpulmonic pleural effusion is the problem that usually mimics diaphragmatic elevation. It should be distinguished from true diaphragmatic elevation with lateral decubitus views.

The most common causes of diaphragmatic elevation are atelectasis, abdominal masses, eventration of the diaphragm, and phrenic nerve paralysis.

Abdominal masses, such as subphrenic abscess and liver masses (including tumors, abscesses, and even echinococcal cysts), must be considered in the differential diagnosis of an elevated right hemidiaphragm.

Traumatic rupture of the diaphragm may mimic elevation of the diaphragm by permitting herniation of the liver into the right hemithorax or stomach, spleen, and bowel into the left hemithorax. This diagnosis should be considered when there is a history of significant abdominal or chest trauma and the appearance of a high hemidiaphragm.

ANSWER GUIDE

Legend for introductory figure

Fig. 6.1 Elevated right hemidiaphragm in this patient with lung cancer could have resulted from phrenic nerve paralysis, but the chest radiograph reveals additional findings of right upper lobe atelectasis. Note increased opacity and elevation of the horizontal fissure.

ANSWERS

1. c   2. b   3. a

7 | SHIFT OF THE MEDIASTINUM

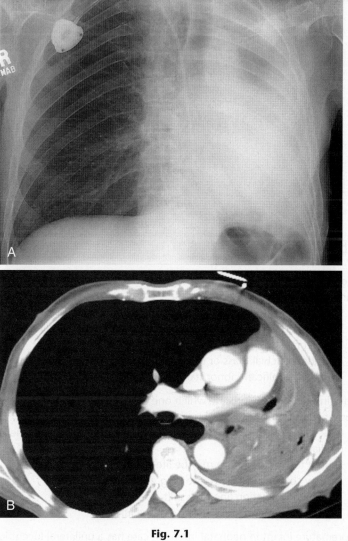

Fig. 7.1

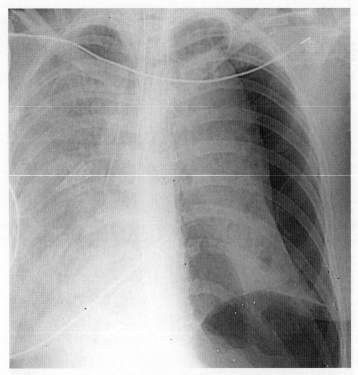

Fig. 7.2

QUESTIONS

1. Regarding the case shown in Fig. 7.1, *A* and *B*, which one of the following statements is incorrect?
   a. The right lung is overinflated.
   b. There is herniation of the right lung in front of the ascending aorta.
   c. Left pleural effusion is compressing the left lung.
   d. An endobronchial mass or mucous plug should be considered.
   e. The most significant abnormality may not be visible on this examination.

2. Referring to Fig. 7.2, indicate which one of the following statements is not true of tension pneumothorax:
   a. Collections of air may mimic the appearance of herniation of the lung through the mediastinum.
   b. Shift of the mediastinum may be life-threatening.
   c. Air may collect medially to the lung.
   d. The anterior junction line may shift.
   e. There is always complete collapse of the lung.

3. A premature infant in neonatal intensive care has a unilateral lucent lung with a contralateral shift of the mediastinum. Which one of the following is the most likely diagnosis?
   a. Congenital pulmonary airway malformation (CPAM).
   b. Bronchogenic cyst.
   c. Congenital lobar overdistention.
   d. Pulmonary interstitial emphysema (PIE).
   e. Bronchial obstruction.

Chart 7.1	SHIFT OF THE MEDIASTINUM

I. Decreased lung volume
   A. Atelectasis
   B. Hypoplastic lung
   C. Postoperative (e.g., lobectomy, pneumonectomy)
II. Pleural space abnormalities[588]
   A. Large unilateral pleural effusion[358]
   B. Tension pneumothorax
   C. Large diaphragmatic hernias (congenital or posttraumatic)
III. Increased lung volume in adults
   A. Asymmetric bullous emphysema
   B. Large masses (e.g., pulmonary, mediastinal, chest wall)
   C. Bronchiolitis obliterans (Swyer-James syndrome; rare)
   D. Bronchopulmonary sequestration (rare)
   E. Bronchogenic cyst (rare)
IV. Increased lung volume in young children
   A. Congenital lobar overdistention
   B. Interstitial emphysema
   C. CPAM
   D. Aspirated foreign body

Discussion

Shift of the mediastinum (Chart 7.1) is identified by displacement of the heart, trachea, aorta, and hilar vessels. Because shift of the mediastinum indicates an imbalance of pressures between the two sides of the thorax, one of the first steps in the evaluation of this problem is to determine which side is abnormal. Associated findings are frequently helpful in making this determination. For example, atelectasis is frequently associated with elevation of the hemidiaphragm and crowding of the ribs, as well as increased opacity of the lung. It is also frequently accompanied by overexpansion of the contralateral side of the chest, which is described as compensatory overaeration. In the absence of diaphragmatic elevation, the possibility that the overexpanded lung is the abnormal one has to be considered; the overexpanded lung could be compressing the normal lung, resulting in increased opacity on the normal side. The radiologist has two important tools for making this determination. The best-known method is the expiratory examination, which will demonstrate that air moves freely from the overexpanded side when it is the normal side and will show that the underexpanded lung is essentially unchanged, confirming the diagnosis of atelectasis. In contrast, air trapping in an overexpanded lung will be exaggerated.

When the patient is unable to cooperate, the best substitute for the expiratory examination is the lateral decubitus view. In this procedure the overexpanded side should be down, with the effect of splinting the down side. The radiologic result is similar to that of the expiratory examination. An overexpanded lung that remains overexpanded in the down position indicates bronchial obstruction with obstructive overaeration. The lateral decubitus examination is particularly helpful in a child who has a foreign body in the bronchus. If the overexpanded lung resumes normal size in the down position, the smaller lung can be assumed to be abnormal.

Fluoroscopy is another method for evaluating a shift of the mediastinum. In the case of atelectasis that has resulted from an endobronchial mass, deep inspiration causes the mediastinum to shift more toward the side of the atelectasis, whereas the diaphragm moves normally on the overexpanded side. Fluoroscopic examination will reveal that air trapping causes a shift of the mediastinum away from the lucent side during forced expiration.

DECREASED LUNG VOLUME

Loss of lung volume is an important cause of a shift of the mediastinum. The case shown in Fig. 7.1, *A* and *B* illustrates a shift of the mediastinum caused by a lung cancer arising in the left main bronchus. There is total atelectasis of the left lung with compensatory overinflation of the right lung and herniation of the lung in front of the anterior mediastinum. There is no evidence of left pleural fluid. (Answer to question 1 is *c*.) The various types of atelectasis, which are considered in Chapter 13, may all result in a shift of the mediastinum. It should also be apparent that lobectomy and pneumonectomy are common causes of a mediastinal shift. In fact, a shift of the heart and mediastinum accounts for much of the thoracic opacity that follows pneumonectomy.

A hypoplastic lung is a rare anomaly that results in a characteristic radiologic appearance consisting of a small hemithorax with crowding of the ribs, elevation of the hemidiaphragm, shift of the mediastinum, and an absent or very small pulmonary artery on the involved side. In addition to the small or absent hilar pulmonary artery, the peripheral vascularity of the involved lung is primarily bronchial with small irregular vessels lacking the normal hilar orientation of pulmonary arteries. This phenomenon is usually referred to as a *hypogenetic lung* or *congenital venolobar syndrome*.[654,670] It is usually seen on the right and is frequently associated with dextrocardia and anomalous pulmonary venous return from the right lung to the inferior vena cava. When the anomalous venous drainage is radiologically visible as a large vein coursing through the right lung to the inferior vena cava, the so-called scimitar syndrome is said to be present. Signs of decreased lung size with a shift of the mediastinum or elevation of the diaphragm need not be present to suggest the diagnosis of hypogenetic lung syndrome when the characteristic vascular changes are present (Fig. 7.3).

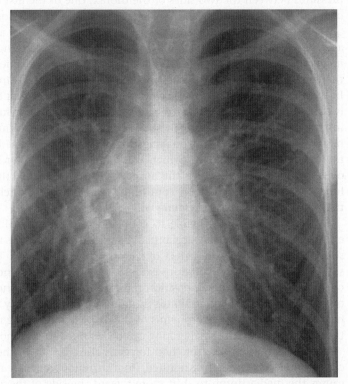

Fig. 7.3 Posterior-anterior chest radiograph shows a shift of the mediastinum to the right. A small right hilum is partially obscured by an overlying anomalous vein from the right, upper lobe. This is an example of a hypogenetic right lung with scimitar syndrome.

PLEURAL SPACE ABNORMALITIES

A massive increase in the content of the pleural space may dramatically compress the lung and shift the mediastinum. This may occur with fluid or air in the pleural space. Pleural effusion may result in a virtually opaque hemithorax before the mediastinum begins to shift (Fig. 7.4, *A* and *B*; see Chapter 4). In these cases, the underlying lung parenchyma will be completely obscured. Correlation with clinical findings is often helpful in identifying the more common causes of effusion, such as metastases, empyema, and congestive heart failure.[358] Thoracentesis is often the most direct method of establishing the diagnosis. If the entire thorax is filled with fluid without a shift of the mediastinum, the mediastinum is probably fixed, which suggests a metastatic tumor, malignant mesothelioma, or extensive fibrosis (as might be seen with fibrosing mediastinitis).

Tension pneumothorax is a medical emergency. It is the result of a leak from the lung into the pleural space. As the patient takes a deep breath, additional air enters the pleural space, and the tension is increased. Total collapse of the lung may be a relatively late

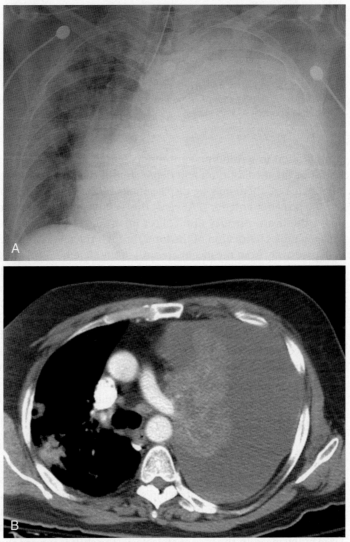

Fig. 7.4   A, Complete opacification of the left thorax with shift of the mediastinum to the right should suggest the diagnosis of tension hydrothorax. **B,** CT confirms the large left effusion with shift of the mediastinum to the right and irregular opacities in the right lung. This is metastatic invasive mucinous adenocarcinoma of the lung with a large left pleural effusion and metastatic nodules in the right lung.

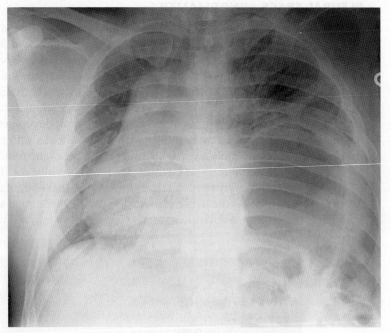

Fig. 7.5 A large dilated stomach is in the left thorax with compression of the left lung and a shift of the mediastinum. The patient had no history of recent injury but gave a history of injury following an automobile accident 4 years earlier.

complication in tension pneumothorax. Often, the first detectable signs of tension are a shift of the mediastinum and depression of the diaphragm (see Fig. 7.2). As the pressure increases, there may be displacement of the anterior and posterior junction lines. On the posterior-anterior (PA) view, this will have the appearance of a large lucent area above the heart. Air may also collect in the azygoesophageal recess behind the heart. This resembles herniation of the lung through the mediastinum, except that the lung is collapsed away from the lucent area. All of the statements in question 2 are true except *e*; there is not always complete collapse of the lung. This is especially true in patients with emphysema, diffuse interstitial disease, diffuse pneumonia, or acute respiratory distress syndrome, any of which may prevent complete collapse owing to abnormal compliance.

Diaphragmatic hernias frequently cause compression of the lung and a shift of the mediastinum. Left diaphragmatic hernias may contain stomach, small bowel, mesentery, spleen, or colon, whereas right hernias usually contain liver, but may contain mesentery or even hepatic flexure of the colon. Diaphragmatic hernias may be congenital or traumatic. Traumatic hernias are usually diagnosed as an acute abnormality, but a careful history will sometimes uncover a traumatic cause of chronic hernias (Fig. 7.5).

INCREASED LUNG VOLUME IN ADULTS

Masses constitute an infrequent cause of a mediastinal shift. When they become large enough to shift the mediastinum, it is often difficult to determine their precise site of origin, and they are often extrapulmonary. Mediastinal masses are the most likely masses to shift mediastinal structures (Fig. 7.6, *A* and *B*). Unusually large lung masses are frequently benign or of low-grade malignancy. It is true that lung cancer often causes shifting of the mediastinum, but the shift is the result of atelectasis rather than a large bulky mass. In the case of atelectasis, the shift is toward the side of the carcinoma, whereas very large masses shift the mediastinum to the side opposite the mass.

Bullous emphysema may be asymmetric and cause considerable overexpansion of one side of the chest.[174,175] This usually assumes a characteristic radiologic appearance

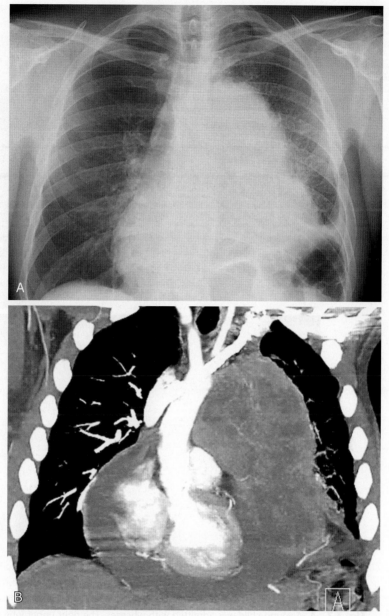

Fig. 7.6   A, A large left mediastinal mass obscures the left heart border and shifts the trachea to the right. **B,** Coronal CT scan confirms that the heart and great vessels are shifted to the right. This is a germ cell tumor with associated pericardial effusion.

because of the large avascular areas of the lung and the thin linear opacities that separate the bullae (see Chapter 22).

Bronchiolitis obliterans[377] is the cause of Swyer-James syndrome, which is a radiologic syndrome of a unilateral, hyperlucent lung (see Chapter 22). The history frequently reveals a previous viral pulmonary infection. Biopsy has shown that these patients have small airway obstructive disease. Some reports have suggested that these patients do not have significant air trapping; however, there have been cases of considerable air trapping resulting in a shift of the mediastinum and herniation of the overexpanded lungs anterior to the mediastinum. CT often reveals that this is actually a bilateral but asymmetric process.

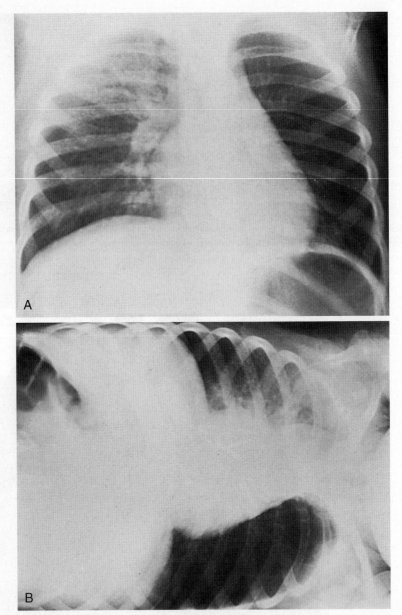

Fig. 7.7   A, A young child was admitted with wheezes. The right upper lobe is abnormally opaque, and the left lung is hyperlucent. A subtle shift of the mediastinum to the right is not diagnostic because right upper lobe collapse or air trapping on the left would shift the mediastinum to the right. **B,** Lateral decubitus examination (carried out with the patient's left side down) emphasizes the shift of the mediastinum and confirms the presence of air trapping on the left, virtually confirming the diagnosis of a foreign body in the left bronchus. (Case courtesy of Jeffrey Blum, M.D.)

INCREASED LUNG VOLUME IN CHILDREN

A foreign body obstructing a mainstem bronchus is a common cause of air trapping in children.[175] This typically leads to a hyperlucent lung with a shift of the mediastinum toward the opaque but normal side (Fig. 7.7, *A* and *B*). In effect, this is a ball valve obstruction of the bronchus that permits air to enter the lung but obstructs outflow. Collateral air drift also appears to contribute to the

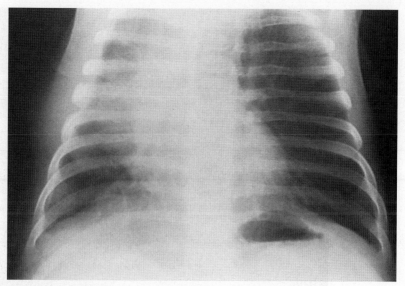

Fig. 7.8 A combination of a hyperlucent left lung, shift of the mediastinum to the right, and flattening of the left hemidiaphragm in this newborn is essentially diagnostic of congenital lobar overdistention.

overexpansion. Collateral air drift through the pores of Kohn and canals of Lambert is not a bidirectional process; it only permits air to enter an alveolus and thus contributes to the hyperexpansion distal to a bronchial obstruction. Incomplete interlobar fissures are common and are another explanation for collateral pathways between lobes.

Congenital lobar overdistention[670] is another entity that causes overexpansion of one lobe and may therefore result in a shift of the mediastinum. It has been observed only in infants. The hyperexpanded lobe frequently herniates through the mediastinum and may lead to serious respiratory insufficiency by compressing the normal lung. There is diminished vasculature in the overexpanded lobe, resulting in a large hyperlucent area (Fig. 7.8). Congenital lobar overdistention usually involves an upper lobe, but has been reported in the right middle lobe. Lobar overdistention should not result in increased opacities unless the entire lobe is homogeneously filled with fluid. In the latter case, the appearance may mimic a large mass lesion with displacement of the mediastinum.

PIE is dissection of air through the interstitium of the lung caused by barotrauma (Fig. 7.9). This is the result of positive pressure ventilation, which is used in the treatment of surfactant deficiency disease. The normal vascular markings are outlined with air, causing a pattern of coarse lines, which should distinguish interstitial emphysema from lobar overdistention. Positive pressure ventilation therapy may be further complicated by pneumothorax, which is an additional contributing cause of the shift of the mediastinum. PIE is the most common cause of unilateral lucent lung with contralateral shift of the mediastinum in a premature infant (answer to question 3 is *d*).

CPAM[357,670] is a complex anomaly consisting of multiple cystic structures that, like sequestration and bronchogenic cyst, may become overdistended with air and appear to herniate through and shift the mediastinum (see Chapter 24). They are almost always diagnosed during the neonatal period or by the age of 2 years, but they have been reported in adults who presented with recurrent pneumonias with computed tomography (CT) features of a complex cystic mass.

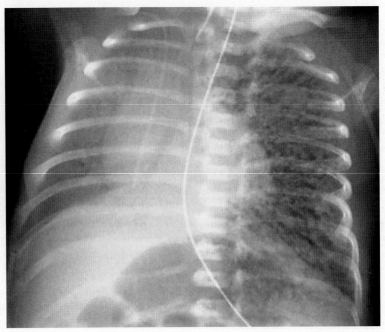

Fig. 7.9   The diffuse lucent lines and overinflation of the left lung with a shift of the mediastinum to the right are the result of pulmonary interstitial emphysema (PIE). This is a complication of positive pressure ventilation, which is used for the treatment of surfactant deficiency disease.

Top 5 Diagnoses: Shift of the Mediastinum

1. Atelectasis
2. Pleural effusion
3. Pneumothorax
4. Large mass
5. Bullous emphysema

Summary

Shift of the mediastinum indicates a severe asymmetry of intrathoracic pressures.

Pulmonary abnormalities that result in shift of the mediastinum include an increase or decrease in lung volume.

Atelectasis is the most common cause of decreased lung volume leading to a shift of the mediastinum.

Increased lung volume in infancy may be due to congenital lobar overdistention or CPAM, but pulmonary interstitial emphysema complicating positive pressure ventilation is more common and may be unilateral, resulting in a shift of the mediastinum.

Tension pneumothorax is a life-threatening emergency that appears with a shift of the mediastinum.

Large pleural effusions result in a shift of the mediastinum when there is nearly complete opacification of one side of the thorax. The absence of a shift implies fixation of the mediastinum by tumor or fibrosis or by a combination of atelectasis and effusion.

A foreign body in a bronchus is the most likely cause of air trapping during childhood.

ANSWER GUIDE

Legends for introductory figures

Fig. 7.1 A, Shift of the mediastinum and complete opacification of the left hemithorax are the result of complete atelectasis of the left lung caused by a bronchogenic carcinoma arising in the left main bronchus. Note the shift of the trachea and the heart. **B,** Axial CT scan confirms complete atelectasis of the left lung with the overinflated right lung extending anterior to the mediastinum into the left hemithorax.

Fig. 7.2 Tension pneumothorax is diagnosed by observing a shift of the mediastinum or depression of the diaphragm in a patient with pneumothorax. The lung may not be totally collapsed, even in the presence of increasing positive pressure.

ANSWERS

1. c   2. e   3. d

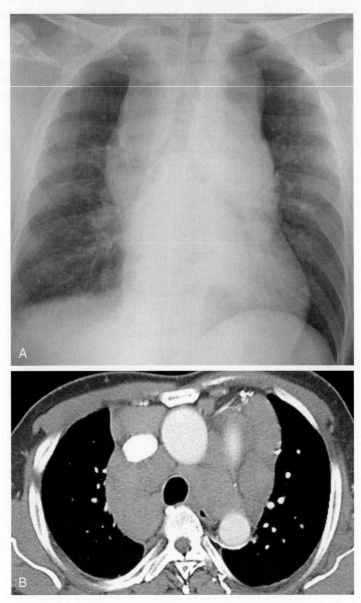

Fig. 8.1

QUESTIONS

1. What is the most likely cause of the mediastinal widening in this patient (Fig 8.1, *A* and *B*)?
   a. Lipomatosis.
   b. Hematoma.
   c. Adenopathy.
   d. Mediastinitis.
   e. Thymoma.

2. Which one of the following statements regarding aortic trauma is true?
   a. The mediastinal width is at least 8 cm.
   b. Mediastinal hematoma is specific for aortic injury.
   c. Ascending aorta is the most common sight of aortic injury.
   d. Computed tomography (CT) angiography is the definitive test for aortic injury.
   e. Right flail chest excludes aortic injury.

3. Which of the following statements about mediastinal hematomas are true?
   a. Often obscure the aortic arch and descending aorta.
   b. May indicate aortic injury.
   c. May be caused by vertebral fractures.
   d. May occur when sternal fractures injure internal mammary vessels.
   e. All of the above.

Chart 8.1	WIDENING OF THE MEDIASTINUM

I. Radiographic technique
  A. Magnification (anteroposterior [AP] supine chest radiograph, low-volume inspiration)
  B. Lordotic position
II. Adenopathy
  A. Neoplasms
    1. Lymphoma
    2. Primary lung cancer (small cell tumors)
    3. Metastases
  B. Inflammatory
    1. *Mycobacterium avium-intracellulare* (in patients with acquired immunodeficiency syndrome [AIDS][314])
    2. Tuberculosis[261]
    3. Coccidioidomycosis
    4. Anthrax[125]
    5. Sarcoidosis
III. Hematoma
  A. Aortic injury[655]
  B. Venous and arterial tears
  C. Sternal fractures
  D. Vertebral fractures (thoracic and lower cervical spine)[115]
  E. Postoperative bleeding
  F. Malposition of vascular catheters (also the cause of hydromediastinum)
IV. Vascular structures (nontraumatic)
  A. Tortuous atherosclerotic dilation of aorta
  B. Aneurysm
  C. Aortic dissection[265,267]
  D. Coarctation of aorta[658]
  E. Congenital, left superior vena cava (SVC) with absent right SVC[622]

Chart 8.1	WIDENING OF THE MEDIASTINUM—cont'd

V. Mediastinitis
   A. Perforated esophagus (Boerhaave syndrome, carcinomas)
   B. Tracheobronchial rupture (traumatic)[165]
   C. Iatrogenic (postoperative, endoscopic)
   D. Pneumonias
   E. Tuberculosis[641]
   F. Coccidioidomycosis
   G. Histoplasmosis[141,492,633]
   H. Actinomycosis[393]
   I. Fibrosing or sclerosing mediastinitis[147,306,371,492]
   J. Extension of extrathoracic infections
     1. Pharyngeal abscess
     2. Abdominal abscess
     3. Pancreatitis or pancreatic pseudocyst
VI. Lipomatosis[251,439,566]
   A. Cushing syndrome
   B. Corticosteroid therapy
   C. Obesity
VII. Other
   A. Chylomediastinum (thoracic duct obstruction or iatrogenic laceration)[165]
   B. Mediastinal edema (allergic)[165]
   C. Penetrating trauma (stab wound)
   D. Achalasia

Discussion

Mediastinal widening (Chart 8.1) is a common observation on the posterior-anterior (PA) chest radiograph. It is more difficult to identify confidently on a supine AP view because of magnification and crowding of normal vascular structures by the splinting effect on the patient's chest. In addition, a lordotic projection distorts and magnifies the superior mediastinum. This is a common problem in the patient who is unable to make a deep inspiratory effort voluntarily, and it is a serious consideration in the emergency department or intensive care unit in which the critically ill patient must be evaluated with portable supine radiography.

Chest radiograph analysis must begin with the identification of as many normal structures as possible, including the ascending aorta, aortic arch, descending aorta, aortic pulmonary window, trachea, paratracheal stripes, carina, main stem bronchi, and paraspinous stripes.[84] Failure to visualize these landmarks requires an explanation and may be an indication for additional procedures, including CT angiography and magnetic resonance imaging (MRI).

Clinical considerations often determine the urgency for a definitive diagnosis. Mediastinal widening after major trauma is strongly suggestive of mediastinal hematoma and requires urgent exclusion of aortic injury. Determining the cause of mediastinal widening in patients without a history of trauma may also be challenging.

Determining the cause of the mediastinal widening is often more difficult than recognizing the presence of an abnormality, especially in older patients with atherosclerotic vascular disease that leads to dilation and tortuosity of the aorta and great vessels. Patients who have had cardiac or vascular surgery are easily recognized by the radiographic identification of surgical clips and metal sutures, but this may further confuse the evaluation of mediastinal widening. These patients may have both tortuous vessels and postoperative abnormalities, including hematomas during the acute convalescent period and, later, mediastinal scarring. A mass lesion that develops subsequent to mediastinal or cardiac surgery may be obscured by postoperative changes.

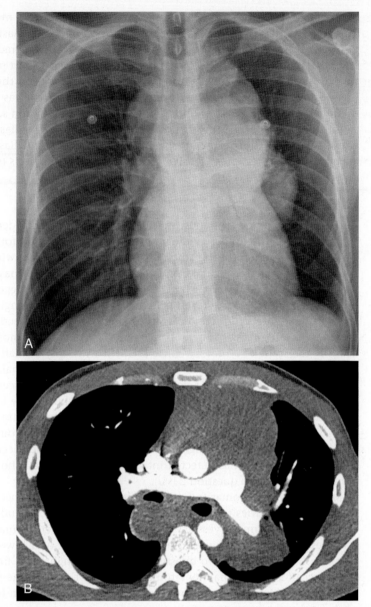

Fig. 8.2 A, Widening of the mediastinum is suggested by the appearance of the upper mediastinum with increased opacity on both sides of the trachea, obscuring the aorta and left hilum with a subcarinal mass. **B,** CT confirms that the mediastinal widening is the result of large soft-tissue masses involving the anterior, middle, and posterior mediastinum. This is extensive adenopathy resulting from B cell lymphoma.

ADENOPATHY

Mediastinal tumors are expected to produce discrete masses, but neoplasms that involve multiple lymph node groups may cause diffuse mediastinal widening. This type of tumor dissemination results from lymphomas and metastases from either primary lung cancer or distant primaries. It is particularly common with poorly differentiated primary tumors, such as small cell lung cancer. Such extensive nodal involvement may also be seen with metastases from retroperitoneal tumors and even from testicular tumors, particularly seminomas.

Lymphoma frequently involves mediastinal lymph nodes and, when the involvement is extensive, numerous large nodes may diffusely widen the mediastinum (Fig 8.2, *A* and *B*). The tumor should regress following chemotherapy, but the nodes may be replaced by extensive fibrosis, which may leave residual mediastinal widening. This is most often recognized by the identification of paramediastinal reticular opacities that result from mediastinal fibrosis. In their early stages, radiation pneumonitis and fibrosis may appear to become more prominent over a short period, requiring further consideration of recurrent tumor. Increasing opacity from the radiation effect on the mediastinum may be further evaluated with MRI, which has been reported to be useful for identifying viable tumor in the midst of postradiation scarring.

Inflammatory adenopathy is not a common cause of mediastinal widening, but granulomatous diseases cause involvement of the hilar and mediastinal nodes, and the adenopathy may become extensive, as in the case of sarcoidosis (see Fig 8.1, *A* and *B;* answer to question 1 is *c*).

HEMATOMA

Aortic injury is one of the most urgent diagnoses to be considered following major trauma. The reported chest radiograph findings include the following: mediastinal widening; obscuration of the aortic arch or descending aorta; widened right paratracheal stripe; left apical pleural cap; deviation of a tracheal or nasogastric tube to the right; and pleural effusion (Fig 8.3).[102,655] These are all signs suggestive of mediastinal hemorrhage, but they are not specific for aortic injury. CT angiography[186] (Fig 8.4, A-C) is required to confirm and classify an aortic injury. Transection of the ascending aorta carries a high risk for hemopericardium. It is likely the most common cause of death at the scene of a motor vehicle accident with only a small number of patients surviving to have diagnosis and treatment via CT. The proximal descending aorta is the most common sight of CT-detected aortic injury. Distal descending aortic injuries are possible but much less frequent. Most patients who survive to reach the hospital have partial transections. CT signs of aortic injury include extravasation of contrast (Fig 8.5), pseudoaneurysms (Fig 8.6), intimal defects, aortic contour abnormalities, and intraluminal thrombus. CT angiography is very sensitive and specific for the detection of aortic injuries and has detected intimal tears in patients who have no associated hematoma (answer to question 2 is *d*).

Mediastinal hematomas following acute trauma have also been well documented to result from injuries to structures other than the aorta, including other great vessels, internal mammary vessels, SVC, and fractures. Hematomas often result from fractures of the sternum, posterior ribs, and thoracic and lower cervical vertebrae (Fig 8.7, A and B; answer to question 3 is *e*). Although these findings may explain the source of a mediastinal hematoma, they do not exclude the possibility of associated aortic injury and should therefore not be used as a reason to avoid or delay CT angiography.

VASCULAR STRUCTURES

Dilation of the aorta and great vessels with tortuosity is most often the result of atherosclerotic disease and is very frequent in older patients. Dilation of the ascending aorta is observed in patients with severe hypertension and may also result from aortic stenosis. The dilated tortuous aorta must be distinguished from aortic aneurysms, aortic dissection, and even mass lesions (Fig 8.8, A-C). When the entire aorta is extremely dilated and tortuous, the abnormality may be regarded as a long fusiform aneurysm.

Dissection of the aorta results from an intimal tear followed by intramural hematoma. Complete dissection occurs when there are multiple tears, permitting blood to flow through the aortic wall and creating a false lumen. The patient may be asymptomatic, but typically presents with retrosternal chest pain, syncope, and signs of peripheral vascular arterial occlusion.

The most frequent radiographic findings in dissection of the aorta include mediastinal widening and enlargement of the aortic arch and descending aorta (Fig 8.9, A and B). Other findings may include enlargement of the ascending aorta, blurring of the aortic

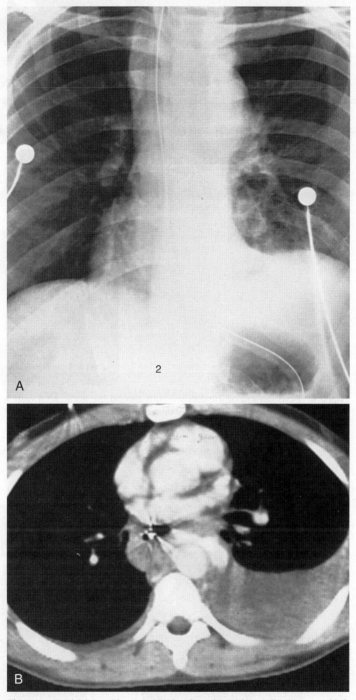

Fig. 8.3   A, This motor vehicle accident victim developed a wide mediastinum and left subpulmonic pleural effusion with deviation of a nasogastric tube to the right. **B,** Contrast-enhanced CT scan shows a large left effusion and extraluminal contrast medium around the descending aorta, indicating severe aortic injury.

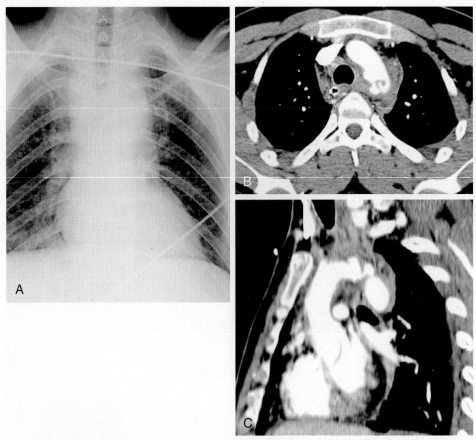

Fig. 8.4   A, Widening of the mediastinum around the aortic arch with a shift of the trachea to the left is very suggestive of a mediastinal hematoma from an aortic injury. **B,** CT angiography confirms a mediastinal hematoma and an irregular filling defect at the arch of the aorta. **C,** Coronal reconstruction confirms a pseudoaneurysm in the proximal descending aorta. This is the most common site for aortic injuries, but such injuries may also occur in the ascending and lower descending portions of the aorta.

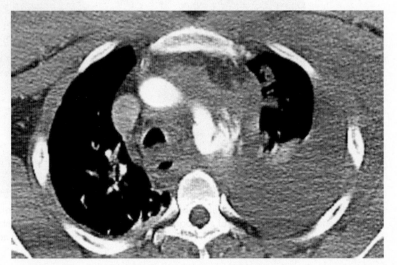

Fig. 8.5   Mediastinal hematoma and a large left pleural effusion with extravasation of contrast on CT angiography are signs of aortic transection requiring urgent treatment.

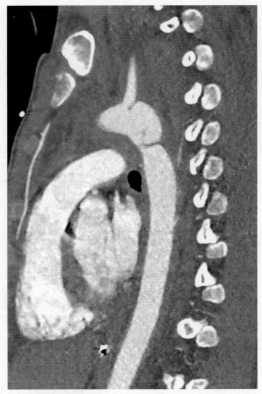

Fig. 8.6   Pseudoaneurysm of the aorta is the result of a contained aortic hemorrhage from a partial transection.

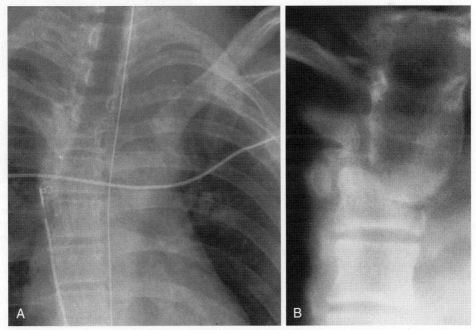

Fig. 8.7   A, Wide mediastinum, loss of definition of the aortic arch, and apical cap indicate mediastinal hematoma, but this patient had a normal aortogram. **B,** Tomogram of the upper thoracic spine better demonstrates the fracture dislocation that caused the mediastinal hematoma.

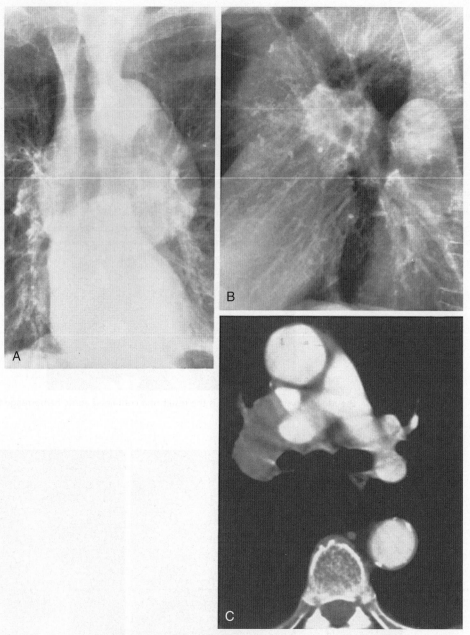

Fig. 8.8 **A,** Large tortuous aorta must be distinguished from an aneurysm and could obscure a mass in the mediastinum or either hilum. **B,** Lateral view reveals dilated ascending aorta and tortuosity of the descending aorta. Also note the increased opacity of the hila projected between the aortic opacities. **C,** This contrast-enhanced CT scan was performed to exclude the diagnosis of aneurysm and confirmed the thoracic aorta to be very tortuous with an upper abdominal aneurysm (not shown). The scan also confirmed right hilar adenopathy caused by small cell carcinoma.

arch, soft-tissue opacity lateral to calcification in the aortic arch, deviation of the trachea or nasogastric tube, a wide paraspinal stripe, and pericardial and pleural effusions. The finding of widening of the mediastinum and aortic arch (Fig 8.10, A-C) should be followed by CT or MRI. CT angiography or conventional aortography may be required for patients who are hemodynamically unstable and are candidates for emergency surgery. Either of these procedures provides precise anatomic detail and permits the application of anatomic classification of the dissection. The Stanford classification[175] is used to

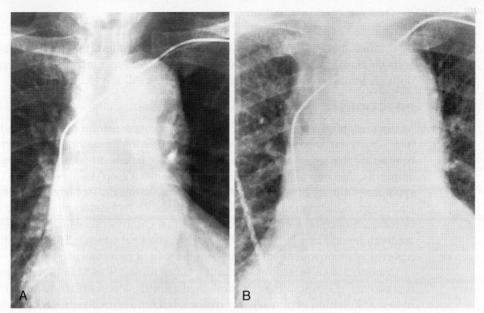

Fig. 8.9 **A,** Tortuous aorta accounts for the wide mediastinum. Observe the sharply defined aortic arch and descending aorta. **B,** This examination was done 13 months later. The patient reported acute chest pain. The widening of the aorta has increased as a result of aortic dissection.

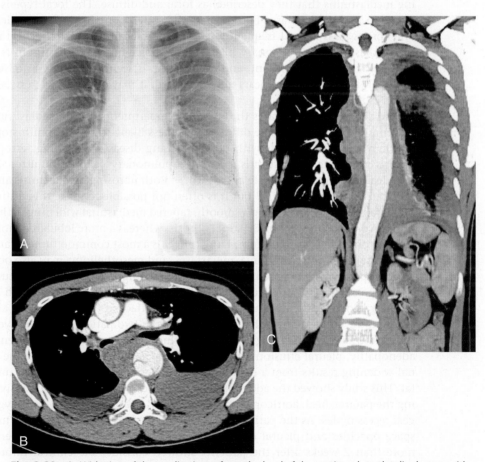

Fig. 8.10 **A,** Widening of the mediastinum from the level of the aortic arch to the diaphragm with a left, subpulmonic pleural effusion should suggest a mediastinal hematoma. The patient had a history of hypertension and presented with severe chest pain. **B,** CT section from just below the carina confirms a mediastinal hematoma around the descending aorta with a lucent curved line through the aorta. The lucent line is the intimal flap and confirms the diagnosis of aortic dissection. **C,** Coronal reconstruction shows the extent of the mediastinal hematoma and confirms that the flap extends from the level of the arch into the abdomen.

determine surgical versus medical management. Dissections that involve the ascending aorta are classified as type A and require urgent surgical treatment, whereas type B dissections are limited to the descending aorta and are medically managed.

INFECTIONS

Mediastinal infection may take the form of diffuse mediastinitis or abscess, and these two forms may even coexist. Acute infections may enter the mediastinum by direct extension from a nasopharyngeal abscess, subphrenic abscess, pancreatic pseudocyst, pneumonia, or empyema. Infection may also result from spontaneous esophageal perforation (Boerhaave syndrome), rupture of an esophageal carcinoma, iatrogenic esophageal perforation from endoscopy, or dilation of an esophageal stricture.[189] Perforation of either the esophagus or tracheobronchial tree also causes mediastinal emphysema, which often precedes the mediastinitis and may be the initial cause of mediastinal widening. Mediastinitis has been reported as an infrequent but serious complication of cardiovascular surgery.

Granulomatous infections, including tuberculosis,[641] coccidioidomycosis, and histoplasmosis, may also produce diffuse mediastinitis. Mediastinal adenopathy is a common manifestation of primary tuberculosis, but diffuse involvement of the mediastinal nodes by tuberculosis is rare, except in patients who are immunologically compromised.

Fibrosing mediastinitis (Fig 8.11, *A* and *B*) may be idiopathic, but is most often caused by histoplasmosis.[147,633,634] Rossi et al.[492] have reported two types of fibrosing mediastinitis that they described as focal and diffuse. The focal type is the most common and presents as a fibrous mass that often contains multiple calcifications. The fibrous mass is most frequently seen in the subcarinal or paratracheal regions of the mediastinum or pulmonary hila. The right side of the mediastinum is the most common area of involvement, and calcification is seen in as many as 63% of cases. Although the focal type appears more localized, it may still occlude vessels, bronchi, or the esophagus.

The diffuse type infiltrates through all compartments of the mediastinum and is less commonly calcified. The diffuse type is less likely to result from histoplasmosis and may occur in patients with other fibrosing diseases, including retroperitoneal fibrosis. Fibrosing mediastinitis may cause pulmonary venous and arterial obstruction, leading to cor pulmonale and death.[634] Both fibrosing mediastinitis and tumors may cause SVC syndrome,[141] but it is often not possible to make this distinction by radiograph. CT scans showing a smooth, tapered mediastinal widening with calcifications favor a diagnosis of mediastinal fibrosis, whereas a more lobulated, noncalcified mass favors a diagnosis of tumor. Lung cancer is a most common tumor, causing SVC syndrome; however, lymphoma, metastases, and mesothelioma may also occlude the SVC. Biopsy may be required to distinguish fibrosing mediastinitis from tumor.

Anthrax is a very rare bacterial infection that has not received much attention in the radiologic literature until the terrorist attacks of 2001. Earls et al.[125] have reported the chest radiograph and CT findings in two patients who survived inhalational anthrax. The radiologic findings include diffuse mediastinal widening, hilar adenopathy, pleural effusions, and air space opacities. CT reveals that the mediastinal widening results from a combination of adenopathy and edema of mediastinal fat. This study showed the adenopathy to be hyperattenuating and extensive, involving the paratracheal, aorticopulmonary window, subcarinal, hilar, and azygoesophageal recess nodes. As the patients in this limited series recovered, the pulmonary air space opacities and pleural effusions improved, but the adenopathy persisted for more than 2 weeks after the patients showed considerable clinical improvement. Their study[125] emphasized the importance of distinguishing the early finding of mediastinal widening from atherosclerotic tortuosity of the aorta. The acute onset of mediastinal widening is also an important feature of anthrax when compared with most other bacterial pneumonias.

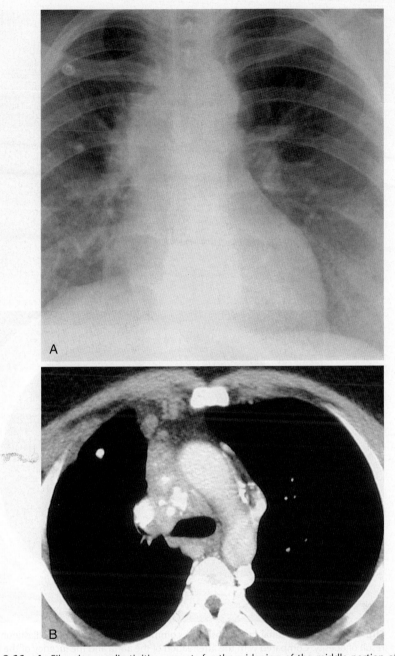

Fig. 8.11 A, Fibrosing mediastinitis accounts for the widening of the middle portion of the mediastinum. Observe the tapered right paratracheal mass that partially obscures the right hilum. There is also an opacity adjacent to the arch of the aorta. **B,** CT confirms a large right paratracheal mass with multiple calcifications. The SVC is occluded and is therefore not seen. Large collateral veins have developed, including a large hemiazygos vein posterior to the aorta and a dilated, superior intercostal vein lateral to the aortic arch.

LIPOMATOSIS

Mediastinal lipomatosis is a benign cause of diffuse mediastinal widening (Fig 8.12, A and B).[195,439,566] Some signs that help suggest this diagnosis include the following: (1) a large mediastinum without indentation on the trachea; (2) smooth contours of pleural lines; and (3) a prominent epicardial fat pad. Although fat appears similar

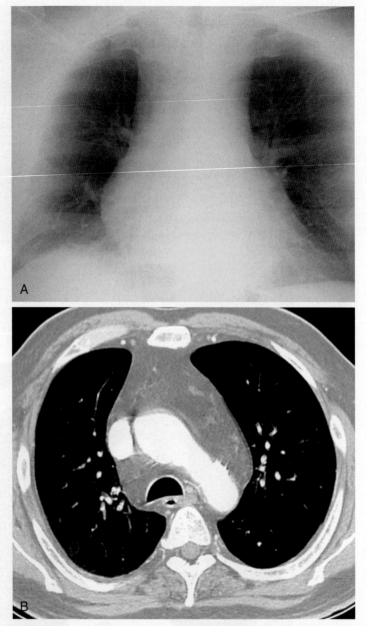

Fig. 8.12   A, Mediastinal lipomatosis is a common cause of a wide mediastinum and is often the result of obesity. Compared with the attenuation of the aorta and the lucency of the lungs, the fat is intermediate in opacity and often does not obscure normal structures, such as the aorta. **B,** CT confirms the diagnosis of mediastinal lipomatosis.

to soft tissue when compared with the opacity of the aerated lung on a chest radiograph, the diagnosis of lipomatosis should be easily confirmed with a CT scan.[251] The condition causes attenuation intermediate between that of the normal soft-tissue structures of the mediastinum and the lower attenuation of the aerated lung. Mediastinal lipomatosis may result from Cushing syndrome, corticosteroid therapy, or exogenous obesity.

Top 5 Diagnoses: Widening of the Mediastinum

1. Hematoma
2. Tortuous aorta
3. Metastases
4. Lymphoma
5. Granulomatous infections

Summary

Acute, posttraumatic mediastinal widening with loss of definition of the aortic arch or descending aorta should be considered suspicious for aortic injury.

Atherosclerotic dilation and tortuosity of the aorta are very common in older adults. A change in aortic size or definition is suggestive of dissection. This diagnosis may be confirmed with the use of contrast-enhanced CT or MRI.

Tortuosity of the aorta and great vessels may obscure mediastinal masses.

Neoplasms that involve mediastinal nodes may diffusely widen the mediastinum.

Mediastinitis may result from bacterial and granulomatous infections, esophageal perforation, and extension of extrathoracic abscesses.

Lipomatosis is a benign cause of mediastinal widening.

ANSWER GUIDE

Legend for introductory figure

Fig. 8.1 **A,** Mediastinal widening usually obscures the normal mediastinal contours. In this case there is mild lobulation, which is suggestive of adenopathy. **B,** CT confirms extensive anterior and middle mediastinal adenopathy. This would most likely be the result of metastases, or lymphoma, but biopsy revealed nonnecrotizing granulomas consistent with sarcoidosis.

ANSWERS

1. c   2. d   3. e

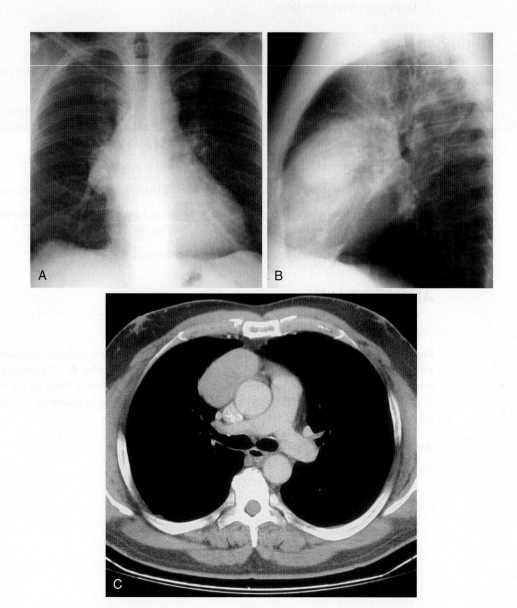

Fig. 9.1

QUESTIONS

1. Which one of the following diagnoses is most likely in a middle-aged adult with the chest radiographs and computed tomography (CT) scan shown in Fig. 9.1, *A-C*?
   a. Goiter.
   b. Thymoma.

   c. Germ cell tumor.

   d. Cystic hygroma.

   e. Pericardial cyst.

2. Which one of the following tumors is most likely to spread contiguously and is unlikely to metastasize to distant sites?

   a. Thymoma.

   b. Thyroid carcinoma.

   c. Germ cell tumor.

   d. Lymphoma.

   e. Thymic carcinoma.

3. Which one of the following is least likely to calcify?

   a. Substernal thyroid.

   b. Thymic cyst.

   c. Thymoma.

   d. Germ cell tumor.

   e. Treated lymphoma.

Chart 9.1	ANTERIOR MEDIASTINAL MASS

I. Thymic lesions[178]
  A. Thymoma (benign and invasive)[509,567,600]
  B. Thymic cyst[276]
  C. Thymolipoma[413,485,583]
  D. Lymphoma
  E. Thymic hyperplasia[413]
  F. Thymic carcinoid tumor[413,567]
  G. Thymic carcinoma[567]
II. Germ cell tumors[486]
  A. Dermoid cyst (mature cystic teratoma)[276]
  B. Teratoma (benign and malignant)[486,582]
  C. Embryonal cell carcinoma
  D. Choriocarcinoma
  E. Seminoma
  F. Mixed germ cell tumor[486]
III. Thyroid
  A. Goiter
  B. Adenoma
  C. Carcinoma
IV. Lymph nodes[67]
  A. Lymphoma (both Hodgkin and non-Hodgkin)[21]
  B. Metastases
  C. Benign lymph node hyperplasia
  D. Angioblastic lymphoid adenopathy
  E. Sarcoidosis and granulomatous infections (rare)
V. Cardiovascular
  A. Epicardial fat pad
  B. Aneurysm of ascending aorta[548]
  C. Aneurysm of sinus of Valsalva[418,470]
  D. Dilated superior vena cava
  E. Pericardial cyst[148]
  F. Cardiac tumors
  G. Traumatic pseudoaneurysm of ascending aorta

Chart 9.1	ANTERIOR MEDIASTINAL MASS—CONT'D

VI. Cysts
    A. Cystic hygroma (lymphangioma)
    B. Bronchogenic cyst
    C. Extralobar sequestration
    D. Thymic and germ cell lesions (see above)
VII. Other
    A. Neural tumors of vagus or phrenic nerves[459]
    B. Paraganglioma (chemodectoma and pheochromocytoma)[459]
    C. Hernia of the foramen of Morgagni[183]
    D. Parathyroid adenoma,[525] adenocarcinoma
    E. Primary bone tumors and metastases to the sternum
    F. Lipoma,[183,195] lipomatosis[339]
    G. Hemangioma[145]
    H. Pancreatic pseudocyst[302]

Chart 9.2	INLET LESION FROM THE NECK INTO THE SUPERIOR MEDIASTINUM

   I. Thyroid masses
  II. Cystic hygroma
 III. Lymphoma
 IV. Metastases

Chart 9.3	RIGHT CARDIOPHRENIC ANGLE MASS

    I. Epicardial fat pad
   II. Pericardial cyst (mesothelial cyst)
  III. Dilated right atrium
  IV. Diaphragmatic lesion
   V. Other anterior mediastinal masses (see Chart 9.1)
  VI. Primary lung mass
 VII. Hernia through the foramen of Morgagni

Discussion

The anterior mediastinum contains the thymus, lymph nodes, vessels, and fat (Chart 9.1). There is considerable variation in the normal width of the mediastinum on the posterior-anterior (PA) chest radiograph and in the size and opacity of the retrosternal clear space on the lateral view.[323] These variations result from differences in the shape and size of vessels and fat content. When there is minimal anterior fat, both lungs extend in front of the ascending aorta, pressing all four layers of pleura together to form the anterior junction line. Masses are visible on the PA and lateral views when they displace the mediastinal pleura and alter the normal mediastinal contour. Visibility is mainly determined by the interface of the mass with the aerated lung, but soft-tissue masses that are surrounded by fat may appear as minimally visible opacities that require CT for confirmation.

Once the presence of a mediastinal mass has been confirmed, precise localization of the mass is the most important aspect of radiologic evaluation. Strict anatomic

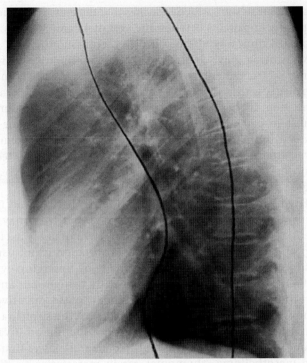

Fig. 9.2   A simplified division of the mediastinum was first described by Felson.[150] The anterior border of the trachea and posterior borders of the heart and inferior vena cava form the line for dividing anterior from middle compartments. A line drawn 1 cm posterior to the anterior border of the vertebral bodies divides the middle and posterior compartments.

divisions of the mediastinum are not easily translated to the lateral chest radiograph. Anatomy texts have divided the mediastinum into four compartments: superior, anterior, middle, and posterior. When this division is applied to the lateral chest radiograph, the radiologist should consider a fifth compartment corresponding anatomically to the posterior gutter, which includes the paravertebral soft tissues. These anatomic divisions of the mediastinal compartments were established before the development of chest radiology. Felson[150] was one of the first to recognize the cumbersome nature of applying anatomic definitions to the lateral chest radiograph and devised a simplified method based on easily identifiable radiologic landmarks. He divided the anterior and middle compartments by drawing a line from the intersection of the anterior border of the trachea with the sternum to intersect the diaphragm. This line follows the posterior border of the heart and the inferior vena cava. A second line, 1 cm posterior to the anterior border of the vertebral bodies, was used to separate the middle from the posterior mediastinum (Fig. 9.2). This method of dividing the mediastinum is not anatomically precise, but it is much less cumbersome to apply to the lateral chest radiograph, and provides the radiologist with a starting point in the evaluation of mediastinal masses. CT permits more precise anatomic localization and reveals the relationship of the mass to normal anatomic structures.[631]

THYMIC LESIONS

Thymomas (see Fig 9.1, *A-C*) are among the most common primary tumors of the anterior mediastinum.[567] Characteristically, they present as a well-circumscribed mass that frequently appears to touch the sternum without being flattened by the compressing effect of the heart and great vessels. This resistance to flattening results in the so-called sulcus sign, which indicates that the mass is very firm. Thymomas occur most frequently in patients between the ages of 45 and 50 years and may have a variety of associated clinical syndromes. (Answer to question 1 is *c*.)

Myasthenia gravis is the most common clinical syndrome associated with thymoma; 15% of patients with this condition have a thymoma, and approximately 40% of patients with a thymoma have myasthenia gravis. Because of this strong clinical association, CT has been advocated as a screening procedure for the detection of thymomas in patients with myasthenia gravis. Autoimmune disorders that have been linked with thymomas include acquired hypogammaglobulinemia, red cell hypoplasia, aplastic anemia, and Cushing syndrome. Other reported associations include systemic lupus erythematosus, rheumatoid arthritis, polymyositis, hyperthyroidism, and Sjögren syndrome.

Thymomas were previously classified as benign and malignant; thymomas do not spread by hematogenous metastases, but they may be locally invasive. Differentiation of benign from invasive thymomas is a challenge for the radiologist, surgeon, and pathologist. This distinction is not usually based on histologic features; rather, the distinction is made by observing evidence of local invasion. Well-encapsulated thymomas are usually benign, but any evidence of local invasion indicates the potential for regional spread. Invasive thymomas spread contiguously, invading other mediastinal structures, pleura, pericardium, and lung. (Answer to question 2 is *a*.) It is not unusual for an invasive thymoma to spread around the pleura and cause multiple pleural masses that resemble mesothelioma. Like mesothelioma, thymomas rarely metastasize to distant sites. In a patient with an anterior mediastinal mass, the presence of hematogenous metastases should suggest another diagnosis, such as thymic carcinoma, germ cell tumor, or lymphoma.

Other abnormalities arising from the thymus include thymolipoma, thymic cyst, lymphoma, thymic carcinoma, and thymic carcinoid tumors. Thymolipoma is a benign tumor with both thymic remnants and fat.[485] These fatty masses are very soft and conform to the shape of surrounding structures. They may simulate an elevated diaphragm or enlarged heart. A right-sided mass makes the cardiac contour appear symmetric; the appearance suggests cardiomegaly or even a large pericardial effusion. The diagnosis of a mixed fatty and soft-tissue tumor may be confirmed with CT. A thymic cyst is also benign and has a chest radiographic appearance that is indistinguishable from that of a thymoma. CT should confirm low-attenuation fluid, which would therefore suggest a thymic cyst (Fig 9.3, *A-C*).

Thymic carcinomas are rare tumors that arise from the epithelial portions of the thymus. A variety of thymic carcinoma cell types include squamous, small cell, mucoepidermoid, adenocystic, clear cell, and sarcomatoid carcinomas. These tumors probably account for cases in which a patient with a diagnosis of thymoma develops hematogenous metastases. There are no associated syndromes with thymic carcinoma. Thymic carcinoid tumors are identical to thymomas in radiologic appearance but have substantial histologic, clinical, and prognostic differences. These tumors are thought to arise from neural crest cells and, unlike thymomas, are of epithelial origin. There have been no reported cases of carcinoid syndrome, but 40% of patients with thymic carcinoid tumors have Cushing syndrome, and 19% of these tumors have been associated with multiple endocrine neoplasia syndromes, including hyperparathyroidism resulting from parathyroid adenoma or hyperplasia. Thymic carcinoid tumors have not been reported to have an association with myasthenia gravis, hypogammaglobulinemia, red cell aplasia, megaesophagus, or collagen vascular disease. Like thymoma, they may be locally invasive, but they tend to be more aggressive. They are more likely to cause superior vena cava obstruction, and they frequently metastasize to distant sites.

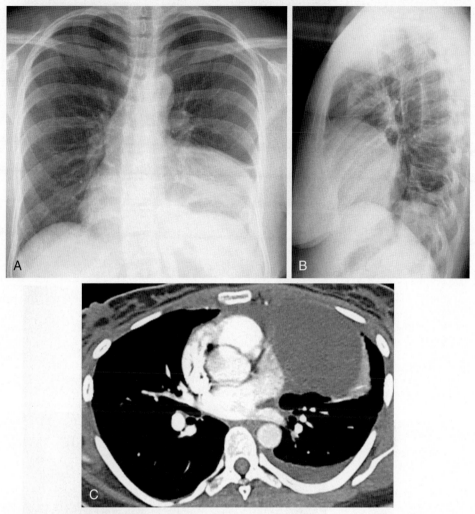

Fig. 9.3 **A,** The large opacity in the left lower chest obscures the heart on the PA view. **B,** The lateral view confirms that the opacity is anterior and likely a mediastinal mass. **C,** CT scan reveals a large, fluid-filled structure around the heart. This appearance is suggestive of a pericardial cyst, but was separate from the pericardium and is a thymic cyst.

GERM CELL TUMORS

Germ cell tumors (Fig 9.4, *A-C*) also present in the middle to lower portions of the anterior mediastinum.[486] These masses tend to be midline structures and, like thymomas, are frequently found between the sternum and heart or great vessels. Mature teratomas are benign and are the most common of the germ cell tumors. They contain elements from all three germ layers with soft tissue, fat, and cystic fluid collections, as well as calcification. When they contain either sebaceous or fatty materials, they are softer than the solid thymomas and tend to flatten against the sternum. The sulcus between the mass and sternum that may be seen on the lateral view in thymomas is therefore encountered less often in the germ cell tumors. CT may demonstrate a characteristic fat-fluid level in cystic teratomas,[180] and magnetic resonance imaging (MRI) usually reveals a mixed signal pattern.[347] Calcification is another feature that might be expected to help identify these entities, but radiographic identification of teeth and bones, as often occurs in dermoid cysts in the pelvis, occurs less frequently in mediastinal teratomas and dermoid cysts. A rim of calcification in the wall of a cystic structure may be seen in a dermoid cyst, but it is also seen in thymic cysts and aneurysms. Other causes of calcification in anterior mediastinal masses include mesenchymal tumor,

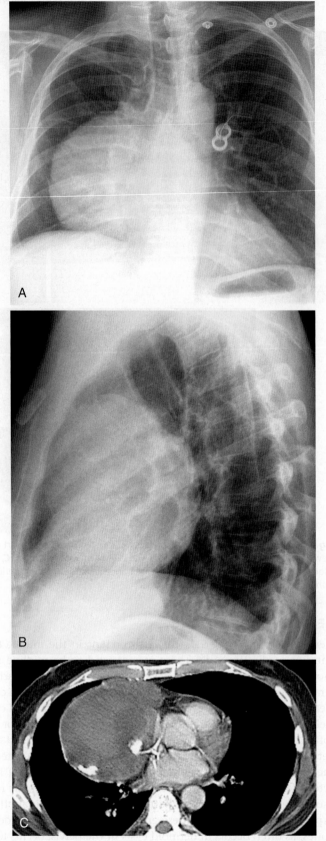

Fig. 9.4 A, Large, well-circumscribed mass projects over the right lower hilum. This is the hilum overlay sign that is seen when a mass is either anterior or posterior to the hilum. **B,** The lateral view confirms the anterior location. An anterior mediastinal mass in a young adult is most likely a germ cell tumor or lymphoma. **C,** CT scan reveals the mass to have mixed soft tissue and fat opacities with the additional finding of calcifications. The diagnosis here is a germ cell tumor.

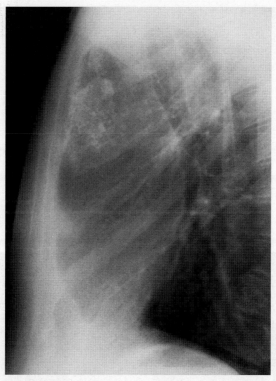

Fig. 9.5   This lateral chest radiograph demonstrates the typical appearance of calcified lymph nodes, which are the late result of a lymphoma that was treated with radiation.

goiter, treated lymphomatous nodes (Fig 9.5; answer to question 3 is *c*), and rarely, untreated lymphoma.[327]

LYMPHADENOPATHY

Lymphoma is another important consideration as a possible cause of an anterior mediastinal mass. Lymphoma arises in both the thymus and lymph nodes and commonly presents as an anterior mediastinal mass. Lymphomas may present as well-circumscribed masses and may be indistinguishable from thymic and teratoid lesions; however, the radiologic signs of malignancy and the differences in the routes of malignant spread are important considerations in the evaluation of anterior mediastinal masses. The only reliable signs that suggest malignancy are signs of spread. Lymphoma is well known for its radiologic appearance, a mass that appears well circumscribed on the frontal view but may be ill defined on the lateral view (Fig 9.6, *A-C*). The lateral view may reveal complete obliteration of the normal retrosternal clear space and silhouetting of normal structures (e.g., the ascending aorta) by a poorly defined mass that involves multiple nodes and thymus. The more occult infiltrating lymphomas may not have the expected appearance of a discrete mass on the frontal radiograph, but may only alter a mediastinal pleural contour. This appearance may also be explained by the tendency for a lymphoma to be locally invasive, although other tumors, including thymomas and teratomas, may also be locally invasive. Both lymphomas and thymomas may spread into the lung, leading to a loss of definition of the borders of the mass. They may even follow the interstitium of the lung, producing a reticular pattern similar to that seen in patients with lymphangitic spread of a carcinoma. Involvement of other node groups, as with hilar adenopathy, may provide a clue for distinguishing lymphomas from the other anterior mediastinal tumors.

Metastases from a variety of primary tumors may involve the anterior mediastinal lymph nodes. Breast cancer involves internal mammary lymph nodes. Lung cancer may metastasize to anterior lymph nodes or may invade the mediastinum directly.

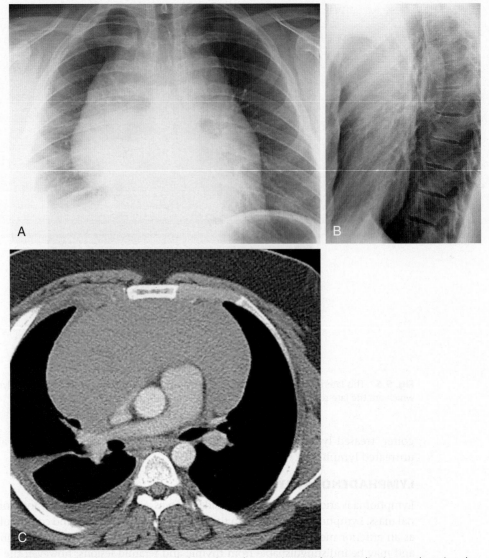

Fig. 9.6   A, This large mass extends from the right superior to inferior mediastinum, obscuring the right heart border, and crosses through the mediastinum, obscuring the left heart border. **B,** The lateral view reveals opacification of the retrosternal clear space above the heart but the opacity is not circumscribed, which is a common observation in patients with lymphoma. **C,** CT scan confirms the presence of a large mass extending across the mediastinum and displacing the great vessels posteriorly. This is a T cell lymphoma that has also spread to the right pleura, causing an effusion.

Melanoma is a tumor that has been reported to rarely metastasize to the anterior mediastinum.[350]

Granulomatous diseases, including tuberculosis, fungal infections, and sarcoidosis, are common causes of mediastinal adenopathy. These diseases rarely present with anterior mediastinal adenopathy in the absence of middle mediastinal or hilar adenopathy.

INLET LESIONS

Once the mass is localized to the anterior mediastinum, its precise location must be considered. Thyroid masses, for example, almost always appear as inlet lesions (Chart 9.2; Fig 9.7, *A* and *B*) and may even be associated with a palpable neck mass; therefore they may appear to extend above the clavicles, in contrast to masses that arise from the anterior mediastinum. They also tend to displace the trachea posteriorly.

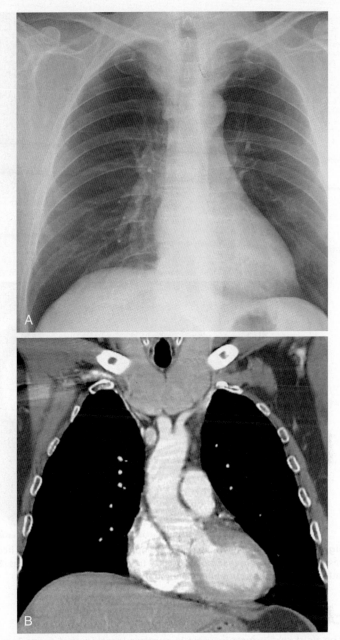

Fig. 9.7   A, The superior mediastinum is widened by a mass with circumscribed right and left borders. **B,** Coronal CT scan confirms that the mass is arising from the thyroid. Large, lobulated thyroid masses are usually the result of nodular goiters.

A mass that appears to extend through the inlet of the thorax from the neck and deviates the trachea suggests a thyroid mass. Occasionally, a thyroid mass may be evident posterior to the trachea with anterior deviation of the trachea and may present in a more posterior location as a result. Careful clinical correlation is essential. An inlet lesion in a child with an associated neck mass is more likely to be a cystic hygroma (lymphangioma). In this case, the physical examination may reveal a soft neck mass and confirm the diagnosis. Ultrasound, CT, or MRI should confirm the cystic character of the lesion. Lymphoma rarely manifests as an inlet lesion, but it should be considered when there are palpable neck or supraclavicular lymph nodes instead of a definite thyroid mass.

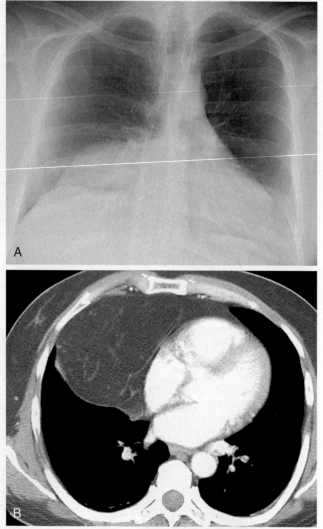

Fig. 9.8   A, The opacity in the right cardiophrenic angle obscures the heart border but not the hilar vessels. This is a common location for fatty tumors and Morgagni hernias. **B,** CT scan confirms a large fatty mass that resulted from herniation of mesenteric fat.

CARDIOPHRENIC ANGLE MASS

The right cardiophrenic angle is another location that suggests a more limited diagnosis (Chart 9.3). Fat collections in this location include an enlarged epicardial fat pad, lipoma, thymolipoma, or Morgagni hernia with mesenteric fat and are the most common causes of a mass in this area (Fig 9.8, *A* and *B*). It is frequently possible to appreciate that the mass is less opaque than the heart but obviously more opaque than the surrounding lung. If there is any doubt about the diagnosis, looking at previous examinations usually confirms the impression of the fat opacity and shows that the mass has not changed in size or configuration. A word of caution is required, however, because fat pads occasionally increase in size. It is well known that there may be growth of fatty tissue in response to treatment with corticosteroids; therefore it is necessary to correlate the radiologic observation of an enlarging mass in this area with the clinical history. In the absence of an obvious reason for the growth, it sometimes becomes necessary to consider further evaluation. Another method used to confirm that the opacity is fat is to measure the attenuation coefficient by CT.

The right cardiophrenic angle is the most common location for a pericardial cyst, which should be of tissue opacity in contrast to the fat pad, but either lesion may be seen in the left cardiophrenic angle. Both ultrasound and CT may reliably confirm the cystic nature of the lesion, but CT offers the added advantage of being able to distinguish the attenuation of fluid, fat, or soft tissue.

ANEURYSM

An aneurysm must be considered if a mediastinal mass cannot be shown to be separate from the aorta.[418] An aneurysm arising from the ascending aorta is likely to appear as an anterior mediastinal abnormality. In the past, angiography provided the only method for excluding the diagnosis of aneurysm, but CT angiography or MRI clearly defines the aorta and provides a less invasive technique for excluding the diagnosis of aneurysm. MRI avoids the risk involved in using a contrast medium and is the procedure of choice for patients with contrast allergy.

Top 5 Diagnoses: Anterior Mediastinal Mass

1. Lymphoma
2. Thymoma
3. Germ cell tumors
4. Thyroid masses
5. Metastases

Summary

Localization to the inlet of the anterior mediastinum strongly suggests a thyroid lesion in an adult or a cystic hygroma in a child.

Anterior mediastinal masses must be distinguished from the aorta. This may require special procedures, including CT angiography and MRI.

Thymomas are most commonly seen after the age of 40 years, whereas lymphoma and teratomas are commonly seen in young adults. Lymphoma also has a second peak incidence in older adults.

Invasive thymomas spread contiguously and rarely beyond the thorax, in contrast to lymphoma and teratomas, which may involve multiple organ systems.

Although a rare finding, the presence of bones or teeth is diagnostic of a teratoid lesion.

Rim-like calcifications are not rare and may be seen in a variety of cystic lesions.

Lymphoma commonly presents with a mass that is ill defined on the lateral view, probably because of its tendency to spread through the mediastinum by infiltration and involvement of multiple node groups.

ANSWER GUIDE

Legend for introductory figure

Fig. 9.1   **A,** Rounded opacity projects over the right hilum and is difficult to localize from the posterior-anterior (PA) view. **B,** Lateral view confirms a well-circumscribed mass in the anterior mediastinum, which has both a superior and inferior sulcus with the sternum. **C,** CT scan confirms a homogeneous soft-tissue mass that is separated from the sternum by some mediastinal fat. This is a noninvasive thymoma.

ANSWERS

1. b   2. a   3. c

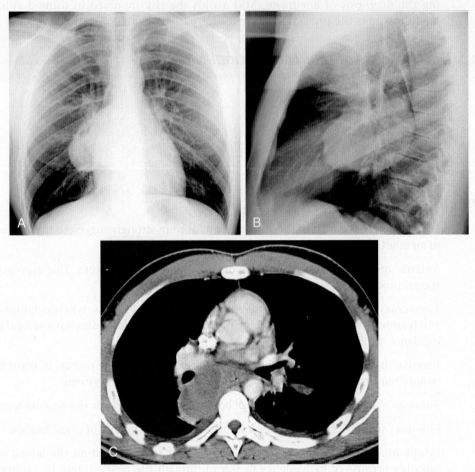

Fig. 10.1

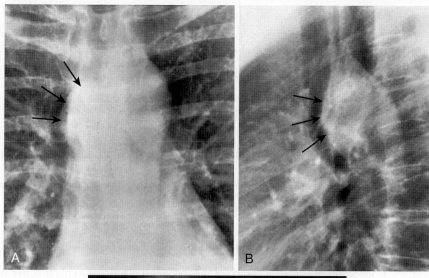

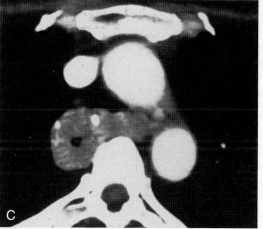

Fig. 10.2

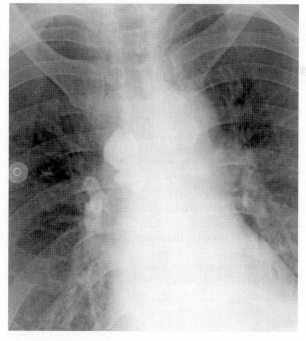

Fig. 10.3

QUESTIONS

1. The most likely diagnosis in the asymptomatic young patient shown in Fig. 10.1, *A-C* is:
   a. Bronchogenic cyst.
   b. Leiomyoma of the esophagus.
   c. Carcinoma of the esophagus.
   d. Lymphoma.
   e. Neurenteric cyst.

2. Which one of the following is the most likely diagnosis for the case illustrated in Fig. 10.2, *A-C*?
   a. Lymphoma.
   b. Metastases.
   c. Primary tuberculosis.
   d. Sarcoidosis.
   e. Leiomyoma of the esophagus.

3. Referring to Fig. 10.3, which of the following diagnoses may result in calcified middle mediastinal masses?
   a. Histoplasmosis.
   b. Tuberculosis.
   c. Sarcoidosis.
   d. Silicosis.
   e. All of the above.

4. What is the most likely cause of mediastinal adenopathy in a patient with acquired immunodeficiency syndrome (AIDS) and a CD4 count of 50?
   a. Persistent generalized adenopathy (PGL).
   b. Tuberculosis.
   c. Lymphoma.
   d. *Pneumocystis jiroveci* pneumonia.
   e. Kaposi sarcoma.

Chart 10.1	**MIDDLE MEDIASTINAL MASSES**

I. Neoplastic adenopathy
   A. Metastasis, including lesions derived from lung primaries[379]
   B. Lymphoma
   C. Leukemia
   D. Angioimmunoblastic lymphadenopathy[292]
   E. Kaposi sarcoma (in patients with AIDS)[111,314]
II. Inflammatory adenopathy
   A. Tuberculosis[225,331,388,394]
   B. Histoplasmosis[97,371,633]
   C. Blastomycosis (rare)[450]
   D. Coccidioidomycosis
   E. Sarcoidosis
   F. Viral pneumonia (particularly measles and cat scratch fever)
   G. AIDS[314]
   H. Infectious mononucleosis[248]
   I. Pertussis pneumonia

Chart 10.1	**MIDDLE MEDIASTINAL MASSES—cont'd**

J. Amyloidosis[246]

K. Plague[544]

L. Tularemia[496]

M. Drug reaction[236,503]

N. Giant lymph node hyperplasia (Castleman disease)[370,611]

O. Connective tissue disease (e.g., mixed, rheumatoid, lupus)

P. Bacterial lung abscess[482]

Q. *Mycobacterium avium* complex (MAC, in patients with AIDS)[314]

R. Anthrax[125]

III. Inhalational disease adenopathy[175]

A. Silicosis

B. Coal worker's pneumoconiosis

C. Berylliosis

IV. Primary tumors

A. Lung cancer[542]

B. Tracheal tumors

1. Carcinoma

2. Adenoid cystic carcinoma

3. Papilloma

4. Metastases

5. Lipoma

6. Leiomyoma[301]

7. Amyloid tumor

8. Granular cell myoblastoma of the trachea (rare)[514]

C. Esophageal tumor[558]

1. Benign (leiomyoma)[530]

2. Malignant (carcinoma, leiomyosarcoma)

3. Solitary fibrous tumor of the pleura[116]

V. Vascular lesions

A. Aneurysms

B. Aortic dissection

C. Distended veins (e.g., superior vena cava, azygos vein, esophageal varices)[326]

D. Hematoma

E. Primary angiosarcoma (pulmonary artery)

F. Left superior vena cava

G. Aberrant right subclavian artery

H. Right aortic arch

VI. Duplication cysts

A. Bronchogenic or respiratory cyst (includes tracheal and some esophageal cysts)[463]

B. Enteric cyst

C. Extralobar sequestration (including esophageal lung)[233]

VII. Other

A. Hiatal hernia

B. Esophageal diverticulum

C. Dilated esophagus (achalasia)

D. Thyroid and parathyroid[121] masses that extend into the mediastinum

E. Cystic hygroma (lymphangioma)

F. Amyloidosis[430]

Chart 10.2	**AIDS-RELATED ADENOPATHY**

I. Neoplastic adenopathy
   A. Non-Hodgkin lymphoma
   B. Kaposi sarcoma
   C. Metastasis, from distant or primary lung tumors
II. Inflammatory adenopathy
   A. Tuberculosis[515,531]
   B. *Mycobacterium avium* complex (MAC)
   C. Fungal infections (histoplasmosis, coccidiomycosis)
   D. Persistent generalized adenopathy (small nodes between 1 and 1.5 cm detectable on computed tomography [CT])

Discussion

The evaluation of a middle mediastinal mass requires careful consideration of the normal structures found in the middle mediastinum.[87,237,443,517,631] Based on the divisions of the mediastinum described by Felson,[150] the middle mediastinum does not correspond precisely with the classic anatomic description of the middle mediastinum. On the lateral chest radiograph, it is the area between the anterior border of the trachea and posterior border of the heart and a line drawn 1 cm posterior to the anterior border of the vertebral bodies. This area includes the trachea, bifurcation of the trachea, arch of the aorta, great vessels, pulmonary arteries, esophagus, and numerous paratracheal and peribronchial nodes. The trachea is outlined with air, and small amounts of air may be detected in the esophagus.[444] The lateral view is especially important in the evaluation of the normally lucent retrotracheal space.[171]

The causes of a middle mediastinal mass can be divided into four broad categories: lymphadenopathy, primary tumors, vascular lesions, and duplication cysts (Chart 10.1). When the various causes of lymphadenopathy are taken together, they are clearly the most common cause of a middle mediastinal mass.

Middle mediastinal lymphadenopathy is most reliably identified by the detection of a mass in an area that is known to have a specific lymph node—for example, a subcarinal, right paratracheal, azygos, or ductal node (Fig 10.4). Because many of the processes to be considered involve multiple nodes in the same area, there is a strong but not invariable tendency for mediastinal adenopathy to result in the appearance of a lobulated mass. The causes of middle mediastinal adenopathy greatly overlap the causes of hilar adenopathy, a condition that further contributes to the lobulated appearance of the masses.

NEOPLASTIC ADENOPATHY

The neoplastic involvement of middle mediastinal lymph nodes is usually metastatic.[379] It must be emphasized that lung cancer usually metastasizes to the middle mediastinal nodes.[542] In fact, nodal metastases frequently constitute the bulk of the masses produced by carcinomas that arise in the mainstem bronchi. Small cell lung cancer (Fig 10.5, *A-C*) commonly presents with extensive middle mediastinal adenopathy, which may involve nodes in the other mediastinal compartments and in the hila.[79] Metastases from peripheral lung tumors and even distant primaries may also produce metastatic deposits in the middle mediastinum.[101]

The challenge of detecting masses that are deep in the mediastinum with minimal contact with the lung, such as subcarinal masses, is similar in all three compartments of the mediastinum. Both CT and magnetic resonance imaging (MRI) are very sensitive methods for detecting small mediastinal masses and are of particular value in staging lymphomas and carcinomas, which have a tendency to metastasize to mediastinal

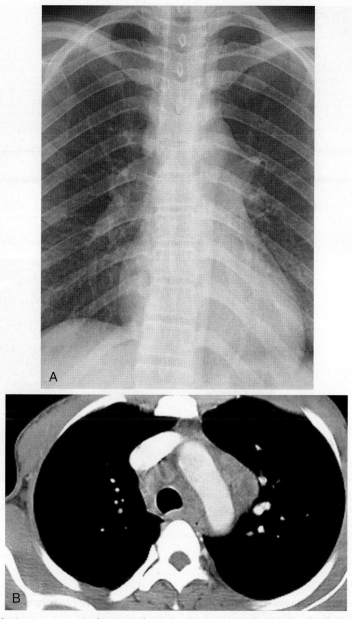

Fig. 10.4   A, A convex opacity between the arch of the aorta and the left pulmonary artery should always be regarded as abnormal. This is the typical appearance of an enlarged ductus node in the aorticopulmonary window. **B,** CT scan confirms the presence of lymph nodes around the aortic arch. In this patient with AIDS, the lymphadenopathy was caused by tuberculosis.

nodes. The two techniques are especially useful for detecting nodal metastases from primary lung cancer and local extensions of esophageal carcinoma.[402,403,550]

Lymphomas, particularly Hodgkin lymphoma, more frequently arise in the anterior mediastinum but are also an important cause of middle mediastinal adenopathy.[21] Lymphoma may arise in the middle mediastinum, and chronic lymphocytic leukemia is a less common hematologic malignancy that involves the middle mediastinal nodes. As many as 25% of patients with leukemia are reported to have mediastinal adenopathy in the late stages of their disease. Like lymphoma, the adenopathy that occurs in patients with leukemia is often not confined to the middle mediastinum, but may also involve the bronchopulmonary (hilar) nodes.

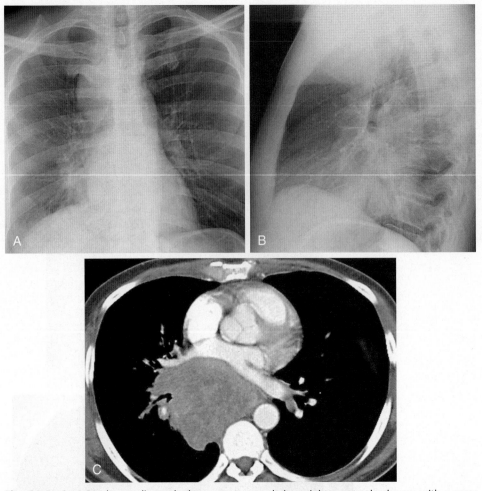

Fig. 10.5 A, A PA chest radiograph demonstrates an obvious right paratracheal mass with a more subtle subcarinal mass. **B,** Lateral view reveals a large subcarinal mass. **C,** Axial CT scan confirms the large subcarinal mass with compression and anterior displacement of the pulmonary arteries. This is a common presentation of small cell carcinoma of the lung.

The diagnosis of a neoplastic condition is frequently suggested by clinical information. When a patient is being followed up for a known primary carcinoma located elsewhere and develops a middle mediastinal mass, a metastatic lesion is the most likely diagnosis. A primary lung tumor should be suspected in patients who have associated hemoptysis and a history of smoking. Patients with primary lung tumors frequently have other indirect radiologic signs of the tumor, including atelectasis or obstructive pneumonia. These signs of an obstructing lesion are helpful for distinguishing primary lung cancer from metastases because endobronchial metastases are infrequent (see Chapter 13). On the other hand, associated pulmonary opacities and even atelectasis are unreliable features for distinguishing a primary lung cancer from lymphoma. Both types of tumor may invade the pulmonary interstitium locally with a resultant ill-defined perihilar opacity that may be associated with a mediastinal mass. This is best known in the case of small cell carcinoma, which can completely mimic the appearance of lymphoma in the chest because of its early metastases to the regional lymph nodes. Small cell carcinoma[57] may even produce massive mediastinal adenopathy before the primary tumor is radiologically detectable.

Calcification of lymph nodes that are enlarged by tumor is very rare. It is reported to occur as a result of bone-forming metastases from malignant bone tumors (osteosarcoma) and even more rarely from primary lung cancer.[360] Calcification has also been observed to develop in nodes affected by Hodgkin lymphoma, usually after treatment with radiation therapy.[51,327] In both cases, serial examinations and the history should permit a correct diagnosis.

INFLAMMATORY ADENOPATHY

A large variety of inflammatory lesions (see Chart 10.1) may result in middle mediastinal adenopathy. Like the neoplastic processes, these diseases commonly cause associated bronchopulmonary adenopathy. Careful correlation of clinical and laboratory information is usually required for their diagnosis.

Primary tuberculosis may present with hilar or mediastinal adenopathy.[54,225,261,641] There is frequently an associated exudative pneumonitis with the radiologic appearance of a localized or even lobar consolidation. This combination of a localized air space consolidation, particularly in the middle or lower lobes, with either hilar or mediastinal adenopathy in a child, is a classic radiologic presentation of primary tuberculosis. The adenopathy results from the formation of tuberculoid caseating granulomas in the lymph nodes. This reaction may resolve completely or heal by fibrosis and calcification. It is therefore a common cause of mediastinal nodal calcification. Although primary tuberculosis is usually expected to occur in children, this combination of localized air space consolidation and mediastinal adenopathy may occur in any age group.[54,225]

The age at onset of primary tuberculosis closely follows geographic distribution. In areas in which tuberculosis is endemic, the age at onset is younger, whereas in areas in which the disease is no longer common, the first exposure and therefore the initial infection may occur at a later age.[394] For example, in eastern Asia, adults do not typically sustain the onset of primary tuberculosis, whereas in the United States, Canada, and Europe, the incidence of primary tuberculosis in adults is greater simply because the number of adults previously exposed to tuberculosis is relatively small. There is also increasing evidence that the radiologic findings associated with primary tuberculosis may be more related to the patient's immune response than to his or her age.[495]

Histoplasmosis is another common cause of middle mediastinal adenopathy (Fig 10.6).[97] The adenopathy in histoplasmosis may be more dramatic in that it presents with bulkier nodes than expected in tuberculosis. The incidence of histoplasmosis as a cause of middle mediastinal masses probably exceeds that of tuberculosis in areas of the world where histoplasmosis is endemic. The radiologic features of lymphadenopathy secondary to histoplasmosis are nonspecific. There is, however, an even higher incidence of calcification in lymph nodes that are enlarged by histoplasmosis granulomas. Skin testing for tuberculosis and histoplasmosis frequently enables a distinction to be made between these two causes of mediastinal node enlargement or calcification.

Other fungal infections, including coccidioidomycosis and blastomycosis, cause mediastinal adenopathy less frequently, although radiologically both these infections may mimic primary tuberculosis. Coccidioidomycosis is particularly well known for this presentation in endemic areas in the desert of the southwestern United States. Blastomycosis rarely causes either hilar or mediastinal adenopathy. Rabinowitz et al.[450] have reported that only 3 of 51 cases that they studied had definite hilar adenopathy.

Sarcoidosis is a common cause of middle mediastinal adenopathy that often has a characteristic radiologic appearance because of the propensity for sarcoidosis to involve the hilar nodes symmetrically in combination with middle mediastinal adenopathy. The middle mediastinal adenopathy in sarcoidosis frequently appears to be asymmetric on the chest radiograph with predominant involvement of the right paratracheal lymph nodes. Because of differences in the anatomy of the mediastinum, CT often reveals that the left lymph nodes are enlarged, which is not readily appreciated on the

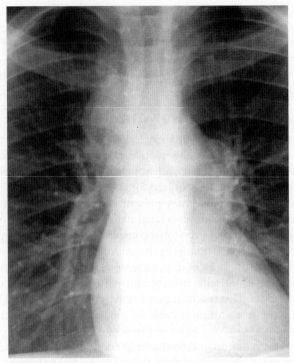

Fig. 10.6 The large right paratracheal and left aorticopulmonary window masses with calcifications are the result of histoplasmosis.

chest radiograph. Middle mediastinal adenopathy without hilar adenopathy is highly atypical in sarcoidosis; in fact, it is so atypical that a patient with middle mediastinal nodes who is believed to have sarcoidosis should have a very careful review of all available histologic material to exclude the possibility of a sarcoid-like reaction around a malignant tumor, such as lymphoma.

Viral pneumonias, particularly measles pneumonias, have also been associated with lymphadenopathy. The combination of pulmonary opacities with adenopathy must be distinguished from primary tuberculosis and the fungal infections previously described. In contrast to primary tuberculosis, this presentation of viral infection is almost always restricted to the pediatric age group. The diagnosis of viral pneumonia with adenopathy should be suspected on the basis of the clinical presentation. An acute febrile response with leukocytosis during an epidemic of viral infection supports the diagnosis. Confirmation requires laboratory testing, including serologic studies and frequently viral cultures.

Infectious mononucleosis[248] is another entity that resembles a viral infection. In contrast to the viral pneumonias, which may mimic primary tuberculosis, infectious mononucleosis does not usually produce a significant pneumonic process. There have been only rare reports of a fine interstitial pneumonitis caused by this disease, but widespread lymphadenopathy is a common observation in infectious mononucleosis and occasionally involves the middle mediastinum or hilum. Laboratory confirmation of the diagnosis is essential to exclude early lymphocytic malignancy, a more common cause of middle mediastinal adenopathy. Splenic enlargement is frequent in patients with infectious mononucleosis, but it also occurs in those with lymphoma and sarcoidosis. Associated splenomegaly is therefore not specific but narrows the differential to these three possibilities.

Silicosis and coal worker's pneumoconiosis are well-known causes of both hilar and mediastinal adenopathy and are considered together. The adenopathy in both silicosis and coal worker's pneumoconiosis is almost invariably associated with the pulmonary disease, which will be discussed elsewhere in the text in the chapters on fine nodular patterns (see Chapter 17), fine reticular opacities (see Chapter 18), honeycomb lung (see Chapter 19), and multiple masses (see Chapter 21). In both diseases, silica particles appear to be picked up by pulmonary macrophages and transported to the lymph nodes. The silica excites a granulomatous and later a fibrotic reaction, which enlarges the nodes. Calcification of the nodes is a late result of this reaction. There is a well-described but unexplained tendency for the calcification to appear in the periphery of the nodes, leading to the distinctive radiologic appearance described as eggshell calcification. Eggshell calcification was once considered a diagnostic finding of silicosis, but a similar appearance has been observed rarely as a late finding in sarcoidosis and tuberculosis. In answer to question 3, all the listed entities may result in calcified mediastinal nodes.

Berylliosis is a rare disease that produces a granulomatous reaction very similar to that of sarcoidosis. The adenopathy is due to the accumulation of granulomas in the nodes. Berylliosis typically involves both the hilar and mediastinal lymph nodes and is often associated with either a diffuse nodular or reticular pulmonary pattern, also resembling that of sarcoidosis. Even histologic distinction of the reactions of berylliosis and sarcoidosis may be impossible. The diagnosis is usually suspected because of a history of exposure, and it is confirmed by spectrographic examination of wet tissue.

AIDS-RELATED ADENOPATHY

Lymphadenopathy is a common occurrence in patients infected with human immunodeficiency virus (HIV). The most likely cause of the adenopathy is determined by the stage of the infection, which is closely related to the CD4 cell count. In early HIV infection, while the CD4 count is in the 300- to 500-cell/μL range, patients may have clinical symptoms of persistent generalized lymphadenopathy (PGL).[563] Biopsy of nodes in patients with PGL reveals reactive lymph node hyperplasia. Although this is a common cause of axillary and inguinal adenopathy, occurring in 50% of patients with acquired immunodeficiency syndrome (AIDS), it is not a common cause of mediastinal adenopathy. PGL may account for nodes that are detectable with CT in the range of 1 to 1.5 cm, but it is not a likely cause of adenopathy detectable by chest radiography. Kuhlman et al.[314] have reported that extensive adenopathy is most likely the result of mycobacterial infections, Kaposi sarcoma, non-Hodgkin lymphoma, fungal infection, or drug hypersensitivity. As the CD4 count decreases below 300 cell/μL, tuberculosis, lymphoma, and Kaposi sarcoma are more likely causes of mediastinal adenopathy.[367,559] *Mycobacterium avium complex* (MAC) and Kaposi sarcoma become more likely causes of mediastinal adenopathy after the CD4 counts has dropped below 200 cell/μL (Fig 10.7, *A and B*). Additionally, the observation of mediastinal adenopathy may be important in the differentiation of *Pneumocystis jiroveci* pneumonia (also known as PCP) from tuberculosis. PCP and tuberculosis are both causes of diffuse lung disease in patients with CD4 counts less than 200 cell/μL. Adenopathy is a rare manifestation of PCP but is a common finding in patients with tuberculosis[515] (answer to question 4 is *b*).

The patterns of tuberculosis in patients with AIDS are closely correlated with the CD4 count.[531] In the early stages of HIV infection, before the CD4 count begins to drop, apical cavitary disease is the expected presentation. As the immune response declines, the patterns are more variable. After the CD4 count has dropped into the range of 50 to 200 cell/μL, the radiologic patterns change to the expected patterns of primary tuberculosis. These findings include asymmetric hilar and mediastinal adenopathy (see Fig 10.4, *A and B*), noncavitary pulmonary air space opacities, miliary nodules, and pleural effusions.[531] This new understanding of the relationship of the immune response and the different presentations of tuberculosis suggest that the classic separation of primary and postprimary tuberculosis is related more to the patient's immune response than to whether it is the first or a later episode of the infection.[495]

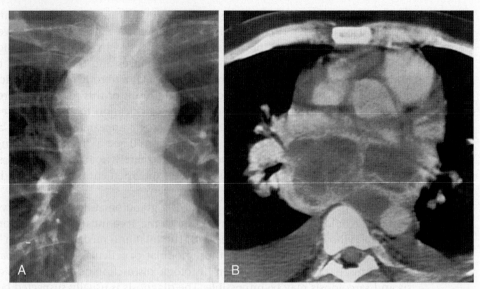

Fig. 10.7   A, This patient with AIDS has a large, right-sided, paratracheal mass that is continuous with a mass of subcarinal nodes. **B,** CT scan confirms a collection of large middle mediastinal nodes with central necrosis. There are also bilateral pleural effusions. Biopsy revealed a mixture of Kaposi sarcoma and *Mycobacterium avium complex* (MAC).

PRIMARY TUMORS

Primary carcinoma of the trachea, a rare tumor, is easily missed on the initial chest radiograph because it may produce a subtle contour abnormality with tracheal narrowing. In the later stages, it may produce a paratracheal mass and may be recognized as a mediastinal mass. In such cases, radiologic distinction of an intrinsic mass from an extrinsic mass compressing the trachea may be difficult. CT is most useful for outlining the contour of the mass. A nodular irregular defect in the trachea indicates an intrinsic mass and nearly confirms the diagnosis of primary tumor. Final confirmation requires bronchoscopy and biopsy. Less common endotracheal masses include carcinoid, leiomyoma,[301] granuloma, papilloma, metastasis, lipoma, fibroma, and amyloid tumor. A history of stridor is often elicited in patients with an endotracheal mass and is an indication for CT. Tracheal stenotic lesions are even more subtle on the chest radiograph. Like the tracheal tumors, they often present with stridor and require CT for confirmation and evaluation. The causes of stricture include postintubation, infections, and posttransplantation stenosis. Systemic diseases such as granulomatosis with polyangiitis, relapsing polychondritis, papillomatosis, relapsing polychondritis, tracheobronchopathia osteochondroplastica, and amyloidosis are some of the other conditions that should be considered.[442]

Esophageal carcinomas are typically seen as constricting lesions of the esophagus with symptoms of dysphagia long before there is a significant mass effect. It is therefore unusual but sometimes possible to identify a primary carcinoma of the esophagus as a middle mediastinal mass (Fig 10.8, *A* and *B*). One middle mediastinal finding that has been observed in an esophageal tumor is thickening of the paratracheal stripe (Fig 10.9). This finding has also been seen in other constricting lesions of the esophagus and may represent either an inflammatory infiltrate or spread of the tumor in the paraesophageal tissues.

Leiomyoma[530] is a primary esophageal tumor that is more likely to present as a mediastinal mass. The tumor grows in the wall of the esophagus and may displace the esophagus, producing a large bulky mass before symptoms of obstruction become significant (Fig 10.10, *A-C*). When the mass forms an annular mass in the wall of

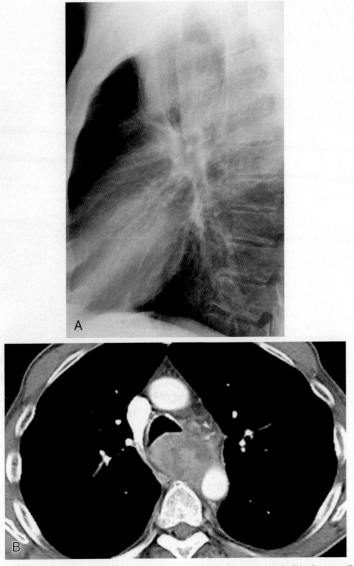

Fig. 10.8 A, The mediastinum appeared to be normal on this patient's PA chest radiograph, but the lateral view reveals an area of increased opacity posterior to the trachea. **B,** CT scan confirms an esophageal mass with anterior displacement of the trachea and bronchi. Biopsy confirmed the suspected esophageal cancer.

the esophagus, it may cause symptoms of obstruction while the mass is smaller and may be more difficult to detect on the chest radiograph (see Fig 10.2, *A-C*; answer to question 2 is *e*).

A solitary fibrous tumor of the pleura[116] is another primary tumor that occasionally mimics a middle mediastinal mass. This tumor arises from the pleura of the mediastinum on the medial aspect of the lung. Although not a true mediastinal tumor, it has the radiologic appearance of such a tumor because of its location. Biopsy is required to make this diagnosis. The radiologist's role is to identify the mass.

Vascular Abnormalities

Enlargement of the great vessels often has a radiologic appearance simulating that of a mediastinal mass. Aneurysm and aortic dissection must be ruled out when a

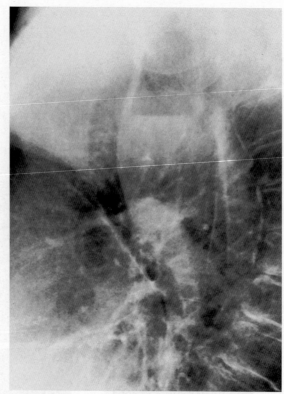

Fig. 10.9 Carcinoma of the esophagus caused obstruction with an air-fluid level in the dilated proximal esophagus. Thickening of the posterior tracheal stripe is another indication of carcinoma of the esophagus.

mediastinal opacity is indistinguishable from the aorta (Fig 10.11, *A* and *B*). Both aneurysms and dissections may involve the anterior, middle, and posterior mediastinum. Distinguishing masses from aneurysms is a common challenge in the evaluation of opacities adjacent to the aorta. CT angiography is the most frequently performed procedure for evaluating a suspected aneurysm or dissection of the aorta (Fig 10.12, *A* and *B*). MRI is the preferred alternative for patients with a contrast allergy or abnormal renal function; catheter angiography is reserved for patients who are candidates for intravascular stent therapy.

Distention of normal veins, in particular the azygos vein and superior vena cava, may occasionally be confused with a mass. The distinction of an enlarged azygos node from a distended azygos vein may be done by comparing flat and upright films that document a change in size or by a Valsalva maneuver that shows the opacity to decrease in size. The latter phenomenon may be observed with fluoroscopy or documented with posteroanterior (PA) chest radiographs (Fig 10.13, *A* and *B*).

Aortic injury following rapid deceleration injury to the chest may produce a false aneurysm with the appearance of a mediastinal mass. The appearance of a mediastinal mass after significant chest trauma should strongly suggest the diagnosis, and CT angiography is necessary to confirm the diagnosis and localize the injury. Usually, the injury of a great vessel results in diffuse mediastinal widening. Extensive hemorrhage into the mediastinum obscures the aortic arch and frequently dissects over the apex of the lung. Apparent asymmetric, apical, pleural thickening after chest trauma is therefore a clue to a significant vascular injury. When the pleura is lacerated, there is associated intrapleural bleeding. In these cases, CT angiography is the definitive emergency procedure.

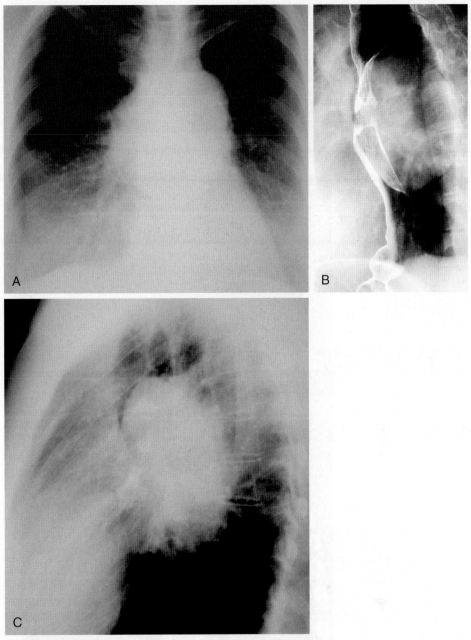

Fig. 10.10 A, A large opacity projects over the right hilum. **B,** The lateral view confirms a large middle mediastinal mass. **C,** Because the patient had difficulty swallowing, a barium swallow was given and revealed a large mass in the wall of the esophagus. Leiomyoma of the esophagus is often large before it causes symptoms.

DUPLICATION CYST

Duplication cysts of foregut origin are relatively rare causes of intrathoracic masses, but the middle mediastinum is their most common location (see Fig 10.1, *A-C*). The dorsal foregut gives rise to the esophagus, and the tracheobronchial tree is derived from the ventral foregut. This probably explains the frequency of a middle mediastinal location for the foregut cyst.

Bronchogenic or respiratory cysts arise from the trachea, mainstem bronchi, or esophagus.[463] They are identified histologically by their characteristic respiratory epithelium,

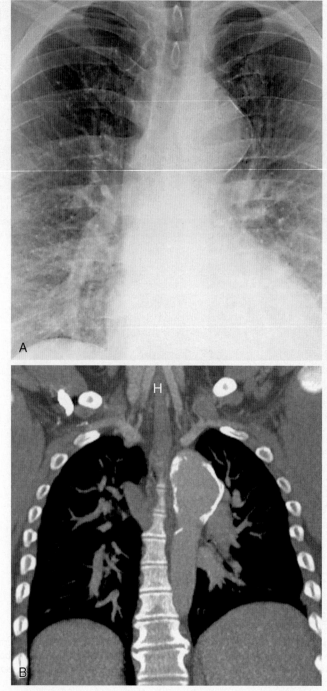

Fig. 10.11   A, The large opacity in the left mediastinum obscures the normal aortic contour and has a rim of calcification suggesting a large aneurysm. **B,** Coronal CT scan confirms a large aortic aneurysm.

presence of seromucous glands, and cartilage plates. The cartilage plates are the most diagnostic feature of these cysts. Some cysts with a respiratory epithelium have actually been dissected from the wall of the esophagus and thus may be named *esophageal cysts* on the basis of their location, although their histologic appearance is that of a bronchogenic cyst. These cysts have also been reported to extend below the diaphragm.[15]

The most common chest radiographic appearance of a duplication cyst is that of a homogeneous opacity. The most common location of the cyst within the

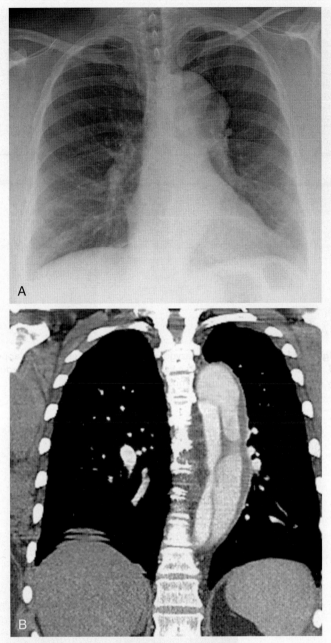

Fig. 10.12   A, This contour abnormality of the aortic arch is also suggestive of an aneurysm but must be evaluated with CT to exclude a mass and evaluate the aorta. **B,** CT angiography reveals an aortic dissection extending from the arch down the descending aorta.

mediastinum is around the area of the carina (Fig 10.14), but such cysts may also be paratracheal and even retrocardiac (Fig 10.15, *A* and *B*). Duplication cysts rarely communicate with the tracheobronchial tree or esophagus, but when communication is established, the fluid in the cyst may drain out, leaving a lucent cystic structure. Infrequently, a thin rim of calcification develops in the wall of the cyst. This feature is also an indication of the cystic character of the lesion; however, distinguishing these cysts from solid masses is not usually possible by chest radiography, and ultrasound is not useful because of interference from bone and aerated lung. CT

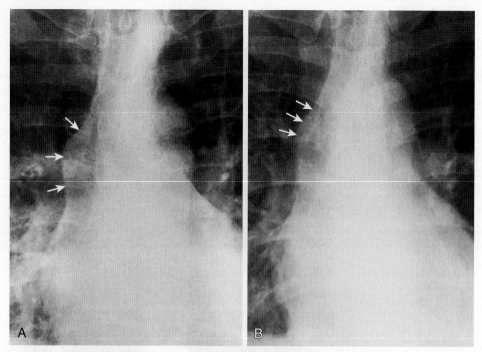

Fig. 10.13   **A,** Opacity in the azygous area *(arrows)* resembles the appearance of the azygos node. **B,** Repeated examination during a Valsalva maneuver demonstrated reduction in the size of the opacity *(arrows).* It is therefore the azygos vein.

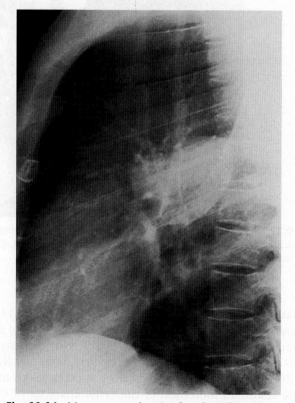

Fig. 10.14   Most common location for a bronchogenic cyst.

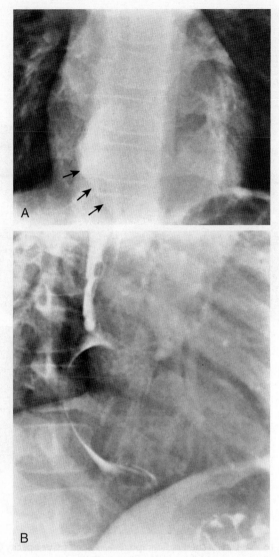

Fig. 10.15   A, Posteroanterior (PA) chest radiograph demonstrates a mass crossing the midline posterior to the heart. Note the tapered inferior border *(arrows),* indicating a mediastinal location. **B,** Lateral view from a barium swallow confirms the presence of a middle mediastinal lesion deviating the esophagus. This appearance suggests that the lesion may be arising from the wall of the esophagus. Based on the chest radiograph and the swallow, this might have been a leiomyoma, but it was actually found to be a more rare esophageal duplication cyst.

can reliably identify most of these cysts as fluid-filled structures when the fluid is of low attenuation[194,315] (see Fig 10.1, *A-C*). However, numerous authors have reported cases in which the cysts are filled with high-attenuation material that resembles a solid mass on the CT scan. MRI is more reliable for determining the cystic character of these lesions[315,347] (Fig 10.16, *A-C*).

Enteric cysts are radiologically very similar to bronchogenic cysts. Occasionally, they also appear as homogeneous opacities in the middle mediastinum, but are more commonly posterior (see Chapter 12).

Extralobar sequestration is a rare cause of a middle mediastinal mass.[484] It is a complex foregut anomaly that contains multiple cysts. The cyst linings resemble both alveoli and bronchioles. When this lesion is closely related to the esophagus, the phenomenon is often called an *esophageal lung.* The extralobar sequestration should have an anomalous feeding vessel identifiable on enhanced CT.

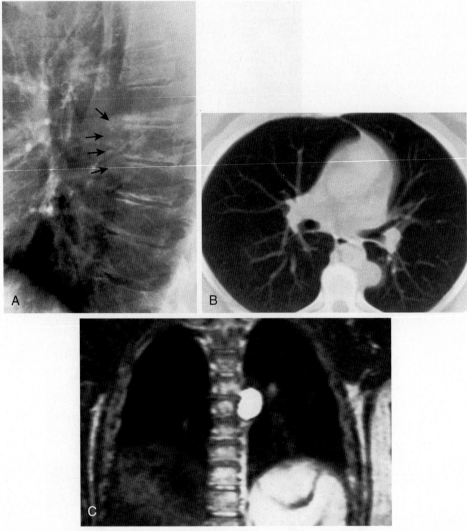

Fig. 10.16   A, Lateral chest radiograph reveals a soft tissue opacity (*arrows*) that overlaps the arbitrary line that divides the middle and posterior mediastinal compartments. **B,** CT scan suggested that this was a homogeneous soft tissue mass. **C,** T2-weighted, coronal MRI scan reveals a bright white lesion, indicating that it is a fluid-filled cystic structure. This is a bronchogenic cyst.

Top 5 Diagnoses: Middle Mediastinal Mass

1. Metastases
2. Lymphoma
3. Granulomatous infections
4. Hiatal hernia
5. Aneurysm

Summary

Lymphadenopathy is the most common cause of a middle mediastinal mass. The azygos, subcarinal, ductus, and paratracheal nodes are located in the middle mediastinum.

Middle mediastinal masses that result from bronchogenic carcinoma are regional nodal metastases.

Lobar consolidation, in combination with mediastinal adenopathy, is a classic radiologic appearance for primary tuberculosis.

Lymph node calcification generally indicates an old inflammatory process such as tuberculosis, histoplasmosis, silicosis, or rarely, sarcoidosis. Lymphomatous nodes sometimes calcify after radiation. There have been rare reports of bone-producing metastases to mediastinal nodes.

The middle mediastinum is a common location for an aortic aneurysm. Masses that are not easily distinguishable from the aorta should be studied by CT angiography or MRI to rule out this diagnosis.

Carcinoma of the trachea, a rare cause of a middle mediastinal mass, is easily missed on the initial chest radiograph, but it should be sought when there is a history of wheezing.

Esophageal tumors typically produce symptoms of obstruction before there is an appreciable mediastinal mass.

A bronchogenic cyst usually presents as a smooth, homogeneous, middle mediastinal mass in an asymptomatic young patient.

ANSWER GUIDE

Legends for introductory figures

Fig. 10.1 A, Bronchogenic cysts typically occur in the middle mediastinum, near the level of the tracheal carina. They usually arise from the tracheobronchial tree but have been reported to arise from the esophagus. **B,** The lateral chest view confirms the location in the middle mediastinum. **C,** CT scan reveals the content to be fluid attenuation, confirming the cystic character of the lesion.
Fig. 10.2 A, Posteroanterior (PA) chest radiograph demonstrates right paratracheal opacity (*arrows*). **B,** Lateral view shows the opacity to be posterior to the trachea (*arrows*) and to indent the posterior wall of the trachea. **C,** CT scan reveals the soft-tissue mass to contain calcifications, surround the esophagus (*central lucency*), and extend across the mediastinum. This is a leiomyoma of the esophagus.
Fig. 10.3 Calcified lymph nodes in the middle mediastinum often occur in combination with hilar nodes and virtually always indicate a granulomatous process. Exceptions are usually suspected on the basis of the history (i.e., treated lymphoma or, rarely, with new calcifications in patients with osteosarcoma).

ANSWERS

1. a   2. e   3. e   4. b

11 | HILAR ENLARGEMENT

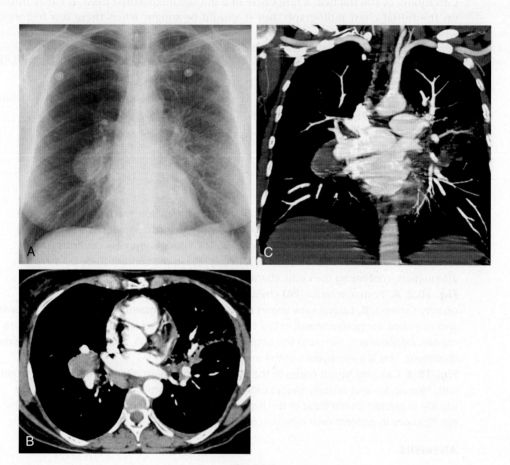

Fig. 11.1

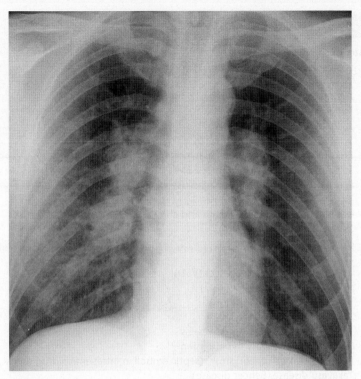

Fig. 11.2

QUESTIONS

1. The most likely cause of unilateral hilar enlargement in the adult in Fig. 11.1, *A-C*, is:
   a. Bronchogenic cyst.
   b. Lung cancer.
   c. Large right pulmonary artery.
   d. Pulmonary varix.
   e. Aneurysm of the descending aorta.

2. The most likely cause of the bilateral hilar enlargement in the asymptomatic young adult in Fig. 11.2 is:
   a. Metastasis.
   b. Primary tuberculosis.
   c. Sarcoidosis.
   d. Lymphoma.
   e. Histoplasmosis.

Chart 11.1	HILAR ENLARGEMENT

I. Large pulmonary arteries
  A. Postcapillary pulmonary arterial hypertension
    1. Left-sided heart failure
    2. Mitral stenosis[75]
    3. Left atrial myxoma
    4. Pulmonary veno-occlusive[529]
    5. Mediastinal fibrosis
  B. Precapillary pulmonary arterial hypertension
    1. Emphysema[368] (see Chapter 22)
    2. Chronic interstitial lung disease (see Chapter 19)
    3. Cystic fibrosis
    4. Pulmonary embolism (acute and chronic)[65,637]
    5. Portal hypertension[71]
    6. Metastatic tumor emboli
    7. Cardiac shunts
      a. Ventricular septal defect (VSD)
      b. Atrial septal defect (ASD)
      c. Patent ductus arteriosus
      d. Truncus arteriosus
      e. Transposition of great vessels
    8. Primary pulmonary hypertension[607]
  C. Pulmonary artery aneurysms[66] (septic emboli in intravenous drug users, Takayasu disease, Behçet disease)
II. Unilateral hilar mass
  A. Neoplasm
  B. Lung cancer[533,542,629]
  C. Bronchial carcinoid[275]
  D. Metastasis[379]
  E. Lymphoma
  F. Inflammation
    1. Tuberculosis[225,388,515]
    2. Nontuberculous mycobacteria[389]
    3. Fungal infection (histoplasmosis,[97] coccidioidomycosis,[373] blastomycosis,[450] infrequently in cryptococcosis)[200,346]
    4. Viral infections (atypical measles)
    5. Infectious mononucleosis (rare)[248]
    6. Acquired immune deficiency syndrome[314]
    7. Drug reactions[236,503] (phenytoin [Dilantin])
    8. Sarcoidosis (infrequent)
    9. Bacterial lung abscess[482]
III. Bilateral hilar masses
  A. Neoplasm
    1. Lymphoma
    2. Leukemia (chronic lymphocytic leukemia)
    3. Metastases[107]
    4. Lung cancer (usually asymmetric)
  B. Inflammation
    1. Sarcoidosis[308,642]
    2. Occupational diseases (silicosis and coal worker's pneumoconiosis)
    3. Inhalational anthrax[125]
  C. Collagen vascular diseases
    1. Lupus (rare)
    2. Polyarteritis nodosa
    3. Mixed
IV. Duplication cysts (bronchogenic cysts)[463]

Discussion

The first problem in the evaluation of hilar enlargement is the distinction of vascular enlargement from hilar masses.[73] The normal hilar contours are formed by the pulmonary arteries. Distinction of enlarged pulmonary arteries from hilar masses often requires careful analysis, followed by computed tomography (CT) scanning for confirmation. In cases with bilateral hilar enlargement, it may be especially difficult to distinguish vascular enlargement from masses. Unilateral hilar enlargement also requires careful evaluation but is more suggestive of a mass. In addition to changes in the contour of the hilum, the finding of added opacity strongly suggests a mass. For precise localization to the hilum, it is important to note whether the increased opacity blends imperceptibly with the normal pulmonary artery shadows and thus obscures their borders, or whether the pulmonary arteries are easily identified in addition to the suspected opacity. When the borders of the pulmonary arteries are clearly identifiable, it must be assumed that the mass is discrete and either anterior or posterior to the hilum. The contour of the pulmonary artery is visible because of the adjacent aerated lung. When the aerated lung is filled or displaced, the border of the pulmonary artery will no longer be detected. An area of increased opacity anterior or posterior to the hilum has no effect on the air adjacent to the pulmonary artery and therefore has no effect on its visibility. Felson[150] has described this phenomenon as the hilum overlay sign (Fig 11.3, A-C). This is very useful for separating true hilar abnormalities from superimposed anterior or posterior opacities. In such cases, the lateral view is usually adequate for verifying that the abnormality is not in the hilum. This separation is easily accomplished with CT scanning.

Once it has been ascertained that a hilum is abnormal, the next step in evaluating hilar enlargement is to determine whether the abnormal hilum is the result of an enlarged vascular structure or a mass (Chart 11.1). This requires detailed understanding of the anatomy of the hilum in at least the posteroanterior (PA) and lateral projections (Fig 11.4, A and B). As noted earlier, the hilar shadows in both projections are produced mainly by the right and left pulmonary arteries. The left pulmonary artery is very characteristic in its appearance on the PA chest radiograph, creating an opacity above the left mainstem bronchus and continuing as an opacity that appears to be lateral to the large bronchi.

In a normal patient, the lateral border of the main pulmonary artery should be smooth and may appear to be superimposed over the proximal left pulmonary artery. On the lateral view, the left pulmonary artery courses over the origin of the left upper lobe bronchus, which is seen as a circle. The left pulmonary artery descends behind the bronchus. On the PA view, the right pulmonary artery casts a shadow that is mainly lateral to the bronchus intermedius and largely inferior to the right upper lobe bronchus. Like the left pulmonary artery, the major portion of the descending right pulmonary artery has a smooth contour. This large smooth portion of the right pulmonary artery parallels the bronchus intermedius. It must be emphasized that both pulmonary arteries are branching structures that result in multiple superimposed opacities. In the lateral view, the right pulmonary artery is seen on end, with its superior portion superimposed over the origin of the left pulmonary artery and its inferior portion anterior and slightly inferior to the circular origin of the left upper lobe bronchus.

Pulmonary veins can best be distinguished from arteries by tracing the course of the vessels, keeping in mind that the veins converge on the left atrium inferior to the hilum. With the exception of a pulmonary varix,[38] pulmonary veins do not make a major contribution to the hilar opacities. The convergence of the pulmonary veins on the left atrium is most easily appreciated on the lateral view. The lower lobe veins can be readily observed on the PA view crossing the arteries and converging on the left atrium. The upper lobe veins tend to be lateral to the arteries and may be identified,

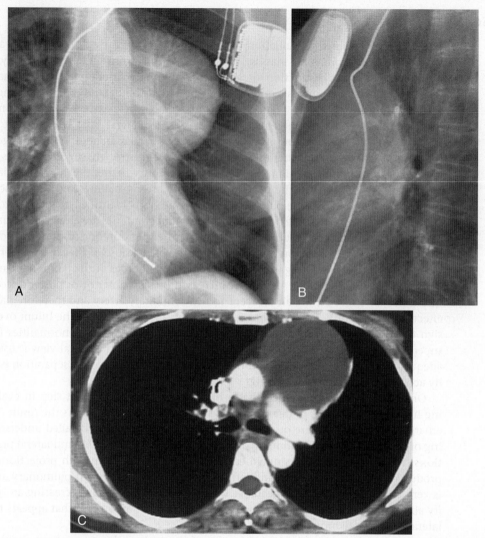

Fig. 11.3   A, This large mass has a well-circumscribed lateral border that is tapered at both the superior and inferior margins. The mass projects over the left hilum but does not obscure the pulmonary artery. This combination of findings indicates that this cannot be a hilar mass. This is an example of the so-called hilum overlay sign. **B,** Lateral view confirms that the mass is anterior to the hilum. **C,** Contrast-enhanced CT scan confirms that the mass arises anterior to the hilum and displaces the pulmonary artery posteriorly. The low attenuation further indicates that it is not a solid mass. This is a large thymic cyst.

especially on the right when their shadows are observed to cross the hilar arteries in a downward direction. The right upper lobe vein characteristically enlarges in left-sided heart failure.

PULMONARY ARTERIAL HYPERTENSION

Pulmonary arterial hypertension is a major cause of bilateral hilar enlargement (Fig 11.5, A-D). The loss of normal arterial tapering results in an abrupt change in caliber between the proximal pulmonary arteries and peripheral pulmonary arteries. There is marked enlargement of the proximal vessels[72] and abrupt tapering or loss of the peripheral vessels. Measurements of the width of the right descending pulmonary artery (>16 mm) and of the left descending pulmonary artery (>18 mm) correlate well with an elevated pulmonary arterial pressure (>20 mm Hg).[368] Other radiologic clues to the diagnosis of pulmonary artery hypertension include enlargement of the main pulmonary artery

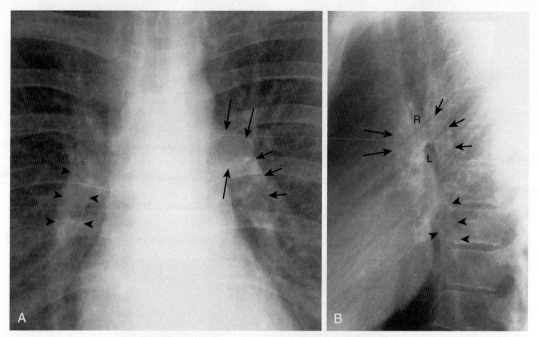

Fig. 11.4 A, *Arrows* outline the normal pulmonary arteries. The right pulmonary artery *(arrowheads)* is lateral to the bronchus intermedius. The left pulmonary artery *(large arrows)* passes posteriorly over the left upper lobe bronchus. The lateral border of the left hilum is formed by the descending left lower lobe artery *(small arrows).* **B,** Normal appearance of the right pulmonary artery on the lateral view is indicated with *large arrows.* The right upper lobe bronchus is marked with *R.* The course of the left pulmonary artery crossing over the left main bronchus *(L)* is outlined with *small arrows. Arrowheads* identify the confluence of lower lobe pulmonary veins.

and enlargement of the right ventricle. The main pulmonary artery produces a bulging rounded shadow that projects over the left pulmonary artery and may appear to enlarge the left hilum on the PA view (see Fig 11.5, *A*). On the lateral view, enlargement of the right ventricle and main pulmonary artery has the effect of producing an opacity over the ascending aorta or sometimes filling in the retrosternal clear space. Main pulmonary artery enlargement is easily confirmed by CT showing that the main pulmonary artery is larger than the diameter of the aorta (see Fig 11.5, *D*).[66]

Postcapillary pulmonary arterial hypertension is usually the result of congestive heart failure. Identification of the anterior segmental bronchus leading to either upper lobe may also be helpful in evaluating suspected pulmonary arterial enlargement. Left-sided heart failure is the most common cause of right heart failure and therefore is a common cause of pulmonary arterial hypertension. This is all preceded by pulmonary venous hypertension; as a result, left heart failure differs significantly from most of the other causes of pulmonary artery hypertension described in this chapter. Congestive heart failure and mitral stenosis both result in enlargement of the upper lobe vessels and constriction of the lower lobe vessels, or cephalization. Identification of the anterior segmental bronchus leading to either upper lobe may also be helpful in evaluating suspected cephalization of flow to the upper lobes. When the bronchus is seen on end, it appears as a ring shadow. The segmental pulmonary artery is adjacent to the bronchus. In the normal patient, the size of this artery is slightly larger than that of the bronchus when seen on end. When the anterior segmental artery is more than twice the caliber of the anterior segmental bronchus, pulmonary arterial enlargement can be inferred. A change in the size of a segmental artery over a short period may provide a helpful clue to the diagnosis of pulmonary arterial hypertension secondary to congestive heart failure (Fig 11.6, *A* and *B*). Cephalization[454] is rapidly followed by

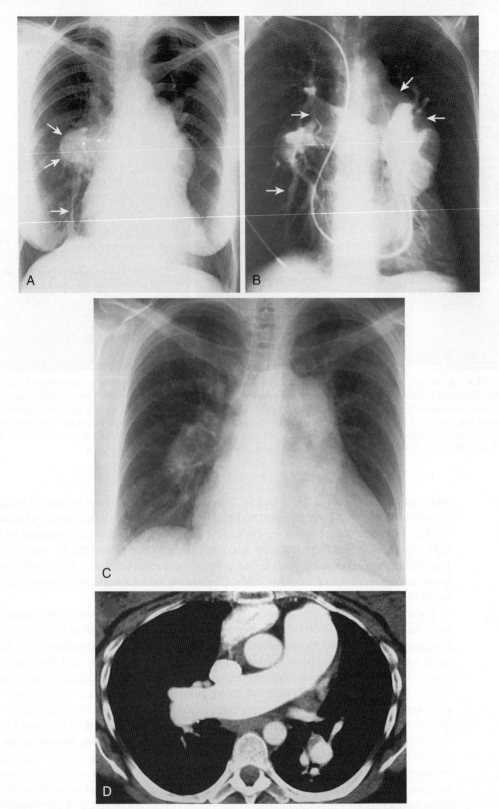

Fig. 11.5 **A,** Bilateral enlargement of proximal pulmonary arteries *(arrows)* with abrupt tapering of peripheral vessels indicates pulmonary arterial hypertension. Linear opacity *(lower arrow)* extending from the hilum to the diaphragm is a scar from a prior infarct. This is pulmonary arterial hypertension secondary to recurrent pulmonary embolism. **B,** Pulmonary arteriogram confirms that hilar opacities represent massively enlarged proximal pulmonary arteries. **C,** Another case of bilateral hilar enlargement resulting from primary pulmonary arterial hypertension shows more symmetric enlargement of the proximal pulmonary arteries. **D,** Contrast-enhanced CT scan shows massive enlargement of the main and proximal pulmonary arteries. Observe that the main pulmonary artery is larger than the ascending aorta. (**B** from Chen JTT. *Essentials of cardiac roentgenology.* Boston, 1987, Little Brown. Used by permission.)

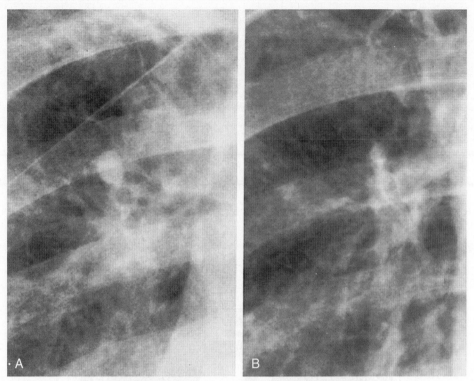

Fig. 11.6 **A,** This segmental artery is larger than its companion bronchus, indicating increased pulmonary arterial pressure in a patient with congestive heart failure. **B,** After treatment, the same segmental artery returned to normal size.

interstitial edema as the intravascular pressure exceeds the osmotic and interstitial pressures, which normally maintain fluid in the vascular compartment. The radiologic result is a fine reticular pattern and increased vascular markings with blurring of the margins of the pulmonary vessels. This may be accompanied by enlargement of the hila, main pulmonary artery, and right ventricle.

Because of the increased markings, this radiologic appearance of postcapillary pulmonary arterial hypertension is in sharp contrast to the appearance of the causes of precapillary pulmonary artery hypertension. Precapillary pulmonary artery hypertension results in enlargement of the hilar vessels with a decrease in the peripheral vessels. In contrast with postcapillary pulmonary artery hypertension, it requires consideration of a larger number of possible causes.

Chronic lung diseases are a major cause of precapillary pulmonary artery hypertension; therefore identification of other signs of lung disease may be key to the correct diagnosis of pulmonary arterial hypertension. In the case of emphysema, the presence of large avascular areas surrounded by thin lines that indicate bullous lesions is helpful in making the diagnosis. The other radiologic signs of emphysema are discussed in Chapter 22. In addition to emphysema, chronic restrictive interstitial diseases from a variety of causes, including idiopathic pulmonary fibrosis, scleroderma, sarcoidosis, and cystic fibrosis, may cause pulmonary arterial hypertension (see Chapter 19).

Pulmonary embolism is another major cause of pulmonary arterial hypertension related to lung disease.[65] An acute, massive pulmonary embolism may produce radiologic signs of pulmonary arterial hypertension with marked prominence of the hilar vessels, obliteration of the peripheral vessels, and right-sided heart enlargement. The diagnosis of chronic pulmonary emboli may be suggested by a clinical history of recurrent episodes of pleuritic chest pain and hemoptysis associated with thrombophlebitis,

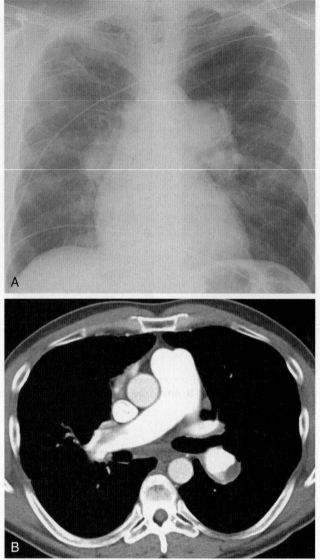

Fig. 11.7 A, The bilateral hilar enlargement is greater on the left because of enlargement of both the left pulmonary artery and main pulmonary artery. **B,** CT angiogram of the pulmonary arteries in this patient with chronic pulmonary emboli shows a filling defect in the proximal left pulmonary artery.

but frequently the history is less dramatic. The diagnosis of pulmonary artery hypertension resulting from a pulmonary embolism is usually confirmed with CT (Fig 11.7, *A-D*).

Metastatic tumor emboli are rarely diagnosed premortem. Increasing size of the proximal pulmonary arteries may be the only chest radiographic finding. Radionuclide lung scans are reported to show multiple, small peripheral defects. Because these emboli are usually very small, they do not produce the segmental and lobar defects expected with thromboemboli. In addition, pulmonary arteriograms typically reveal small tortuous vessels typical of pulmonary arterial hypertension and fail to demonstrate the very small tumor emboli. Because of the severe pulmonary arterial hypertension, pulmonary arteriography is a high-risk procedure in patients with tumor emboli. The diagnosis is sometimes confirmed by lung biopsy or at the postmortem examination.

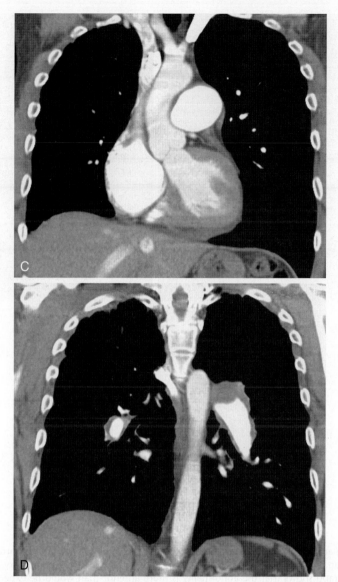

Fig. 11.7, cont'd C, Coronal reconstruction shows the main pulmonary artery to be significantly larger than the ascending aorta, indicating pulmonary arterial hypertension. **D,** The enlarged, descending left pulmonary artery accounts for the left hilar enlargement.

Congenital heart disease is another important cause of pulmonary arterial hypertension (Fig 11.8, *A-C*). It is most commonly secondary to severe left-to-right shunts that remain undiagnosed and untreated for a long time. These include VSDs, ASDs, patent ductus arteriosus, and, less frequently, the admixture lesions—transposition of the great vessels and truncus arteriosus. These heart lesions are usually suspected from clinical signs, particularly when characteristic murmurs are detected. The VSD, ASD, and patent ductus arteriosus are acyanotic lesions until the pulmonary arterial hypertension becomes severe enough to reverse the shunts. This is in contrast to the admixture lesions, which are a cause of early cyanosis. Definitive diagnosis of the cardiac causes of pulmonary hypertension may be made by echocardiography, CT, magnetic resonance imaging (MRI), or catheterization.

The remaining cause of pulmonary arterial hypertension is referred to as *idiopathic* or *primary*.[476] Although this is a diagnosis reached by exclusion, it is not a rare condition, and it has an unfavorable prognosis. Of the causes of pulmonary arterial hypertension

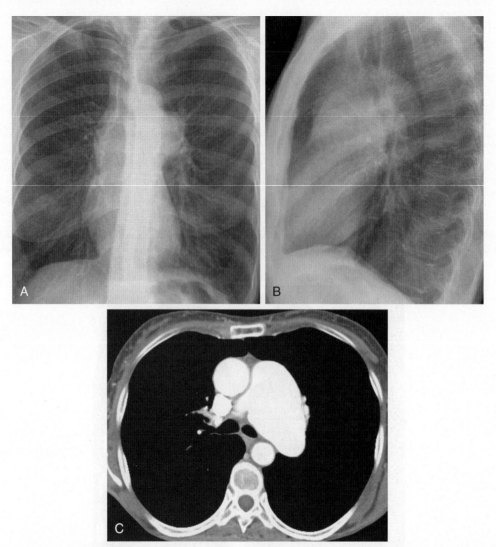

Fig. 11.8   A, Left hilar enlargement in this case is the result of a large main pulmonary artery. This patient was not diagnosed with an atrial septal defect (ASD) until late in life and has severe pulmonary artery hypertension. **B,** The lateral radiograph shows that the abnormality is more anterior than would be expected from a left hilar mass. Note that the opacity has an anterior border projecting over the ascending aorta. **C,** CT scan with contrast confirms massive enlargement of the main pulmonary artery.

considered in this chapter, chronic pulmonary emboli are the most difficult to distinguish from primary idiopathic pulmonary hypertension. Only the characteristic plexiform arterial changes seen in histologic sections of the lung permit the definitive diagnosis of idiopathic pulmonary arterial hypertension[607]—plexogenic pulmonary arteriopathy.

PULMONARY ARTERY ANEURYSMS

Pulmonary artery aneurysms are a rare cause of proximal pulmonary artery enlargement but do occur in patients with right heart endocarditis, especially in intravenous (IV) drug users. They may also be the result of systemic diseases that cause vasculitis. Behçet disease is a rare systemic disease that causes oral and genital ulcers, uveitis, and a systemic vasculitis. The vasculitis affects arteries and veins of all sizes and may cause aneurysms of the pulmonary arteries (Fig 11.9, *A-D*).[602]

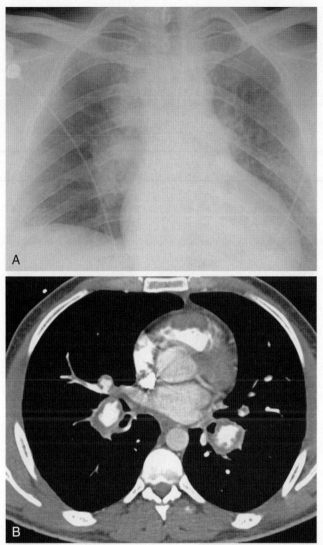

Fig. 11.9 **A,** Bilateral hilar enlargement is more obvious on the right with prominence of the upper portion of the right hilum that is not easily separated from a paratracheal mass. **B,** CT scan with contrast shows that the pulmonary arteries are enlarged with low-attenuation peripheral opacities and localized dilations, which are consistent with aneurysms. The pulmonary artery aneurysms are the result of Behçet disease.

Continued

HILAR ADENOPATHY

The contour of the hilum must be carefully evaluated to distinguish hilar lymphadenopathy from pulmonary artery enlargement. As suggested earlier, a diffuse smooth enlargement of the pulmonary arteries with abrupt tapering of peripheral vessels is characteristic of pulmonary artery enlargement. This is in contrast to the appearance of lumpy nodular hila that are typical of hilar adenopathy. The description makes the problem appear simple, but many cases present a diagnostic dilemma. These cases often require either CT with IV contrast or MRI. CT provides excellent discrimination of hilar nodes from pulmonary vessels. Because MRI is sensitive to blood flow through the pulmonary arteries, it also provides a clear distinction of pulmonary vessels from any surrounding soft tissue opacity nodes.

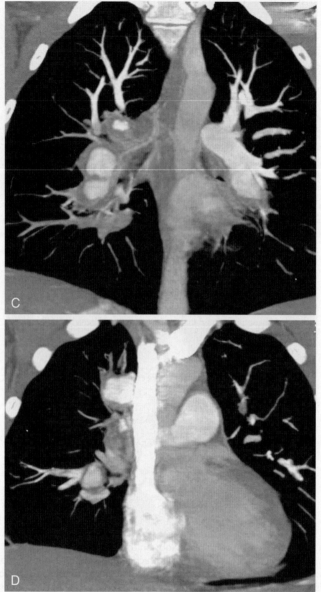

Fig. 11.9, cont'd   C, Coronal reconstruction of the CT scan through the level of the pulmonary arteries shows the lobulated appearance of the pulmonary artery aneurysms. **D,** A more anterior-superior, right pulmonary artery aneurysm accounts for the opacity that resembles a right paratracheal mass on the posteroanterior (PA) view.

UNILATERAL HILAR ADENOPATHY

The vast majority of cases of hilar adenopathy are of inflammatory or neoplastic origin. Many of these cases have associated middle mediastinal adenopathy with involvement of the subcarinal, azygos, ductus, or paratracheal lymph nodes; therefore this differential overlaps considerably with the differential of middle mediastinal masses.

Lung cancer (see Fig 11.1, *A-C*) is the most common neoplastic cause of hilar adenopathy. It should be emphasized that the presence of a hilar mass secondary to lung cancer is an indication of metastatic spread to the hilar nodes.[533,542] Most central primary carcinomas produce endobronchial masses that may spread along the wall of the bronchus or occlude the bronchus, resulting in atelectasis. These endobronchial masses may produce a minimal mass effect before involving the regional hilar lymph nodes. The detection of hilar adenopathy in a case of primary lung cancer is extremely important in staging the tumor, and it is a primary indication for CT in the evaluation of a known primary lung tumor. These regional metastases are usually unilateral in their early phases. When they become extensive, they may involve the mediastinal nodes and later evolve to bilateral hilar adenopathy. In these advanced cases, the adenopathy continues to be asymmetric, particularly in some left-sided tumors, which may metastasize to the right paratracheal nodes. Small cell lung cancer is notorious for this radiologic presentation.

As indicated in Chapter 10, distant, primary tumors may metastasize to the mediastinal nodes with some frequency, but true hilar involvement with no mediastinal involvement is unusual, with the occasional exception of metastatic renal cell carcinoma.[101] This is in contrast to lymphomas, and particularly Hodgkin lymphomas, which may present with asymmetric hilar adenopathy and only minimal mediastinal involvement.

Granulomatous infections are also important causes of asymmetric hilar enlargement. Asymmetric hilar and mediastinal adenopathy is a common presentation of primary tuberculosis.[225] In the past, primary tuberculosis was considered a childhood disease, and this is still true in areas of the world where tuberculosis is endemic, but in North America and Europe, a large population of people who are well into their adult years are at risk for tuberculosis with adenopathy. This is especially true for patients with impaired immunity. The diagnosis is often confirmed at biopsy because the risk for tumor is so much greater. Fungi such as *Histoplasma spp.* are also well known for producing asymmetric hilar adenopathy. Granulomatous nodes resulting from tuberculosis or histoplasmosis are radiologically confirmed only when they lead to the development of hilar lymph node calcification. When the hilar lymph nodes are essentially replaced by calcium, the diagnosis may be confirmed by chest radiography; however, often the appearance of hilar enlargement on the radiograph is less specific, and CT may be required to confirm that the nodes are calcified and therefore the result of a benign, prior, granulomatous infection (Fig 11.10, *A* and *B*).

Other causes of hilar lymphadenopathy include viral pneumonias (measles, in particular), infectious mononucleosis, silicosis, coal worker's pneumoconiosis, and drug reactions. These entities all require careful clinical correlation. Silicosis and coal worker's pneumoconiosis are possibly the easiest to confirm when a history of exposure is obtained, and the lymph nodes are calcified. The calcification may even assume a characteristic appearance with a thin rim of calcification.

BILATERAL HILAR ADENOPATHY

Sarcoidosis produces the classic example of bilateral hilar adenopathy (see Fig 11.2).[308] (Answer to question 2 is *c*.) In contrast to all the causes of hilar adenopathy that have been considered so far, the adenopathy of sarcoidosis is typically bilateral, symmetric, and frequently associated with mediastinal node (paratracheal and ductus) enlargement. This cause of hilar adenopathy often assumes such a characteristic radiologic appearance that radiologists and clinicians will lean strongly toward it as the diagnosis. Even when the patient is asymptomatic, it is prudent to obtain a biopsy for confirmation. Although it is rare, bilateral, symmetric hilar adenopathy resembling the appearance of sarcoidosis can result from lymphoma (Fig 11.11, *A-D*) and even chronic lymphocytic leukemia (Fig 11.12).

Sarcoidosis frequently involves the supraclavicular nodes, liver, and interstitium of the lung. The interstitium of the lung may be extensively involved with minimal granulomas that are too small for radiologic detection but may be easily detected on transbronchial biopsy. Therefore transbronchial biopsy may be an effective method for

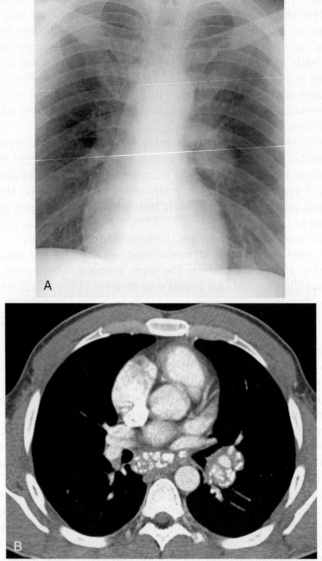

Fig. 11.10   A, The enlargement of the left hilum is suggestive of a hilar mass, which could be the result of neoplastic or inflammatory adenopathy. **B,** CT scan confirms a calcified node in the left hilum and the additional finding of a calcified subcarinal node in the mediastinum. This is diagnostic of a prior granulomatous infection that could have resulted from tuberculosis or histoplasmosis.

confirming the diagnosis of sarcoidosis, even in the absence of radiologically demonstrable interstitial disease.

Bilateral hilar adenopathy may occasionally be associated with other radiologic abnormalities, including the following: (1) fine nodular interstitial opacities; (2) large, multifocal, ill-defined opacities; (3) confluent opacities suggestive of pulmonary edema; (4) diffuse interstitial reticular disease; and (5) even pleural effusion. Its combination with these must be carefully evaluated. Both sarcoidosis and lymphoma may result in such combinations. Of the combinations, bilateral, symmetric hilar adenopathy with pleural effusion is perhaps the least common presentation of sarcoidosis. No more than 3% of patients with sarcoidosis are reported to have significant pleural effusion. Therefore, the presence of pleural effusion should be an additional reason for biopsy confirmation of the diagnosis of sarcoidosis. In fact, the presence of pleural effusion with asymmetric hilar adenopathy could support a number of diagnoses, including

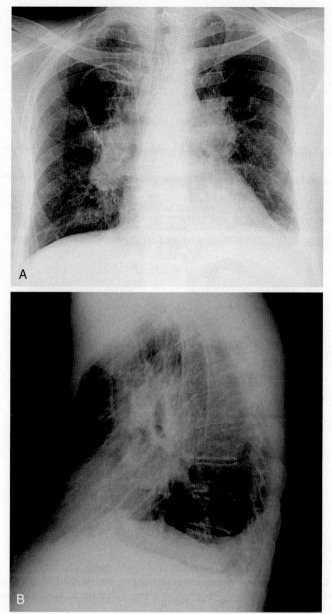

Fig. 11.11   A, Bilateral, symmetric hilar adenopathy resulting from lymphoma may resemble the appearance of adenopathy from sarcoidosis. **B,** The lateral view further confirms hilar enlargement but also reveals blunting of the posterior costophrenic angle, which is suggestive of associated pleural effusion. This makes sarcoidosis an unlikely diagnosis.

Continued

carcinoma of the lung, metastases from a distant site, lymphoma, tuberculosis, and, least likely, sarcoidosis.

Calcified bilateral hilar nodes could be the result of treated lymphoma, but they are almost always the result of chronic granulomatous diseases. Histoplasmosis and tuberculosis are the most common causes of hilar and mediastinal nodal calcifications. The calcifications are usually amorphous and scattered throughout the nodes. Infrequently, peripheral or so-called eggshell calcifications are seen in enlarged nodes that have resulted from silicosis, coal worker's pneumoconiosis, or less frequently, sarcoidosis (Fig 11.13).

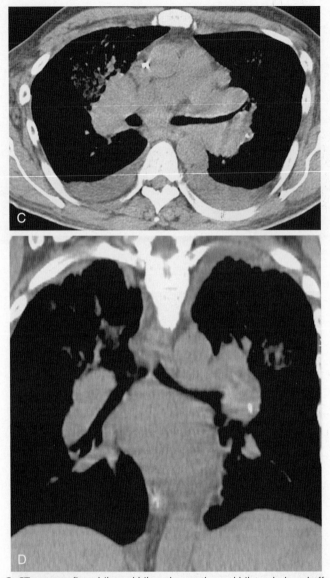

Fig. 11.11, cont'd **C,** CT scan confirms bilateral hilar adenopathy and bilateral pleural effusions. **D,** Coronal CT reconstruction confirms the bilateral hilar adenopathy and reveals subcarinal adenopathy. Biopsy confirmed the suspected diagnosis of lymphoma.

Top 5 Diagnoses: Hilar Enlargement

1. Pulmonary artery hypertension
2. Lung cancer
3. Metastases
4. Sarcoidosis
5. Lymphoma

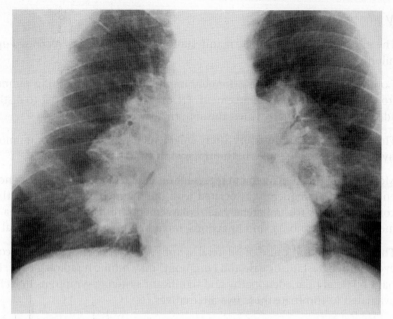

Fig. 11.12   Hematologic malignancies, including lymphoma and leukemia, are common causes of middle mediastinal masses. This patient, who has a late stage of chronic lymphocytic leukemia, has extensive hilar adenopathy.

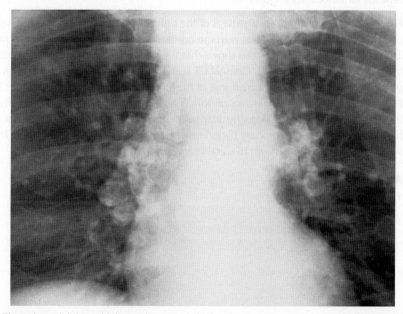

Fig. 11.13   The enlarged, bilateral hilar nodes are calcified with a unique pattern of calcification. This rim-like, peripheral calcification has been described as eggshell calcification and is seen in patients with sarcoidosis, coal worker's pneumoconiosis, and silicosis. This patient has silicosis.

Summary

The most common radiologic manifestation of a hilar mass is increased opacity of the hilum.

Contour abnormalities are extremely important in distinguishing pulmonary artery from hilar lymph node enlargement. CT or MRI may be essential to distinguish hilar adenopathy, particularly when the abnormality is minimal.

The differential for pulmonary artery enlargement is the same as for pulmonary arterial hypertension and includes both primary lung and cardiac diseases.

Most cases of hilar enlargement represent unilateral or bilateral hilar adenopathy. Hilar enlargement is frequently associated with middle mediastinal adenopathy. The most common causes for unilateral hilar enlargement are primary carcinoma of the lung, metastases, lymphoma, and infections, including tuberculosis and fungal infection.

The most common cause of bilateral symmetric hilar adenopathy is sarcoidosis; however, both metastatic disease and lymphoma may mimic it radiologically. Patients who have bilateral hilar adenopathy and significant systemic symptoms must be rigorously evaluated to eliminate these two alternatives.

ANSWER GUIDE

Legends for introductory figures

Fig. 11.1 **A,** Unilateral enlargement of the right hilum is typical of hilar adenopathy. Note that the rounded opacity blends with the borders of the pulmonary artery. Left pulmonary artery is normal. **B,** Axial CT scan shows that the mass is between two inferior branches of the right pulmonary artery. **C,** Coronal CT scan shows the smooth mass to be lateral to the pulmonary artery. Small cell carcinoma of the lung has metastasized to the right hilar nodes.
Fig. 11.2 Lobulated appearance of both hila with normal peripheral vascularity is characteristic of bilateral hilar adenopathy. Normal peripheral vascularity is an important radiologic finding that excludes pulmonary hypertension as a cause of hilar enlargement. This is a classic example of sarcoidosis with bilateral hilar adenopathy.

ANSWERS

1. b   2. c

12 | POSTERIOR MEDIASTINAL MASS

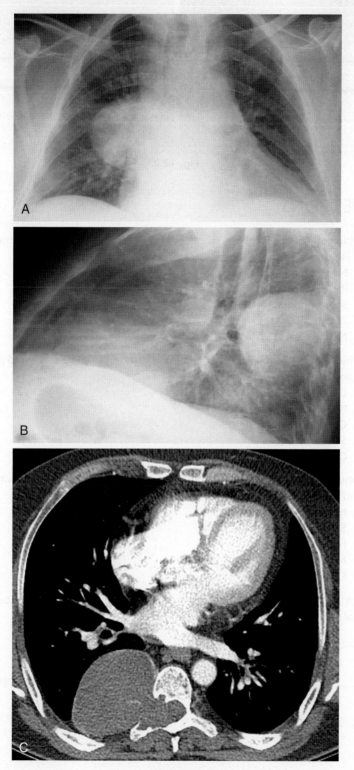

Fig. 12.1

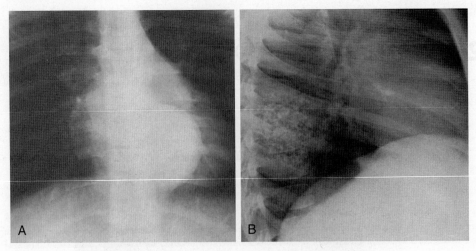

Fig. 12.2

QUESTIONS

1. Which one of the following diagnoses is most likely for the case illustrated in Fig. 12.1, *A-C*?
   a. Neuroblastoma.
   b. Paraspinal abscess.
   c. Schwannoma.
   d. Paraganglioma.
   e. Neurenteric cyst.

2. Which one of the following neural tumors is most likely in a 6-year-old patient (Fig. 12.2, *A* and *B*)?
   a. Ganglioneuroma.
   b. Neurofibroma.
   c. Ganglioneuroblastoma.
   d. Schwannoma.
   e. Chemodectoma.

3. Which one of the following is most likely a vertical elongated mass with rib spreading and erosion of multiple ribs?
   a. Neurofibroma.
   b. Schwannoma.
   c. Hemangioma.
   d. Neuroblastoma.
   e. Chemodectoma.

Match the following descriptions with the list of diagnoses that might cause a posterior mediastinal mass:

4. _____ Congenital hereditary spherocytosis   a. Neurenteric cyst

5. _____ Alcoholism with elevated amylase level   b. Extramedullary hematopoiesis

6. _____ Hemivertebra   c. Pancreatic pseudocyst

Chart 12.1	**POSTERIOR MEDIASTINAL MASSES**

I. Neoplasms
  A. Neural tumors459
    1. Ganglion series tumors (e.g., neuroblastoma, ganglioneuroblastoma, ganglioneuroma)
    2. Nerve root tumors (e.g., schwannoma, neurofibroma, malignant nerve sheath tumor)
    3. Paragangliomas (e.g., chemodectoma, pheochromocytoma)
  B. Metastases
  C. Lymphoma
  D. Mesenchymal tumors (e.g., fibroma, lipoma, muscle tumors, leiomyoma)
  E. Hemangiomas
  F. Thyroid tumors
  G. Vertebral tumors (e.g., osteoblastoma, giant cell tumor, multiple myeloma)
  H. Solitarily fibrous tumor of the pleura[116]
II. Germ cell tumors, including seminoma (rare in the posterior mediastinum)[453]
III. Inflammation
  A. Paraspinal abscess (e.g., tuberculosis, staphylococcus)
  B. Mediastinitis[147,165]
  C. Lymphoid hyperplasia
  D. Sarcoidosis
IV. Vascular lesions
  A. Aneurysm or dissection of the descending aorta[265,267,467]
V. Trauma
  A. Traumatic pseudoaneurysm
  B. Hematoma[115,165]
  C. Loculated hemothorax
  D. Traumatic pseudomeningocele
VI. Developmental lesions
  A. Enteric cysts[463]
  B. Neurenteric cysts[463]
  C. Bronchogenic cysts[463]
  D. Extralobar sequestration
VII. Abdominal diseases
  A. Bochdalek hernia (thoracic kidney)[351]
  B. Pancreatic pseudocyst or abscess[302]
  C. Retroperitoneal masses (e.g., germ cell tumors, sarcomas, metastases)
VIII. Other
  A. Loculated pleural effusion (e.g., empyema)
  B. Lateral meningocele
  C. Lipoma and lipomatosis[251]
  D. Extramedullary hematopoiesis[282]

Discussion

This discussion follows the divisions of the mediastinum described by Felson.[150] The middle and posterior compartments of the mediastinum are divided by a line that follows the curvature of the spine and is located 1 cm posterior to the anterior border of the vertebral bodies. Therefore, most of the masses that are considered herein might be classified by other authors as posterior gutter masses. Very large masses often extend into the anatomic posterior mediastinum. It may be difficult to determine the origin of a very large mass and therefore to appreciate that it did arise in the posterior gutter.

NEURAL TUMORS

The neural tumors constitute the largest group of posterior mediastinal and posterior gutter masses (Chart 12.1)[61] and are derived from nerve roots, intercostal nerves, or sympathetic ganglia. Nerve root tumors are schwannomas or neurofibromas. The sympathetic ganglion tumors include the neuroblastomas, ganglioneuroblastomas, and ganglioneuromas. Paragangliomas, including chemodectoma and pheochromocytoma, are infrequent causes of posterior mediastinal masses.[459]

Schwannomas are derived from the sheath of Schwann, which forms the connective tissues of the nerve root. There are no nerve cells in a schwannoma. This is in contrast to the true neurofibroma, which contains both Schwann cells and nerve cells. Before 1955, distinction between these two tumors was not generally made. This suggested that neurofibromas are the most common cause of posterior mediastinal masses. The schwannomas are much more common than true neurofibromas and are the most common of all the neural tumors. Most schwannomas and neurofibromas are benign tumors. The very rare malignant nerve root tumors were previously classified as a malignant schwannoma, regardless of the presence of nerve cells in the tumor, but have been reclassified as malignant nerve sheath tumors.

Neuroblastomas are highly malignant, undifferentiated, small round cell tumors that originate from the sympathetic ganglia. In contrast, the ganglioneuromas, which are also derived from the sympathetic ganglia, are completely benign.[123] Mature connective tissues, which resemble the connective tissues of schwannomas, are the primary tissues in ganglioneuromas. The presence of mature ganglion cells is the histologic feature that distinguishes schwannomas from ganglioneuromas. Ganglioneuroblastomas are mixed cell tumors that not only contain mature, well-differentiated ganglion cells, but also connective tissues and undifferentiated round cells. In other words, ganglioneuroblastomas have features of both ganglioneuromas, which are completely benign, and neuroblastomas, which are highly malignant. These tumors have a better prognosis than the neuroblastomas, but must be regarded as malignant tumors. It is true, however, that cases of spontaneous maturation have been observed. Cushing and Wolbach[105] have described a case that matured from a neuroblastoma to a completely differentiated ganglioneuroma; unfortunately, this is a very rare event.

The radiologic presentation of most neural tumors is a homogeneous opaque mass in the posterior mediastinum. A small percentage of these tumors contain calcification.[127,459] Calcification should be evenly distributed through a mass when the lesion is viewed in both the posteroanterior (PA) and lateral projections. The calcification often assumes a speckled pattern and may vary considerably in quantity (Fig. 12.2, *A* and *B*).

There is a striking difference between the shape of nerve root tumors and tumors of the ganglion series.[61,459,586] Of nerve root tumors, 80% appear as round masses (see Fig. 12.1, *A-C*), whereas 80% of ganglion series tumors appear as vertically oriented, elongated masses (Fig. 12.3). An additional feature that is helpful in distinguishing these masses is a tapered border, which suggests a ganglion series tumor. In contrast, round nerve root tumors tend to have a sulcus, which may indicate a more lateral position. This may suggest that the tumor is arising from the intercostal nerve. In Chapter 2, schwannoma was mentioned as a possible cause of a chest wall mass. (Answer to question 1 is *c*.)

A variety of bone abnormalities may be observed with the neural tumors, including rib spreading, erosion, and destruction. Neural foramina enlargement indicates extension of the mass into the neural canal (see Fig. 12.1, *A-C*). These tumors have been described as dumbbell lesions.[138] Patients with neural foramina enlargement typically have neurologic deficits caused by compression of the spinal cord.[8] This complication usually results from benign nerve root tumors, but it may also occur when a large neuroblastoma extends posteriorly.[34] Slow-growing benign tumors tend to erode bone, whereas malignant tumors invade and destroy bone. Erosion caused by a benign tumor may lead to a scalloped sclerotic defect in the posterior aspect of the vertebral body. Scoliosis is seen with very large masses, both benign and malignant, but rib spreading with erosion should suggest a malignant tumor (Fig. 12.4).

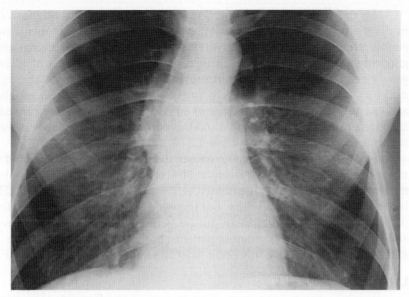

Fig. 12.3   Elongated, tapered, homogeneous, posterior mediastinal mass has the typical appearance for a ganglion series tumor. Ganglioneuromas are the benign member of this group of tumors and are most likely to occur in adults.   (From Reed JC, Hallet KK, Feagin DS. Neural tumors of the thorax: subject review from the AFIP. *Radiology.* 1978;126:9-17. Used by permission.)

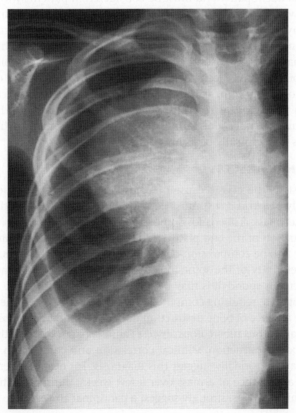

Fig. 12.4   Large ganglioneuroblastoma has eroded and spread multiple ribs. Pleural effusion is an additional sign suggesting malignancy.   (From Reed JC, Hallet KK, Feagin DS. Neural tumors of the thorax: subject review from the AFIP. *Radiology.* 1978;126:9-17. Used by permission.)

Age is the most important clinical feature in the differential diagnosis of posterior mediastinal masses. In patients younger than 1 year, a posterior mediastinal mass is almost certainly a neuroblastoma. After 10 years of age, neuroblastomas are rare. Ganglioneuroblastomas typically occur in children between the ages of 1 and 10 years; ganglioneuromas typically occur in those in the 6- to 15-year-old age group. All the ganglion series tumors are relatively infrequent in adults, although ganglioneuromas are observed in people up to the age of 50 years. In contrast, schwannomas and neurofibromas are infrequent in childhood, occurring most frequently in the third and fourth decades.[459] (Answer to question 2 is *c*.)

Neurofibromatosis (von Recklinghausen disease) may also be associated with posterior mediastinal masses.[383] As many as 30% of patients with true neurofibromas may have neurofibromatosis. As mentioned earlier, the overall incidence of malignancy in the nerve root tumors is very low, but there is a trend to malignant transformation in patients with von Recklinghausen disease. Schwannomas and ganglioneuromas have also been reported in this group of patients, but the association is less frequent. Ganglioneuromas more commonly occur as isolated, posterior mediastinal masses.

LYMPHADENOPATHY

Lymphadenopathy should not be overlooked as a cause of a posterior mediastinal mass. Lung cancer may metastasize to the posterior lymph nodes and should be considered in the presence of other signs of a primary tumor, such as atelectasis or hilar or paratracheal masses. The mass may be quite large and involve both the middle and posterior compartments. Lymphoma is an uncommon but important cause of posterior mediastinal adenopathy and must be considered in patients with systemic symptoms, including weight loss and low-grade fever. The additional finding of associated hilar adenopathy in these patients could be strongly suggestive of lymphoma. Conversely, the combination of a paraspinal mass and bilateral, symmetric hilar adenopathy in an asymptomatic patient raises the possibility of sarcoidosis. Paraspinal masses in patients with sarcoidosis have been reported, but are rare. Often, the differentiation of sarcoidosis from lymphoma can be made by considering the clinical presentation of the patient. In the patient with lymphoma, it is unlikely for her or him to have extensive hilar and mediastinal adenopathy and remain asymptomatic, whereas the patient with sarcoidosis may typically be asymptomatic.

PARASPINAL ABSCESS

Tuberculosis is the classic cause of paraspinal abscess, but other bacterial infections (particularly *Staphylococcus*) must be considered in the differential diagnosis of a posterior gutter mass. Tuberculosis and staphylococcal infections may cause spondylitis with destruction of the end plates of the vertebral bodies and intervertebral disk space. There may also be compression deformity of the vertebral bodies, which is described as the Pott deformity of the spine in cases of tuberculosis. The bone changes of bacterial and tuberculous spondylitis may be minimal and sometimes are not detectable on the chest radiograph, requiring computed tomography (CT) or magnetic resonance imaging (MRI). The absence of bone destruction does not eliminate the possibility of spondylitis. The subligamentous tuberculous abscess causes a paraspinal soft tissue mass without the expected bone destruction. Clinical correlation and comparison with previous examinations may occasionally suggest this diagnosis. For example, serial examinations that reveal the appearance of a mass over a few weeks, during which time the patient has fever and night sweats, strongly suggest a paraspinal abscess (Fig. 12.5, *A-C*).

PARASPINAL HEMATOMA

Fractures of the thoracic, lower cervical, and upper lumbar spine may be associated with bleeding and the development of paraspinal hematoma (Fig. 12.6, *A* and *B*).

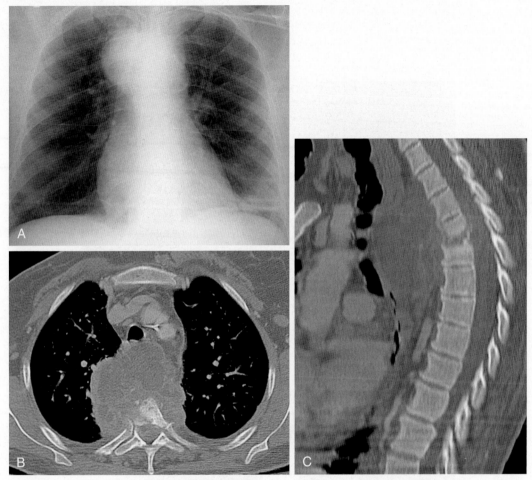

Fig. 12.5   A, Circumscribed, right superior mediastinal mass has tapered inferior borders. **B,** Axial CT scan confirms a large posterior mass with destruction of a vertebral body. **C,** Sagittal CT reconstruction reveals that the mass has destroyed a thoracic disk space and involves two vertebral bodies. This makes a neoplastic process unlikely and makes paraspinal abscess with osteomyelitis and discitis the most likely diagnosis. This may be seen with tuberculosis, but in this case, it was the result of staphylococcus.

Occasionally, even posterior rib fractures may also cause posterior mediastinal hematomas. Because these fractures indicate serious injury, it is important to exclude major vascular injuries as the cause of the mediastinal hematoma. CT angiography is often required to exclude coexisting aortic injury.

DUPLICATION CYSTS

Duplication cysts[463] are rare and typically occur in the mediastinum. The classic location for the bronchogenic cyst is the middle compartment, whereas enteric and neurenteric cysts are more typically found in the posterior compartment. Enteric and neurenteric cysts are histologically indistinguishable. These cysts are lined by a gastric epithelium that secretes gastric juices, and because of this epithelium, the masses tend to be large and symptomatic.

In contrast to bronchogenic cysts, which usually occur as an asymptomatic mass in young adults, enteric and neurenteric cysts typically appear in children. A neurenteric cyst is distinguishable from an enteric cyst because it is accompanied by vertebral body abnormalities, including hemivertebrae and butterfly vertebrae. On occasion, the mass may actually have to be dissected from the vertebral body. It is important to realize

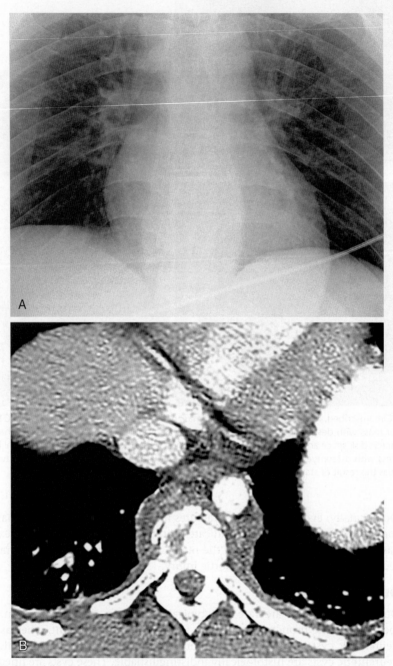

Fig. 12.6 **A,** Bulging, bilateral, retrocardiac paraspinal lines are a clue to the diagnosis of paraspinal hematoma in a patient with a history of a motor vehicle accident. **B,** Axial CT scan confirms a comminuted vertebral body fracture with associated hematoma.

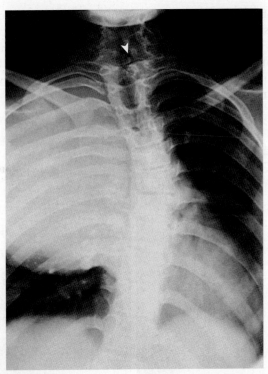

Fig. 12.7 This very large mass has associated skeletal abnormalities that provide the clue to diagnosis. Scoliosis may be associated with a variety of very large posterior mediastinal masses and is therefore not diagnostic. The diagnostic finding is the hemivertebra *(arrowhead)* in the cervical spine. This is a neurenteric cyst. (From Reed JC, Sobonya RE. Morphologic analysis of foregut cysts in the thorax. *AJR Am J Roentgenol.* 1974;120:851-860. Used by permission.)

that the vertebral body abnormality may occur cephalad to the mass (Fig. 12.7). Calcification may occur in the wall of these cystic structures and is useful in distinguishing a cyst from neural tumors such as neuroblastoma or ganglioneuroblastoma.

ANEURYSM

An aneurysm is another important cause of a posterior mediastinal mass. Oblique views may be helpful in evaluating posterior mediastinal masses because the mass can sometimes be clearly distinguished from the shadow of the descending aorta, thus excluding the possibility of an aneurysm. When the mass is indistinguishable from the aorta, the possibility of an aneurysm must be considered, particularly in older adults. Curvilinear calcification similar to that seen in the wall of the cyst may also occur in the wall of an aortic aneurysm. Therefore a posterior mediastinal mass with curvilinear calcification in a 20-year-old patient most likely represents an enteric cyst, whereas the same radiologic presentation in a 70-year-old patient most likely represents an aneurysm. The diagnosis should be confirmed by angiography, CT scanning with contrast enhancement (Fig. 12.8, *A-C*), or MRI.

ABDOMINAL DISEASES

A Bochdalek hernia must be considered as the cause of a posterior mediastinal mass when the mass is continuous with the contour of the diaphragm. The structures that commonly herniate through the diaphragm are retroperitoneal fat and kidney.[336]

A pancreatic pseudocyst[302] is an infrequent cause of a middle or posterior mediastinal mass. It is likely to have associated pleural effusion. A pancreatic pseudocyst should be suspected when a mass develops over a short period of time in a patient with the clinical diagnosis of pancreatitis. A history of alcoholism with recurrent pancreatitis and laboratory test results demonstrating elevated amylase levels strongly support the diagnosis. (Answer to question 5 is *c*.)

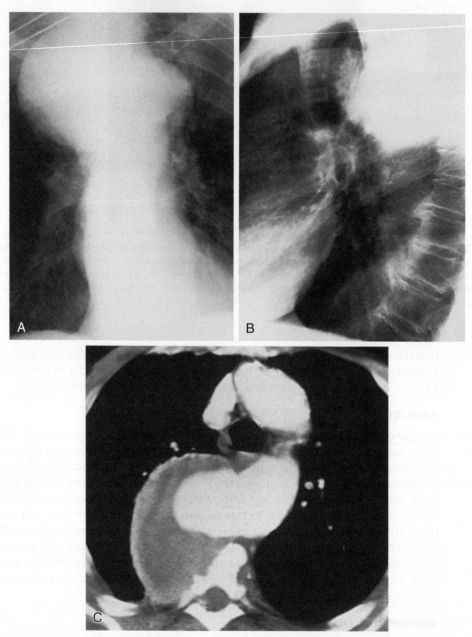

Fig. 12.8   A, Large, superior mediastinal opacity projects to the right and requires consideration of an aneurysm versus a mass. This is above the ascending aorta, which is the most likely origin for a right-sided aneurysm, but it is adjacent to an enlarged aortic arch. **B,** Lateral view shows the opacity to be posterior and to project over the posterior portion of the aortic arch. **C,** Contrast-enhanced CT scan confirms a large aneurysm with thrombus and erosion of the vertebral body.

Teratomas and seminomas that present as primary mediastinal tumors produce anterior mediastinal masses and are not expected in the posterior mediastinum. However, these germinal tumors also present as primary testicular neoplasms that may metastasize to the retroperitoneal nodes. Extension of a retroperitoneal mass into the chest produces the radiologic appearance of a posterior paraspinal mass (Fig. 12.9, *A-D*).

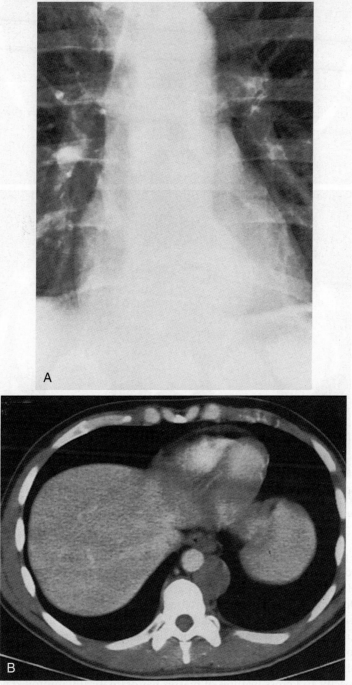

Fig. 12.9   A, Metastatic testicular carcinoma caused this smooth, well-circumscribed retrocardiac mass with a tapered superior border. This appearance is similar to that of a ganglioneuroma. **B,** CT scan at the level of the mass confirmed a homogeneous paraspinal mass that extended anteriorly around the aorta.

Continued

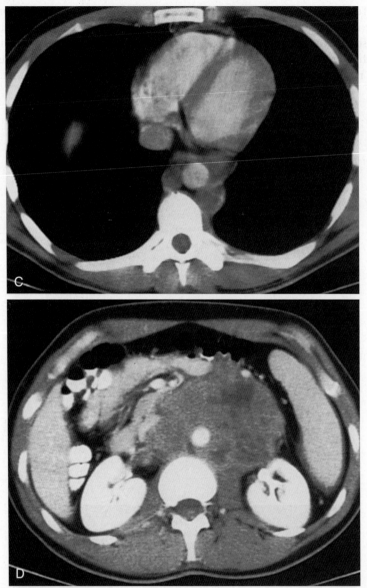

Fig. 12.9, cont'd   C, Additional CT sections taken above the level of the paraspinal mass revealed involvement of additional paraaortic nodes. The aorta is surrounded by enlarged nodes. **D,** Abdominal CT scan revealed a much larger mass of nodes surrounding the aorta. A testicular ultrasound examination detected the primary tumor.

A lateral meningocele is another rare cause of a mediastinal mass and, like nerve root tumors, may have the additional radiologic feature of enlarged neural foramina. The diagnosis should be considered in patients with neurofibromatosis; it is confirmed by MRI (Fig. 12.10, *A* and *B*).

Occasionally, chest wall, vertebral, and pleural tumors may present with the appearance of a posterior mediastinal mass (Fig. 12.11, *A* and *B*). Other rare tumors, including mesenchymal tumors and hemangiomas, which cannot be diagnosed by radiologic criteria, may be encountered. The diagnosis of these tumors is made only by histologic examination of the mass; however, the ability to detect subtle variations in opacity and gross features of masses has dramatically improved with the use of CT scanning. For example, fatty tumors such as lipoma and hibernoma, which could not be diagnosed by chest radiographic criteria, may now be recognized by detecting the low opacity of fat with a CT scan. Steroid-induced mediastinal lipomatosis may be

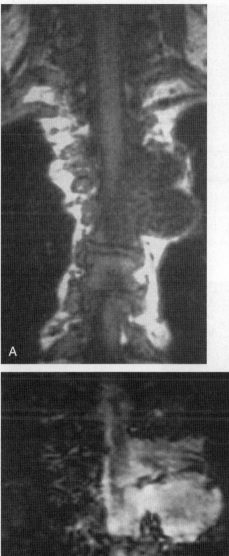

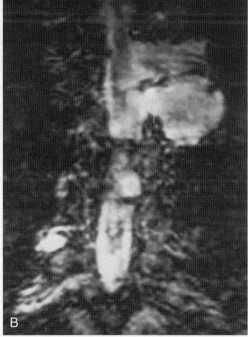

Fig. 12.10   A, T1-weighted coronal MRI scan of a patient with known neurofibromatosis reveals a low-signal abnormality surrounded by high-signal mediastinal fat. **B,** T2-weighted coronal MRI shows a high signal pattern, indicating that the abnormality is fluid-filled, and confirms the diagnosis of meningocele.   (From Reed JC. Schwannoma. In: Siegel BA, Proto AV, eds: *Chest disease (fifth series) test and syllabus.* Reston, VA, 1996, American College of Radiology; pp. 213-236. Used by permission.)

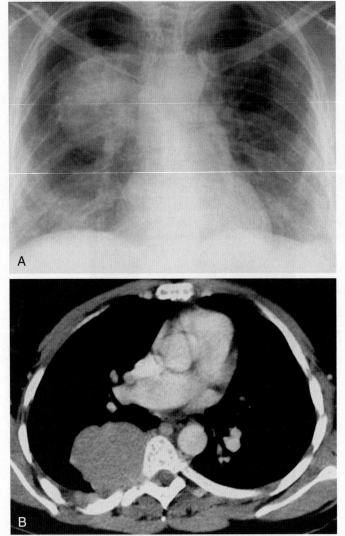

Fig. 12.11   A, Multiple myeloma is the cause of this large medial mass that resembles a posterior mediastinal mass. There are also multiple lytic rib lesions that suggest metastases or multiple myeloma. **B,** CT scan shows a homogeneous mass in a paraspinal location, which is still indistinguishable from a posterior mediastinal mass.

suspected when a patient on steroid therapy develops paraspinal masses (Fig. 12.12, A and B). Studies by Streiter et al.[566] have illustrated how this diagnosis may be confirmed by CT.

Extramedullary hematopoiesis[282] (Fig. 12.13, A-C) is an infrequent cause of a posterior mediastinal mass but should be considered in patients with a hereditary anemia. In fact, it may cause multiple or lobulated masses. Other associated abnormalities may include distinctive bone changes, such as enlargement of the ribs from long-standing increased activity of the marrow. Associated splenomegaly may provide another radiologic clue to the diagnosis. (Answer to question 4 is *b*.)

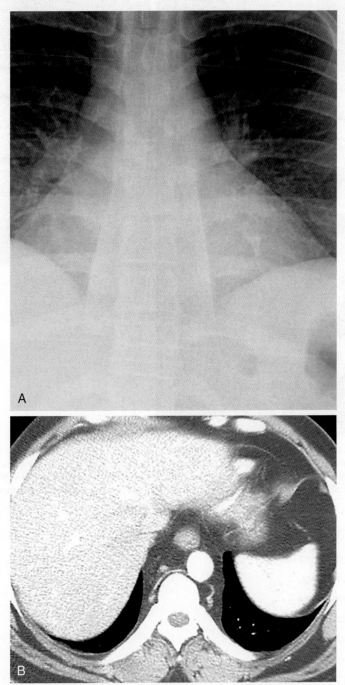

Fig. 12.12   A, Retrocardiac lateral displacement of paraspinal lines could result from a mass, abscess, or hematoma. Mediastinal fat may also cause this appearance. **B,** CT scan confirms the presence of an excessive accumulation of paraspinal fat. This may result from obesity but may be iatrogenic following steroid therapy.

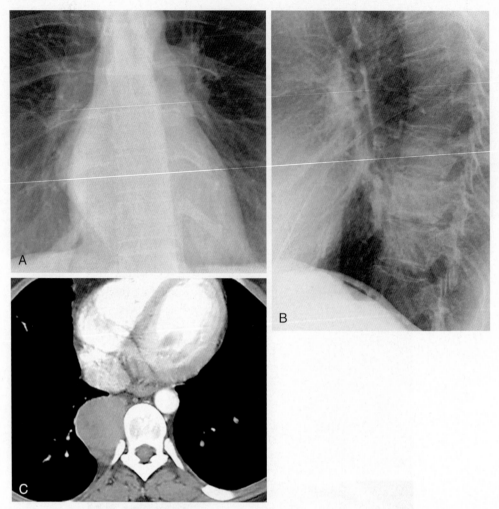

Fig. 12.13 **A,** This circumscribed tapered opacity projecting over the right hilum is similar to a neural tumor. **B,** The increased opacity over the lower thoracic spine is poorly defined because of the shape of the mass. **C,** CT scan confirms the presence of a posterior mediastinal mass with a tapered appearance that is most suggestive of a neural tumor. This patient had a history of chronic severe anemia; the mass was caused by extramedullary hematopoiesis.

Top 5 Diagnoses: Posterior Mediastinal Mass

1. Neural tumors
2. Metastases
3. Hematoma
4. Aneurysm
5. Paraspinal abscess

Summary

The most common cause of a posterior mediastinal mass is a neural tumor.

Nerve root tumors, schwannoma, and neurofibroma usually occur in adults and are benign.

Neuroblastoma and ganglioneuroblastoma are malignant ganglion series tumors that usually occur in children.

Calcification throughout a mass is most suggestive of a ganglion series tumor. It cannot be used to distinguish benign from malignant tumors.

A thin rim of calcification around the periphery of an apparent mass suggests an aneurysm or a cyst.

Rib erosion of a single rib with sclerosis of the rib border, as described in Chapter 2, is compatible with a benign tumor, but the spreading of multiple ribs with erosion or destruction suggests a malignant ganglion series tumor.

The vertebral anomalies of hemivertebrae or butterfly vertebrae, with a posterior mediastinal mass on the chest radiograph, are diagnostic of a neurenteric cyst.

A paraspinal abscess with intervertebral disk destruction is classic for tuberculosis, but staphylococcal organisms are now the most likely infectious cause. The bone abnormality may be minimal to absent.

The gross morphologic features of a posterior mediastinal mass may appear to be nonspecific, but when careful analysis of these features is combined with the clinical presentation of the patient, a precise diagnosis may be made in most cases. Differences in opacity that result from subtle gross differences may be detected with CT scans and should further improve the diagnostic ability of the radiologist.

ANSWER GUIDE

Legends for introductory figures

Fig. 12.1   A, A homogeneous round mass projects over the right hilum but does not obscure the hilar vessels or right heart border. **B,** The lateral view confirms a posterior location. **C,** CT scan confirms a large posterior mass with erosion of the contiguous vertebra and extension through the neural foramen. This is the expected presentation of a nerve root tumor. This tumor was histologically confirmed to be a schwannoma.
Fig. 12.2   A, Distribution of calcium through the mass indicates a solid mass. This is a ganglioneuroblastoma. **B,** Lateral view from case illustrated in **A** confirms the distribution of calcium throughout a solid mass. (From Reed JC, Hallet KK, Feagin DS. Neural tumors of the thorax: subject review from the AFIP. *Radiology.* 1978;126:9-17. Used by permission.)

ANSWERS

1. c   2. c   3. d   4. b   5. c   6. a

PART 2

Pulmonary Opacities

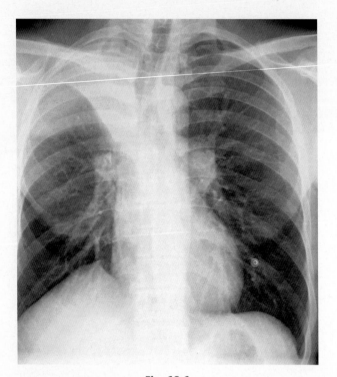

Fig. 13.1

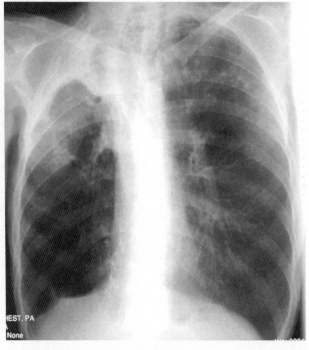

Fig. 13.2

QUESTIONS

1. Which of the following abnormalities are present on the posteroanterior (PA) chest radiograph in Fig. 13.1?
   a. Right upper lobe opacification.
   b. Juxtaphrenic peak.
   c. Displacement of the horizontal fissure.
   d. Deviation of the trachea.
   e. All of the above.

2. Which one of the following is most likely to cause atelectasis?
   a. Metastasis.
   b. Adenocarcinoma.
   c. Lymphoma.
   d. Squamous cell carcinoma.
   e. Sarcoidosis.

3. The case illustrated in Fig. 13.2 is an example of which of the following types of atelectasis?
   a. Compressive.
   b. Obstructive.
   c. Cicatrizing.
   d. Relaxation.
   e. Adhesive.

Match the following types of atelectasis with the disease entities listed in the right column:

4. ____ Obstructive   a. Carcinoid

5. ____ Compressive   b. Surfactant deficiency

6. ____ Passive   c. Bullous emphysema

7. ____ Adhesive   d. Tuberculosis

8. ____ Cicatrizing   e. Pneumothorax

Chart 13.1	ATELECTASIS

I. Resorption atelectasis—large airway obstruction[656,657]
   A. Tumor
      1. Lung cancer (squamous cell)[234]
      2. Carcinoid[39,275]
      3. Metastasis[40,113]
      4. Lymphoma[120,507]
      5. Less frequent (e.g., lipoma, leiomyoma,[301] granular cell myoblastoma)[514,584]
   B. Inflammatory
      1. Tuberculosis (e.g., endobronchial granuloma, bronchial stenosis, broncholith[221,527])
      2. Sarcoidosis, endobronchial granuloma (rare)[240]
   C. Other
      1. Large left atrium
      2. Foreign body (including malpositioned endotracheal tube)
      3. Amyloidosis[246]
      4. Granulomatosis with polyangiitis (formerly Wegener granulomatosis)
      5. Bronchial transection[603]
II. Resorption atelectasis—small airway obstruction[656,657]
   A. Mucous plugs[192]
      1. Severe chest or abdominal pain (particularly in the postoperative patient)
      2. Respiratory depressant drugs (e.g., morphine)
      3. Asthma
      4. Cystic fibrosis
   B. Inflammatory[488]
      1. Bronchopneumonia
      2. Bronchitis
III. Compressive atelectasis[175]
   A. Large pulmonary masses
   B. Air trapping in adjacent lung (e.g., bullous emphysema, lobar emphysema, interstitial emphysema, bronchial obstruction by foreign body)[175]
IV. Passive atelectasis—pleural space–occupying processes[175]
   A. Pneumothorax
   B. Hydrothorax, hemothorax
   C. Diaphragmatic hernia
   D. Pleural masses (e.g., metastases, mesothelioma)
V. Adhesive atelectasis[175]
   A. Surfactant deficiency disease of the newborn (respiratory distress syndrome or, formerly, hyaline membrane disease)
   B. Pulmonary embolism[396]
   C. Intravenous injection of hydrocarbon
VI. Cicatrization atelectasis[175]
   A. Tuberculosis[298]
   B. Histoplasmosis
   C. Coal workers' pneumoconiosis
   D. Silicosis
   E. Scleroderma
   F. Usual interstitial pneumonia (includes scleroderma, rheumatoid and idiopathic pulmonary fibrosis)
   G. Radiation pneumonitis (late phase)[425]

Discussion

Atelectasis is loss of lung volume[221] that may involve all or parts of the lung. Chest radiographic findings of atelectasis include the following: (1) increased opacity; (2) crowding and reorientation of pulmonary vessels[445]; (3) displacement of fissures[253]; (4) elevation of the diaphragm; (5) displacement of the hilum; (6) crowding of ribs; (7) compensatory overinflation of the normal lung; (8) shift of the mediastinum; (9) cardiac rotation[287]; (10) bronchial rearrangement[627]; and (11) juxtaphrenic peak (Fig. 13.3).[112] On occasion, the change in position of an abnormal structure, such as a calcified granuloma, may also provide additional clues to the diagnosis.[481] As with other pulmonary problems, the radiologic signs of atelectasis are variable, ranging from nonspecific signs such as increased opacity to specific signs such as displacement of the fissures and a shift of the mediastinum.[287] Perhaps the most specific sign is displacement of the fissures, indicating a loss of volume in a specific lobe.[656,657]

Right upper lobe atelectasis (see Fig. 13.1) is usually recognized by observation of findings that include right upper lobe opacity with elevation of the horizontal fissure. The horizontal fissure may even appear to be bowed or rotated upward and medially. The mediastinum may shift toward the opacity with deviation of the trachea. Elevation of the right hemidiaphragm and a juxtaphrenic peak are frequently observed additional findings of right upper lobe atelectasis. The juxtaphrenic peak is a triangular opacity extending upward from the diaphragm. It may be caused by traction on either an inferior accessory fissure or the inferior pulmonary ligament[221] (answer to question 1 is *e*). The lateral view shows upper anterior opacity with upward shift of the horizontal fissure, anterior shift of the oblique fissure, and compensatory overinflation of the middle and lower lobes.

Right middle lobe atelectasis causes a combination of increased opacity that silhouettes the right heart border[349] with inferior displacement of the horizontal fissure. The lateral view often shows anterior shift of the lower portion of the oblique fissure

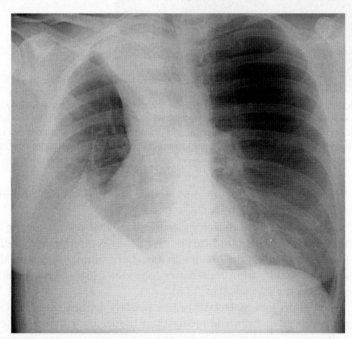

Fig. 13.3 Opacification of the right upper thorax is associated with elevation of the minor fissure and right hemidiaphragm with a juxtaphrenic peak. The juxtaphrenic peak is a triangular opacity at the dome of the hemidiaphragm that indicates upper lobe volume loss. This is a common finding with right upper lobe atelectasis.

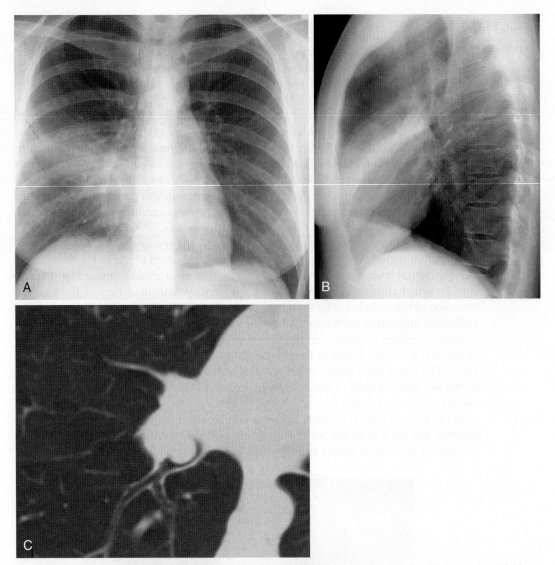

Fig. 13.4   A, Right middle lobe atelectasis causes a lower thoracic opacity that usually silhouettes the right heart border. This sign may be absent in cases that are limited to the lateral segment. **B,** The lateral view shows a narrow strip of anterior opacity defined by the horizontal and oblique fissures. The displacement of the fissures confirms the right middle lobe loss of volume. **C,** Computed tomography scan reveals an endobronchial mass, and a transbronchial biopsy made the diagnosis of carcinoid.

(Fig. 13.4, *A* and *B*). Right middle lobe atelectasis is most often caused by bronchial obstruction (see Fig. 13.4, *C*).

Right lower lobe atelectasis causes increased opacity in the lower thorax without silhouetting of the right heart border. There is inferior and medial shift of the oblique fissure. Remember, the oblique fissure is not normally seen on the PA view,[230] but the shift that results from right lower lobe atelectasis often causes the fissure to become visible on the PA view (Fig. 13.5).

Left upper lobe atelectasis causes a poorly defined left perihilar opacity that appears to be separated from the mediastinal border by a hyperlucency or air crescent (the Luftsichel sign) that highlights the aortic arch.[45] Compensatory overaeration of the superior segment of the left lower lobe accounts for the hyperlucency that is interposed between the mediastinum and opaque upper lobe (Fig. 13.6, *A-C*). Left upper lobe atelectasis assumes a very characteristic appearance on the lateral view with an

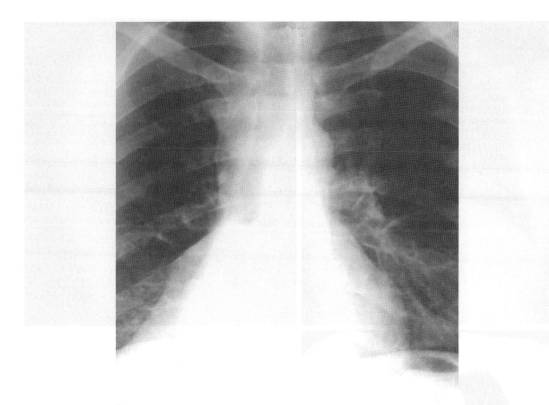

Fig. 13.5 Right lower lobe atelectasis causes inferior displacement of the major fissure so that it becomes visible on the posteroanterior chest radiograph. The sharp lateral border of this opaque atelectatic lower lobe is produced by the major fissure. Note that lower lobe atelectasis does not silhouette the heart border.

anterior opacity that is sharply defined posteriorly by the oblique fissure, which is displaced anteriorly (see Fig. 13.6, *B*). Because of compensatory overinflation of the right upper lobe, which may give the appearance of herniating across the midline, the opacity of left upper lobe atelectasis does not obliterate the retrosternal clear space.

Left lower lobe atelectasis causes a triangular opacity behind the heart (Fig. 13.7). The lateral border is sharp because of the inferior medial shift of the oblique fissure. This often produces the appearance of a line that parallels the heart border. The lateral view confirms a poorly defined opacity that projects over the lower vertebral bodies and silhouettes the left leaf of the diaphragm.

Complete opacification of a hemithorax with a shift of the mediastinum toward the opacity is classic for atelectasis (Fig. 13.8). In these cases, the shift of the mediastinum toward the opaque side confirms the atelectasis, but the opacification obscures the lung and any underlying abnormalities. The diagnostic signs of complete atelectasis of the right lung are not significantly different from those of complete atelectasis of the left lung. In contrast with atelectasis, the completely opaque hemithorax with shift of the mediastinum away from the opacity is most often due to a large pleural effusion.

Because the right lung has three lobes, combinations of atelectasis of two lobes may cause some unique radiologic appearances.[330] Right upper and right middle lobe atelectasis causes a large opacity involving the right upper thorax, obscuring the right upper lobe vessels and silhouetting the heart border, and the diaphragm is elevated with the appearance of a juxtaphrenic peak.[112] The lateral view holds the key to the correct diagnosis (Fig. 13.9, *A* and *B*). The entire oblique fissure is shifted anteriorly to resemble the left oblique fissure position in left upper lobe atelectasis. The horizontal

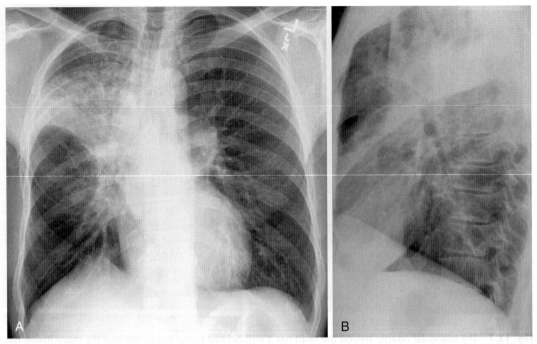

Fig. 13.9   A, The right upper lobe is opacified with elevation of a fissure, indicating atelectasis, with an additional finding of obscuration of the right hilum and upper right heart border. **B,** The lateral view reveals anterior displacement of the entire oblique fissure. The overinflated lung shown on the posteroanterior view is the right lower lobe. The lateral view confirms the diagnosis of right upper and middle lobe atelectasis.

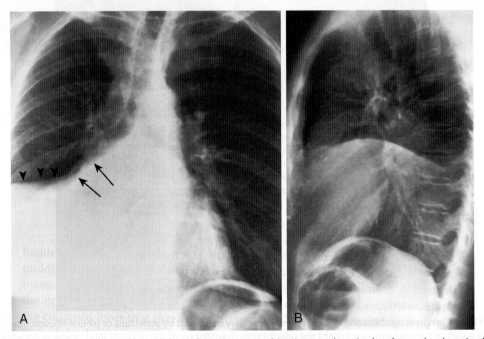

Fig. 13.10   A, Right middle and lower lobe atelectasis as a combination may be mistaken for a subpulmonic pleural effusion. Note the inferior-medial displacement of the major fissure *(arrows)* and the low position of the minor fissure *(arrowheads).* **B,** The depressed fissures produce a sharp interface with the overaerated upper lobe. This could also be confused with an elevated diaphragm.

Several types of atelectasis may be grouped according to their respective causes, as suggested by Fraser et al.[175]: (1) obstructive, (2) compressive, (3) passive, (4) adhesive, and (5) cicatrizing. Furthermore, since airway obstruction is produced by a wide variety of causes (Chart 13.1), this category may be subdivided into large and small airway obstructions, as proposed by Felson.[150] Airway obstruction is by far the most common cause of atelectasis; it can occur as the result of a foreign body, aspiration, endobronchial tumor, or inflammatory reactions such as tuberculosis. Compressive atelectasis is caused by intrapulmonary abnormalities (e.g., a large lung mass or large bulla) that compress the surrounding lung, whereas lung collapse with passive atelectasis develops because of changes in intrapleural pressure (e.g., pneumothorax). Adhesive atelectasis occurs when the luminal surfaces of the alveolar walls stick together. This occurs in surfactant deficiency disease of the newborn because of a deficiency of surfactant in the alveoli. Finally, cicatrizing atelectasis is the result of scarring by fibrosis, with the loss of volume being a secondary effect. Frequently, this is a late sequela of tuberculosis.

LARGE AIRWAY OBSTRUCTIVE LESIONS

Squamous cell carcinoma of the lung is one of the most important causes of large airway obstruction (answer to question 2 is *d*). Approximately two-thirds of squamous cell carcinomas of the lung occur in large airways as endobronchial masses. Although carcinoma of the lung is usually expected to present as a mass, the chest radiograph often shows signs of obstruction with either atelectasis or obstructive pneumonia. When endobronchial masses are small, they are frequently not detectable on the chest radiograph. The abnormalities that do appear while the tumor is small are frequently either segmental or lobar opacities. Adenocarcinoma of the lung most often presents as a peripheral nodule or mass and is not an expected cause of atelectasis.

An outpatient presenting with the unexpected finding of lobar atelectasis must be evaluated to exclude an endobronchial lung cancer. Patients with lung cancer frequently have histories that are complex and in some cases difficult to interpret. These histories often include persistent atelectasis, recurrent atelectasis, or recurrent pneumonia. For example, a patient may have a history of a low-grade fever when the chest radiograph shows segmental or lobar opacities. This might even appear to suggest the diagnosis of pneumonia. Subsequent treatment with antibiotics may even temporarily reduce the severity of the airway obstruction and also diminish the radiologic signs of atelectasis, thus supporting the original diagnosis. However, most cases of bronchial tumor do not show complete clearing of the radiologic abnormality with such therapy. These cases require follow-up examinations until the abnormality has completely cleared. Persistent abnormality on the chest radiograph is an indication for further evaluation with computed tomography (CT) or bronchoscopy.

The combination of a hilar mass and lobar atelectasis is strongly suggestive of a primary lung tumor (Fig. 13.11). When the primary tumor is relatively large and obstructs a main-stem bronchus, the chest radiograph may reveal a "bronchial cutoff," or a "rat tail bronchus."[150] Such tumors, however, are not commonly seen, perhaps because they may be small or hidden by the superimposition of shadows from other structures. Although primary carcinomas arising in the hilum are not rare, the hilar masses seen on the chest radiograph often represent metastases to the regional lymph nodes from an endobronchial tumor. The obstructing tumor is best diagnosed by CT and bronchoscopy with biopsy.[650]

Central primary carcinomas are frequently lobulated, particularly when multiple nodes are involved. When the nodal metastases are extensive, they may involve hilar and mediastinal nodes. If the patient has no evidence of extrathoracic metastases, chest CT should be used as a staging procedure. Because of the high incidence of liver and adrenal metastases, the examination should be extended into the abdomen.

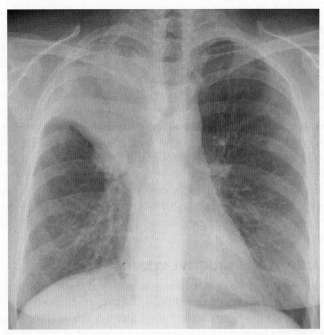

Fig. 13.11 Right upper lobe atelectasis with an associated hilar mass is a common presentation for primary lung cancer with bronchial obstruction.

The combination of atelectasis and bronchial obstruction most frequently indicates the presence of a primary lung cancer, but other lesions can also be responsible for this combination of findings. Bronchial carcinoid tumor is an infrequent tumor but is frequently found in large bronchi, rarely has calcification on the chest radiograph, and often presents with atelectasis (answer to question 4 is *a*).[79] Although metastatic tumors to the bronchi are not common,[36] they can develop from renal cell carcinoma, breast carcinoma, melanoma,[433] carcinoma of the colon,[40] and various sarcomas. Rare benign tumors, such as granular cell myoblastoma, amyloid tumor, lipoma, leiomyoma,[301] and even fibroepithelial inflammatory polyps, all require biopsy for diagnosis. Lymphoma[507] is another tumor that occasionally invades the bronchi with resultant atelectasis; however, this is usually a late stage of the disease and is almost always accompanied by hilar and mediastinal lymphadenopathy. This presentation of lymphoma frequently represents a recurrence of previously treated lymphoma and is not a diagnostic problem.

Infectious diseases are seldom the basis of bronchial obstruction, but historically, tuberculosis was an important cause of obstructive atelectasis. In fact, many cases of right middle lobe syndrome (chronic right middle lobe atelectasis) were caused by tuberculosis. Bronchial obstruction in tuberculosis most commonly results from peribronchial inflammation, endobronchial granulomas, compression by hilar nodes, and rarely, broncholiths,[221] which are calcified lymph nodes that erode into the bronchus (Fig. 13.12).

Sarcoidosis is a common cause of hilar adenopathy (see Chapter 11), yet obstructive atelectasis is very rarely associated with sarcoidosis. In those rare cases of sarcoidosis that do develop atelectasis, the atelectasis is often due to endobronchial granulomas. All of the entities offered as answers to question 2 may cause atelectasis, but unfortunately, squamous cell carcinoma of the lung is the most common.

Left atrial enlargement from mitral stenosis is an occasional cause of left lower lobe atelectasis. The diagnosis is easily made when other findings of mitral stenosis are present, such as a large left atrium and the cephalization of vessels. The lateral radiograph

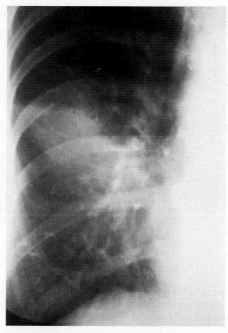

Fig. 13.12 Posteroanterior chest radiograph shows right middle lobe opacity and right hilar calcification. The right middle lobe atelectasis is the result of a broncholith, which is a calcified lymph node that has eroded into a bronchus and may be secondary to tuberculosis or histoplasmosis. The diagnosis may be confirmed by computed tomography or bronchoscopy.

frequently shows the left atrium to be pushing the compressed left main and left lower lobe bronchi posteriorly.

The diagnosis of foreign body obstruction of a bronchus is usually straightforward in adults because it is commonly associated with the aspiration of food, such as a large piece of meat. Endotracheal intubation is another possible cause of large airway obstruction. Malposition of the tube is usually the result of advancing the tube too far. The tube most often enters the right mainstem bronchus, causing obstruction of the left bronchus with atelectasis of the left lung. In contrast to the adult with a foreign body aspiration, a child is often unable to give a definite history and more commonly presents with overaeration of the lung distal to the obstruction rather than with atelectasis. This is presumably due to collateral air drift that permits air to get into the lung distal to the obstruction. Therefore, an endobronchial foreign body will most likely result in atelectasis in an adult patient, whereas it more frequently causes air trapping in the pediatric patient.

SMALL AIRWAY OBSTRUCTION

Mucous plugging is a common cause of both large and small airway obstruction. The bronchial tree branches for approximately seven generations. Bronchi have cartilage in their walls. The airways distal to the seventh generation and without cartilage are defined as *bronchioles.* Mucus production occurs mainly within the bronchial tree in nonsmokers. Bronchioles in nonsmokers have a ciliated lining and lack mucus-secreting glands, whereas the bronchioles of smokers lose their cilia and have increased numbers of mucus-secreting goblet cells. Although the discussion of large airway obstruction was limited to diseases that occur in the proximal main bronchi, mucous plugging may involve multiple small bronchi and bronchioles. Mucous plugs may form in the small bronchi of a patient with an otherwise normal tracheobronchial tree in various clinical settings such as during general anesthesia, after administration of respiratory-depressant drugs, or during central nervous system (CNS) illnesses that

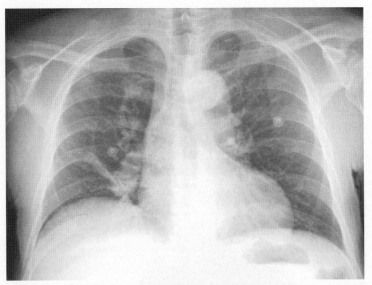

Fig. 13.13   The linear opacity extending from the right hilum into the right lung base is a common appearance for subsegmental atelectasis. Linear scars may resemble the appearance of subsegmental atelectasis, but serial examinations should document the transient nature of subsegmental atelectasis.

produce respiratory depression. Mucous plugging of multiple bronchi is a frequent challenge in the management of intensive care patients. Especially after abdominal or thoracic surgery, atelectasis is very common in the left lower lobe but may be more scattered with lobar, segmental, and subsegmental distributions. Subsegmental linear opacities (Fig. 13.13) most commonly measure from a few millimeters to a centimeter wide and up to several centimeters long. The exact basis for subsegmental atelectasis has been questioned; some authors believe that collateral air drift should prevent the development of subsegmental atelectasis. However, normal collateral air drift may not be present in patients with impaired bronchial clearance. Rather, when clearance is depressed to the point at which mucus obstructs the small bronchi and bronchioles, the even smaller passages between sections of lung, such as the canals of Lambert and pores of Kohn, are likely to become obstructed. The transient nature of these subsegmental opacities also further supports the concept that these linear opacities are the result of subsegmental atelectasis.[404]

Atelectasis is not one of the commonly expected presentations of bronchopneumonia, but infections can produce bronchial inflammation, which may then lead to small airway obstruction followed by atelectasis. This presentation has been occasionally referred to as *atelectatic pneumonia*. Clinical and laboratory correlations are extremely important in establishing this diagnosis over that of other causes of atelectasis. Patients with bronchopneumonia are usually febrile and have an elevated white blood cell counts. Bacteriologic confirmation of the diagnosis is obtained with positive sputum and blood cultures. Atelectasis may also complicate viral and mycoplasma pneumonias, presumably because of the associated bronchial and bronchiolar involvement.[404]

Atelectasis from the obstruction of bronchioles may develop during the course of certain chronic obstructive diseases such as chronic bronchitis, asthma, emphysema, and bronchiolitis obliterans. The atelectasis may develop because many small bronchi and bronchioles become obstructed as a result of chronic changes in the airway walls that lead to narrowing of the lumen, increased mucus formation, and reduced clearing of secretions. Although the radiologic findings in these diseases are frequently minimal, acute exacerbations may result in lobar, segmental, subsegmental, or a more diffuse peripheral pattern of atelectasis. The latter appearance sometimes resembles diffuse pneumonia and requires careful clinical correlation to make this distinction.

A changing appearance with rapid clearing of the opacities followed by recurrences should suggest the diagnosis of atelectasis, especially in the intensive care environment.

COMPRESSIVE ATELECTASIS

The radiologic appearance of compressive atelectasis is often distinctly different from that of obstructive atelectasis. Compressive atelectasis is a secondary effect of compression of normal lung by a primary, space-occupying abnormality. The primary abnormality is often a large peripheral lung tumor that collapses the adjacent lung.

Extensive air trapping can also compress the adjacent normal lung. This type of compression may occur in bullous emphysema, lobar emphysema, and often after an acute bronchial obstruction. The radiologic appearance of bullous emphysema is that of a large lucent area surrounded by a thin wall. These lucent areas are usually in the periphery of the lung. This presentation of bullous emphysema is so characteristic that it is not often a diagnostic problem (answer to question 5 is *c;* see Chapter 22).

In view of the preceding discussion, the finding of distal air trapping with acute bronchial obstruction may appear paradoxical and can be a diagnostic challenge. Presumably, air trapping may result from a ball-valve effect or collateral air drift that allows air to enter the portion of the lung distal to the bronchial obstruction but does not allow air outflow. This unidirectional airflow is a property of the collateral air passages and results in overexpansion of the lung beyond the obstructed bronchus. As the obstructed lung expands, it may compress the normal lung, and it shifts the mediastinum and heart, leading to volume loss in the normal lung (compressive atelectasis). In such cases, it is necessary to determine which is the primary abnormality, the lucent lung or the opaque lung. Expiratory views that reveal persistent overexpansion of the lung confirm that the bronchus to that lung is obstructed. Clinical correlation is also important. Obstructive overinflation is most often encountered in a child after an acute bronchial obstruction by a foreign body.

PASSIVE ATELECTASIS

Although separating atelectasis into passive (relaxation) and compressive categories may seem somewhat artificial, it does focus attention on the source of the primary problem producing collapse. With compressive atelectasis, the problem is intrapulmonary, whereas in the passive form, the problem is intrapleural. Two of the most important causes of passive atelectasis are pleural effusion (see Chapter 4) and pneumothorax (Fig. 13.14; answer to question 6 is *e*).

Probably the most important radiologic consideration in the diagnosis of pneumothorax is documentation of the problem. An extensive pneumothorax produces several obvious radiologic abnormalities, including increased opacity of the collapsed lung, the appearance of a pleural line, and a large lucent space between the pleural line and the chest wall. The pleural space lacks normal pulmonary markings. When the pneumothorax is minimal, the pleural line and lack of normal pulmonary markings may be more difficult to identify. In the upright patient, the small pleural line over the apex of the lung frequently appears to parallel the cortex of the ribs. However, close inspection usually shows that the pleural line only partially parallels the rib cortex and crosses the cortex of the ribs laterally. When there is strong clinical suspicion of a pneumothorax, but the inspiratory exam fails to confirm it, an expiratory exam may be more useful. Expiration enhances the appearance of the pneumothorax because the increased opacity of the lung during expiration effectively increases the contrast between the trapped air in the pleural cavity and the lung.

When the patient cannot stand up and only supine views are possible, the diagnosis of pneumothorax can be especially difficult.[596,667] Superimposed skinfolds on supine chest radiographs may be easily confused with the increased opacity of a pleural line.[161] However, skinfolds can be differentiated from pleural lines because lines

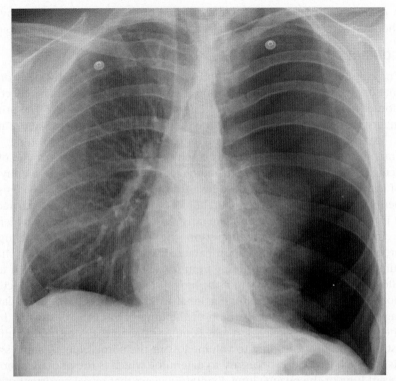

Fig. 13.14   A large left pneumothorax has almost completely collapsed the left lung. The collapse of the lung is the result of relaxation atelectasis.

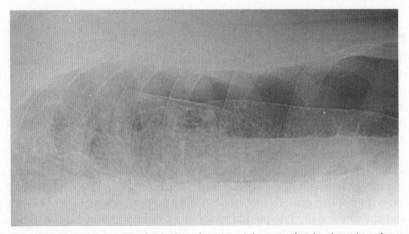

Fig. 13.15   Lateral decubitus view is a good substitute for an upright exam for the detection of pneumothorax.

formed by the folds appear to cross the ribs and thus may be traced off the area of the lungs. A small pneumothorax collects anteriorly in the supine patient, and the pulmonary markings extend to the lateral chest wall. In this instance, the best way to confirm a small pneumothorax is to use either an upright view or a lateral decubitus view, in which the side with the suspected pneumothorax is up (Fig. 13.15).

ADHESIVE ATELECTASIS

Adhesive atelectasis occurs when the luminal surfaces of the alveolar walls stick together. This type of atelectasis is an important component of two prominent

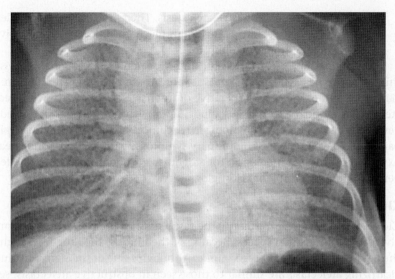

Fig. 13.16 Diffuse, fine, granular opacities with air bronchograms are not the expected radiologic appearance of atelectasis. The diagnosis in this premature newborn is surfactant deficiency disease. This is diffuse bilateral adhesive atelectasis.

pulmonary diseases: (1) respiratory distress syndrome of the newborn (hyaline membrane disease); and (2) pulmonary embolism. In both diseases, the basis for adhesion is presumed to be a deficiency of surfactant.

Surfactant deficiency disease of the newborn (Fig. 13.16), formerly known as respiratory distress syndrome or hyaline membrane disease, causes a pattern of opacities ranging from diffuse fine granular opacities to diffuse ground-glass opacities with air bronchograms in severe cases. The surfactant deficiency reduces surface tension causing acinar atelectasis that may lead to diffuse alveolar collapse (answer to question 7 is *b*).

Pulmonary embolism may also result in radiologic opacities that are typical of atelectasis. An appearance remarkably like that of subsegmental atelectasis is sometimes observed following pulmonary embolism, and occasionally, lobar opacities may also be observed in combination with displacement of fissures and elevation of the diaphragm. Such an appearance indicates lobar atelectasis.

The exact mechanism for atelectasis following pulmonary embolism is not clearly known. Numerous authors have reported that areas of increased opacity following pulmonary embolism often do not represent actual infarction or death of lung tissue. Heitzman[235] has emphasized that the radiologic opacities developing after pulmonary embolism are frequently the result of hemorrhagic edema; as such, they are pleural based and larger than the opacities usually attributed to atelectasis. Experimental studies have shown that the parenchymal opacities seen on chest radiographs may represent either edema and hemorrhage or atelectasis. In the discussion of the respiratory consequences of pulmonary embolism, Moser[396] described two possible mechanisms leading to atelectasis after pulmonary embolism:

1. When an embolus blocks blood flow to an alveolar area, the volume of alveolar dead space increases; in turn, this initiates reflex constriction, leading to a reduction in total lung volume. Reduced lung volume would also help explain the diaphragmatic elevation that often follows pulmonary embolism.
2. The reduced blood supply may also reduce the availability of surfactant. Surfactant levels may be critically reduced 24 hours after the embolism and

may contribute to adhesive atelectasis. There is experimental evidence that a deficiency of surfactant is the major mechanism leading to adhesive atelectasis following pulmonary embolism.

Because atelectasis is a nonspecific finding, careful clinical correlation is essential for this finding to be useful as a diagnostic indicator of pulmonary embolism. This is especially true in the case of postoperative or intensive-care patients, who frequently have atelectasis secondary to mucous plugging but who are also at increased risk for the development of pulmonary embolism. A clinical history that includes pleuritic chest pain, rapid development of pulmonary symptoms with dyspnea, or decrease in arterial oxygen tension is an indication for a definitive workup that may include ventilation-perfusion lung scanning or CT angiography.

CICATRIZING ATELECTASIS

Cicatrizing atelectasis is primarily the result of fibrosis and scar tissue formation in the alveolar and interstitial spaces. Because of the fibrosis, the lung loses compliance, and the end result is reduced lung volume. Although some of the signs of volume loss with cicatrizing atelectasis are similar to those seen in obstructive atelectasis, several important characteristics allow differentiation of the two conditions.

Similar features of cicatrizing and obstructive atelectasis are displacement of the hila and fissures, elevation of the diaphragm, and possibly displacement of the mediastinum. Distinctive of cicatrizing atelectasis are the associated coarse reticular opacities and sometimes even pleural scarring. Tuberculosis is the classic cause of cicatrizing atelectasis (see Fig. 13.2; answer to question 3 is *c*). Tuberculosis typically involves the development of upper lobe opacities, which may have associated cavities or chronic cysts. Late-stage scarring from tuberculosis may cause a shift of the mediastinum with retraction of the trachea, elevation of the hilum, and distortion of the fissures. Entities that can mimic this aspect of tuberculosis are primarily other granulomatous infections such as histoplasmosis. (Answer to question 8 is *d*.)

Usual interstitial pneumonitis produces a more generalized loss of lung volume and may be caused by diseases such scleroderma, rheumatoid lung, and idiopathic pulmonary fibrosis (IPF). In contrast to tuberculosis and histoplasmosis, these diseases do not usually result in segmental or lobar opacities. The volume loss tends to be bilateral and more uniform with the radiologic appearance of increased basilar opacity, crowding of vessels, and elevation of the diaphragm. Interstitial pneumonitis generally results in loss of volume in the lung bases with elevation of the diaphragm, which is often mistaken for poor voluntary inspiratory effort and is not usually recognized as atelectasis.

Coal worker's pneumoconiosis (CWP) and silicosis are somewhat different from the other types of interstitial pneumonitis because they tend to be more localized to the upper lobes, which results in the retraction of both hila toward the upper lobes. An exposure history usually confirms the diagnosis.

Radiation pneumonitis is another form of interstitial disease that leaves scarring in the lung with significant volume loss during its later stages.[78,425] It may occur in patients who have undergone radiation therapy for a variety of cancers but it is limited to the areas of the lung that are in the field of radiation. The most distinctive aspect of radiation pneumonitis is the peculiar nonanatomic distribution of the pathologic finding. It is frequently localized by sharply defined lines that coincide with the portals of the radiation therapy beam to which the patient was exposed (Fig. 13.17, *A* and *B*). Depending on the specific area irradiated, the retracting fibrosis may displace the hilum and interlobar fissures. As with tuberculosis, the late stage of radiation pneumonitis frequently assumes a reticular pattern that is most easily identified around the periphery of the opacity. The diagnosis can be confirmed by knowledge of previous radiation therapy.

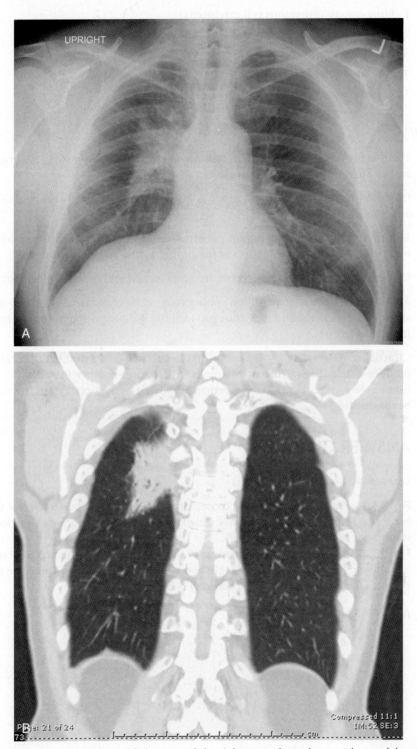

Fig. 13.17 A, The opacity in the medial aspect of the right upper lung does not have a lobar distribution. **B,** Coronal computed tomography scan confirms an angular, sharply defined opacity in the right upper lung. This geographic shape corresponds to the portal for the patient's prior radiation therapy.

Top 5 Diagnoses: Atelectasis

1. Lung cancer (squamous cell carcinoma)
2. Mucous plugs
3. Pneumothorax
4. Aspirated foreign body
5. Tuberculosis

Summary

The five major categories of atelectasis are obstructive, compressive, passive, adhesive, and cicatrizing.

Obstruction of large or small airways is the most commonly recognized cause of atelectasis.

Recurrent atelectasis is a common presentation for central lung cancers and may be an indication for further evaluation of the bronchi with bronchoscopy or CT.

Compressive and passive atelectasis are rarely segmental or lobar atelectasis.

Adhesive atelectasis may follow pulmonary embolism as a result of a localized surfactant deficiency and may thus produce the radiologic appearance of lobar or segmental atelectasis.

Cicatrizing atelectasis may occur during the late stages of a number of conditions that produce extensive scarring of the lung. In the case of tuberculosis, other associated findings (e.g., pleural thickening, reticular scarring of the upper lobes, cavitation) may be diagnostic.

ANSWER GUIDE

Legends for introductory figures

Fig. 13.1   Right upper atelectasis causes lobar opacification with elevation of the horizontal fissure. Other findings may include shift of the mediastinum, elevation of the diaphragm, and a juxtaphrenic peak.

Fig. 13.2   Apical opacity with elevation of the right hilum and lateral pleural scarring has resulted from tuberculosis. Hilar elevation indicates volume loss. This is the result of chronic scarring—thus, the term *cicatrizing atelectasis.*

ANSWERS

1. e   2. d   3. c   4. a   5. c   6. e   7. b   8. d

SEGMENTAL AND LOBAR CONSOLIDATIONS

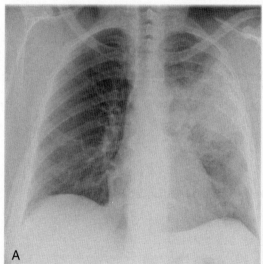
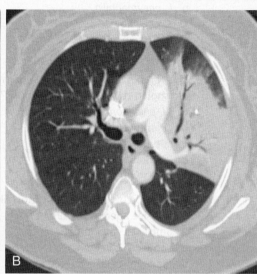

Fig. 14.1

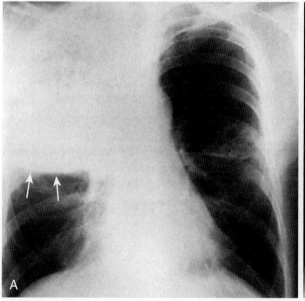
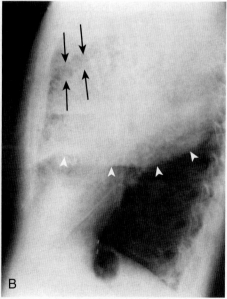

Fig. 14.2

QUESTIONS

1. Homogeneous, left lower lobe consolidation, as seen in Fig. 14.1, *A* and *B*, is the typical radiologic manifestation of community-acquired lobar pneumonia. What is the most likely causal agent?
   a. *Mycoplasma pneumoniae.*
   b. *Streptococcus pneumoniae.*

    c. *Mycobacterium avium intracellulare.*

    d. *Legionella pneumophilia.*

    e. *Klebsiella pneumoniae.*

2. Refer to Fig. 14.2, *A* and *B*. An expanded lobe with interspersed lucent spaces (shown by the *black arrows* on the figure), which are suggestive of multiple cavities, is a classic appearance for pneumonias caused by which of the following agents?

    a. *S. pneumoniae.*

    b. *L. pneumophilia.*

    c. *K. pneumoniae.*

    d. *M. pneumoniae.*

    e. Adenovirus.

3. The combination of hilar adenopathy and right middle lobe consolidation in a 15-year-old should suggest which diagnosis?

    a. *M. pneumoniae.*

    b. Gram-negative pneumonia.

    c. *S. pneumoniae.*

    d. Respiratory syncytial virus.

    e. Primary tuberculosis.

4. Which type of lung cancer is most likely to cause an expanded lobe?

    a. Invasive adenocarcinoma.

    b. Small cell carcinoma.

    c. Large cell carcinoma.

    d. Squamous cell carcinoma.

    e. Semi-invasive adenocarcinoma.

Chart 14.1   LOBAR CONSOLIDATION

  I. Lobar pneumonia
    A. *Streptococcus pneumoniae*[92,273,286]
    B. *Klebsiella pneumoniae*[50]

  II. Bronchopneumonia
    A. *Pseudomonas*[50]
    B. *K. pneumoniae*
    C. *Bacillus proteus*
    D. *Escherichia coli*
    E. Anaerobes (*Bacteroides* and *Clostridia*)
    F. *Legionella pneumophila*[140,461,498]
    G. *Staphylococcus aureus*
    H. Nocardiosis[50,208] and actinomycosis[164,300]
    I. *S. pneumoniae*[286]
    J. *Serratia*[28]

  III. Aspiration pneumonia

  IV. Tuberculosis[388,528] and atypical mycobacteria

  V. Pulmonary embolism[266]
    A. Hemorrhage and edema
    B. Infarction

  VI. Neoplasms
    A. Obstructive pneumonia (endobronchial tumor)
    B. Invasive mucinous adenocarcinoma (formerly bronchioloalveolar cell carcinoma)[134]
    C. Lymphoma[245,543]

  VII. Mitral regurgitation with pulmonary edema localized to the right upper lobe[213]

  VIII. Lung torsion[152,395]

Chart 14.2	**LOBAR EXPANSION**

    I. *Streptococcus pneumoniae*[175]
   II. *Klebsiella pneumoniae*[50]
  III. *Pseudomonas*[50]
  IV. *Staphylococcus*[50]
   V. Tuberculosis[528]
  VI. Carcinoma with obstructive pneumonia (drowned lung)

Discussion

LOBAR CONSOLIDATION

Lobar consolidation results from alveolar filling with fluid, exudate, or tumor that solidifies the lung.[221] The radiologic appearance of a consolidated lobe is a homogeneous confluent opacity that obliterates the normal vascular markings and often contains air bronchograms (see Fig. 14.1, *A* and *B*). Lobar pneumonia is the most common cause of lobar consolidation (Charts 14.1 and 14.2). The opacity is frequently bounded by the fissures, and stretched fissures may even lead to the appearance of an expanded lobe (see Fig. 14.2, *A* and *B*). Because the airways are frequently air filled and surrounded by airless lung, air bronchograms are another component of the classic appearance of lobar consolidation.

From the foregoing description, the distinction of lobar consolidation from atelectasis would appear to be simple. Fraser et al.[175] have emphasized that consolidation of a lobe with fluid is the antithesis of lobar atelectasis. Therefore, bulging fissures that indicate lobar expansion are unequivocal evidence of consolidation. As mentioned in Chapter 13, the displacement of fissures together indicates volume loss in the involved lobe. The problem with applying this approach to the evaluation of a lobar opacity for the purpose of distinguishing atelectasis from consolidation is not in the evaluation of the lobe that is expanded, but rather in the evaluation of the lobe of diminished size. It will become apparent in this discussion that a number of the processes that consolidate the lung also produce small airway obstruction, so that the volume loss produced by the process may be greater than the quantity of fluid that is consolidating the lung. Thus, a consolidating process may also be the cause of atelectasis. For example, bronchopneumonia, which causes air space consolidations, also leads to small airway obstructions that may result in atelectasis.

LOBAR PNEUMONIA

The distinction between lobar pneumonia and bronchopneumonia has been deemphasized in favor of a bacteriologic classification of pneumonias, which is more relevant in determining appropriate therapy. However, knowledge of the gross morphologic distinctions between the two types of pneumonia is important for understanding the variety of radiologic patterns that may be encountered in acute pneumonias.

The pathogenesis of lobar pneumonia is the key to understanding the spectrum of radiologic patterns. Experimental evidence indicates that the pathogens, in the form of small, infected, mucous particles, are inhaled to the periphery of the lung, where they set up foci of reaction. Initially, the tissue reaction involves the exudation of watery edema fluid into alveolar spaces. The exudate then spreads into the air passages and their alveoli. As the alveoli fill, the exudate spreads into adjacent lobules and segments. This movement of the exudate occurs via the pores of Kohn, canals of Lambert, and small airways, but does not appear to spread via the bronchovascular bundle or interstitium of the lung. The watery edema fluid serves as a culture medium for the rapid

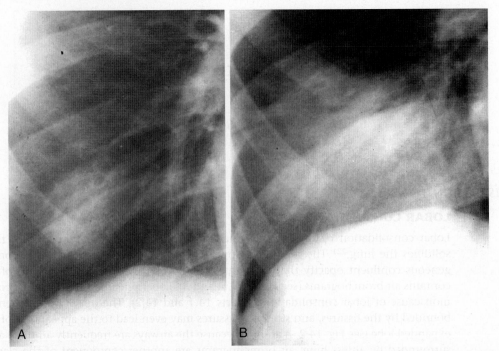

Fig. 14.3 A, Localized rounded opacity with air bronchograms is the result of pneumococcal pneumonia. This has been described as *round pneumonia.* **B,** Examination carried out 24 hours later shows extensive air space consolidation. Note the nonsegmental distribution, the result of contiguous spread of pneumonia via collateral channels.

multiplication of the bacteria. The alveolar walls respond to the organisms by releasing polymorphonuclear leukocytes. The spread of the process through the collateral channels, rather than the bronchioles, explains why lobar pneumonia often does not follow a segmental distribution. Rather, lobar pneumonia produces opacities that appear to involve multiple segments early in the course of the process. During these early phases, the radiologic appearance is that of a nonsegmental sublobar consolidation, which may appear rather sharply circumscribed because of the uniform involvement of contiguous alveoli. This leads to so-called round pneumonia.[608] Round pneumonia is more commonly seen in children but may occur as an early stage of lobar pneumonia in adults (Fig. 14.3, *A* and *B*). Fully developed, classic lobar consolidation is less commonly encountered because early diagnosis of bacterial pneumonia followed by appropriate antibiotic therapy frequently arrests the process in its early phases. Since the initial focus of infection is the periphery of the lung, it is not surprising that pleural effusion and empyema are potential complications. However, the occurrence of these complications is also drastically reduced by early antibiotic therapy.

Streptococcus pneumoniae, formally *Diplococcus pneumoniae,* is the most common bacteriologic cause of community-acquired lobar pneumonia (answer to question 1 is *b*), but the organism involved cannot be determined from the radiologic appearance. *K. pneumoniae* is another cause of lobar pneumonia that tends to follow a more aggressive course than *S. pneumoniae.* It is more likely to expand a lobe and produce necrosis of lung tissue with cavitation (see Chapter 23; answer to question 2 is *c.*)

The clinical course of lobar pneumonia is characterized primarily by nonspecific symptoms, such as productive cough and temperature elevation, so additional history should be obtained. For example, is the patient debilitated by alcoholism or immunologic suppression? Considering the radiologic appearance of an expanding lobar consolidation with cavitation and a history of alcoholism allows the diagnosis of *K. pneumoniae* to be proposed with confidence, but the definitive diagnosis of a bacterial pneumonia can be made only by analysis of smears and cultures of the sputum, blood, and lung aspirate.

BRONCHOPNEUMONIA

In comparison to the limited number of radiologic presentations of lobar pneumonia, the spectrum of radiologic patterns associated with bronchopneumonia (lobular pneumonia)[235] is much more diverse. Bronchopneumonia is the most likely presentation for hospital-acquired and opportunistic pneumonias.

In bronchopneumonia, the primary sites of injury are the terminal and respiratory bronchioles. The disease starts as an acute bronchitis and bronchiolitis. As it progresses, ulcers are formed in the large bronchi by destruction of the epithelial lining, and the bronchial walls become infiltrated with polymorphonuclear leukocytes. These ulcers are covered with a fibrinopurulent membrane that contains large quantities of multiplying organisms. With the more virulent organisms such as *Staphylococcus* and *Pseudomonas*, necrotic bronchitis and bronchiolitis can lead to thrombosis of the lobular branches of the small pulmonary arteries. This inflammatory reaction also spreads through the walls of the bronchioles to involve the alveolar walls. This is followed by exudation of fluids and inflammatory cells into the acinus to produce lobular consolidations. The alveoli become filled with edematous fluid, blood, polymorphonuclear leukocytes, hyaline membranes, and bacteria.

The foregoing description suggests that the specific radiologic pattern depends on both the virulence of the organism and the host defenses. A mild bronchopneumonia in an otherwise healthy individual may lead only to inflammatory peribronchial infiltration and the radiologic appearance of peribronchial thickening with "increased markings." The peribronchial infiltrate may also account for the radiologic appearance of multiple, small (i.e., 5 mm), fluffy, or ill-defined nodules, resembling acinar nodules. These nodules differ from the expected appearance of miliary nodules mainly in their lack of definition or fluffy borders. As the inflammatory process spreads, the nodules enlarge. The number of areas involved is highly variable, ranging from a few localized opacities in one area of the lung to diffuse opacities involving both lungs. Bronchopneumonia may therefore present as multifocal ill-defined opacities and, as such, is considered further in Chapter 16.

Although the concomitant appearance of both lobar and segmental opacities may seem paradoxic in the discussion of bronchopneumonia, the combination is consistent with the diagnosis. Recall that bronchopneumonia involves both bronchioles and bronchi. Patients with bronchopneumonia occasionally have narrowing of the bronchi and mucous plugging; both processes can lead to airway obstruction. Therefore, in contrast to lobar pneumonia, which is characterized by a nonsegmental distribution of opacities and infrequent atelectasis, bronchopneumonia is a common cause of segmental or lobar opacities accompanied by volume loss. With this presentation, bronchopneumonia has occasionally been referred to as *atelectatic pneumonia*. If multiple opacities are present in the other lobes, the radiologic appearance is nearly diagnostic. If atelectasis is the only radiologic abnormality, careful clinical and laboratory correlations are required to distinguish bronchopneumonia from the other causes of atelectasis considered in Chapter 13.

ASPIRATION PNEUMONIA

Aspiration pneumonia is another important cause of segmental consolidation that may lead to complete consolidation of a lobe. The radiologic feature of aspiration pneumonia that distinguishes it from other causes of segmental consolidation is its distribution. Aspiration pneumonia characteristically occurs in the dependent portions of the lung (see Chapter 15) and is frequently bilateral. However, unilateral involvement can occur; in fact, right middle lobe or right lower lobe involvement with sparing of the left side is not rare because of the anatomy of the bronchus intermedius. The diagnosis can often be confirmed on clinical grounds.

Occasionally, a patient is observed to aspirate gastric contents or food, and subsequently the chest radiograph confirms pneumonia. Other cases can be diagnosed on the basis of a radiologic demonstration of segmental consolidation in a dependent portion of the lung and a history of predisposing conditions such as alcoholism, recent anesthesia, head and neck surgery, mental retardation, seizure disorders, and esophageal motility disturbances. In cases of chronic aspiration, segmental consolidation may be a recurring process that never completely clears. On occasion, serial radiographs may document progression from a localized consolidation to interstitial scarring that may even end with the development of an end-stage scar similar to that appearing in honeycomb lung. Pneumonia caused by chronic aspiration is usually distinguished from the other entities that result in honeycomb lung by its localized appearance. A history of mineral oil use is strongly suggestive of chronic aspiration pneumonia (mineral oil or exogenous cholesterol pneumonia). Identification of fat-laden macrophages in the sputum may confirm the diagnosis of mineral oil or lipoid pneumonia.

GRANULOMATOUS INFECTIONS

Tuberculosis is the most common granulomatous infection to cause segmental or lobar air space consolidations. The initial reaction to the tubercle bacillus (primary tuberculosis) is the exudation of inflammatory cells, including macrophages and polymorphonuclear leukocytes from alveolar capillaries into the alveolar spaces. Initially, the alveoli are intact during this exudative phase, but over a period of about 1 month, the exudative reaction is gradually replaced by chronic inflammatory cells as the phase of hypersensitivity reaction begins. After 6 weeks, changes typical of tuberculosis, including caseation necrosis, can be identified in the center of the lesion. This pathogenesis has significant radiologic implications when the air space consolidation of the primary exudative phase of tuberculosis is contrasted with lobar pneumonia. It should be obvious from the preceding description that conventional antibiotic treatment will not clear primary tuberculosis, whereas adequately treated pneumococcal or *K. pneumonia* should clear in a few days to 2 weeks. Even with antituberculous therapy, primary tuberculous exudates may require several weeks for complete clearing. Another feature of primary tuberculosis, which is extremely important in radiologically differentiating tuberculosis from lobar pneumonia, is the presence of hilar or mediastinal adenopathy (see Chapters 10 and 11; answer to question 3 is *e.*)

Fungal infections have many similarities to tuberculosis, including a variety of radiologic patterns. Histoplasmosis, coccidioidomycosis, and blastomycosis[142] are organisms that exist in the soil and cause human infection. The initial infection with these fungi often causes segmental or patchy, sublobar, air space consolidations (Fig. 14.4, *A* and *B*). These fungal infections may clinically and radiographically be indistinguishable from an acute bacterial pneumonia and sometimes resemble primary tuberculosis.

PULMONARY EMBOLISM

Pulmonary embolism is an important but infrequent cause of segmental and lobar consolidation. The consolidation results from edema and hemorrhage with or without infarction[55] (Fig. 14.5, *A-D*). Jacoby and Mindell[266] emphasize that although these opacities can result from the infarction and necrosis of lung tissue, they more commonly represent incomplete infarction with hemorrhage and edema in the surrounding air spaces. The radiologic appearance of this type of consolidation is remarkably similar to that of lobar pneumonia. The hemorrhagic edema produces air space consolidation with a radiologic appearance of confluent opacities with ill-defined borders, peripheral acinar opacities, and even air bronchograms. Radiologic criteria are frequently inadequate for distinguishing between cases in which the opacities are the result of hemorrhage and edema versus those in which they are the result of necrosis with infarction. In cases of proven pulmonary embolic disease, the radiologic diagnosis

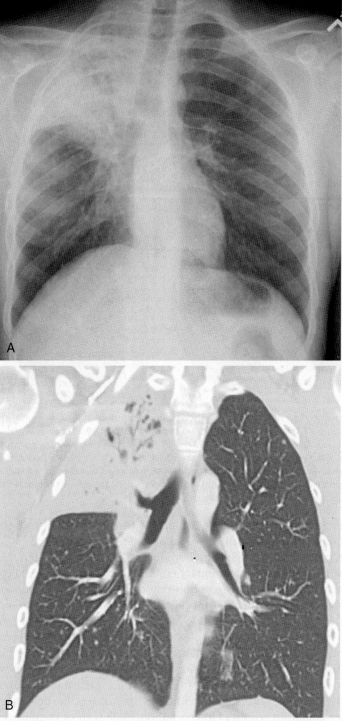

Fig. 14.4 A, Right upper lobe consolidation has the appearance of lobar pneumonia, but the patient did not respond to antibiotics. **B,** Computed tomography scan confirmed right upper lobe consolidation with air bronchograms and small lucent areas suggestive of cavitation. The patient had a persistent low-grade fever and developed skin lesions. Skin biopsy revealed blastomycosis.

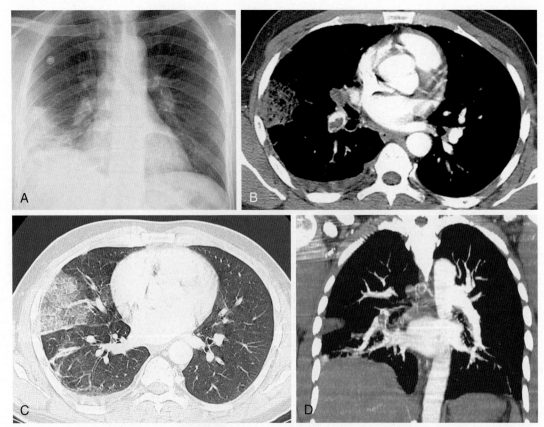

Fig. 14.5 **A,** Posteroanterior chest radiograph shows peripheral, right basilar air space opacity. **B,** Computed tomography (CT) angiogram confirms a filling defect in the right pulmonary artery and reveals a peripheral, pleural-based opacity with a nodular-appearing center. **C,** Axial CT image with lung window confirms peripheral, wedge-shaped, right middle lobe, ground-glass and air space opacities, which are pleural based. These are the result of hemorrhage and edema. **D,** CT coronal reconstruction reveals a more localized opacity that is pleural based. This is suggestive of a pulmonary infarct, but confirmation of an infarct is difficult and usually requires follow-up studies that demonstrate a residual nodular opacity, linear scar, or cavity.

of infarction can be made with confidence when the area of consolidation undergoes subsequent resolution with a residual nodular or linear scar.

The combination of segmental or lobar consolidations with pleural effusion might suggest the diagnosis of pulmonary embolism, but this radiologic combination is also not useful in distinguishing pulmonary embolism from lobar pneumonia. Like the radiologic findings, the clinical findings and laboratory tests for a pulmonary embolism are frequently nonspecific. Even the classic clinical triad of dyspnea, chest pain, and hemoptysis is seen in only 20% of cases, but the additional radiologic findings of peripheral segmental consolidation with pleural effusion would make the diagnosis more likely. A history of fever, leukocytosis, and purulent sputum with lobar consolidation and pleural effusion constitutes strong evidence for pneumonia. Because the clinical symptoms and radiologic findings are nonspecific, definitive diagnosis of pulmonary embolism requires either a radionuclide scan or computed tomography (CT) angiography.

NEOPLASMS

Obstructive pneumonia is a result of a long-standing, large airway obstruction that may have been preceded by atelectasis. Atelectasis is the expected result of acute airway obstruction, but with chronic obstruction, the collapsed lung re-expands with edema, inflammatory cells, and cholesterol-laden macrophages. This produces the radiologic

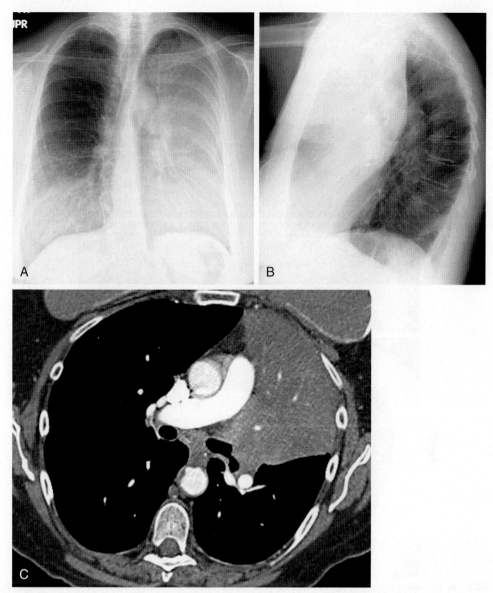

Fig. 14.6 A, The left lung opacification obscures the heart and appears to be diffuse on the posteroanterior view. **B,** The lateral view reveals that the opacity is anterior and displaces the major fissure posteriorly. The left lower lobe is aerated. The posterior bulging of the fissure indicates expansion rather than atelectasis. This has been described as a *drowned lung*. **C,** Computed tomography scan confirms consolidation of the left upper lobe with posterior bulging of the fissure. The left upper lobe bronchus is obstructed by squamous cell lung cancer.

appearance of an expanded lobe and is often described as "drowned" lung or endogenous cholesterol pneumonia (Fig. 14.6, *A-C*). When secondary bacterial infection occurs, patients usually experience a febrile response and leukocytosis that is clinically typical of pneumonia. The radiologic presentation of an associated hilar mass must be considered as strongly suggestive of obstructive pneumonia. In fact, the combination of a persistent segmental or lobar consolidation with hilar adenopathy in a middle-aged patient strongly suggests an underlying endobronchial lung cancer. Radiologic documentation of a lobar opacity that fails to clear completely in response to antibiotic therapy constitutes sufficient clinical grounds for CT or bronchoscopic examination to exclude an underlying tumor. Cavitation is another moderately frequent complication of obstructive pneumonia. A persistent abscess following treatment of pneumonia may

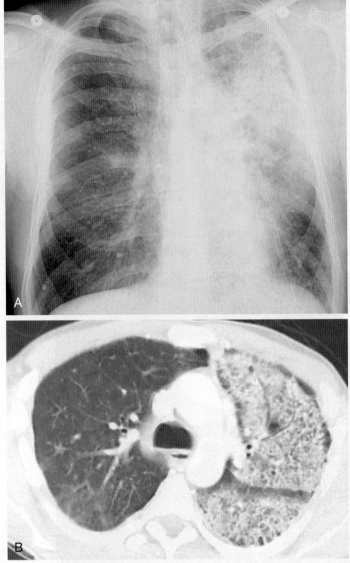

Fig. 14.7   A, Left upper lobe air space consolidation would be compatible with pneumonia, but the patient has a cough with large quantities of thin watery sputum. The absence of fever and other evidence of pneumonia should suggest the possibility of invasive mucinous adenocarcinoma. **B,** Computed tomography scan confirms extensive air space consolidation of the left upper lobe and superior segment of the lower lobe. There was no evidence of bronchial obstruction. This is one of the manifestations of bronchioloalveolar cell carcinoma that has been pathologically reclassified as invasive mucinous adenocarcinoma.

also be a clue to an underlying, obstructive bronchial tumor. Squamous cell carcinoma is the most common tumor that causes a proximal bronchial obstruction that will initially cause atelectasis but may progress to obstructive pneumonia with an expanded lobe (answer to question 4 is *d*).

Invasive mucinous adenocarcinoma (formerly one manifestation of bronchioloalveolar cell carcinoma[597]; Fig. 14.7, *A* and *B*) frequently causes alveolar filling with lobar air space consolidations. These tumors spread through the airways and produce a large amount of mucoid secretions. This often has the radiologic appearance of lobar pneumonia, but carcinoma should be considered in patients with a history of cough and large quantities of sputum but no symptoms of infection.

LUNG TORSION

Torsion[152,395] is a rare cause of lobar atelectasis or consolidation. It is important because of the risk of complicating infarction and necrosis. Torsion should be suspected when lobar opacities are identified in an unusual position or are associated with unusual hilar displacement. For example, right middle lobe atelectasis with elevation of the right hilum should suggest torsion. A major change in the position of an opacified lobe on serial examinations is also evidence to suspect torsion. Torsion has been reported as a complication of thoracic surgery, chest trauma, pneumonia, and both benign and malignant endobronchial tumors.

Top 5 Diagnoses: Segmental and Lobar Opacities

1. Lobar pneumonia
2. Lung cancer (obstructive pneumonia and invasive mucinous adenocarcinoma)
3. Aspiration pneumonia
4. Tuberculosis
5. Infarction

Summary

The classic radiologic appearance of a consolidated lobe is an increased opacity that is homogeneous or confluent, obliterates the normal pulmonary markings, and abuts the fissures. Pure consolidation should not result in volume loss; frequently, it even leads to expansion of the lobe.

The classic cause of community-acquired lobar pneumonia is *S. pneumoniae,* formerly known as *D. pneumoniae.* Other causes of lobar consolidation include *K. pneumoniae;* primary tuberculosis; aspiration pneumonia; pulmonary embolism with edema, hemorrhage, or infarction; and obstructive pneumonia.

The terms *bronchopneumonia* and *lobular pneumonia* are synonyms. The classic appearance of this type of pneumonia is that of multifocal opacities, as described in Chapter 16. There is extensive bronchial involvement; therefore segmental and lobar opacities with volume loss are not rare. A similar mechanism probably accounts for the segmental and lobar opacities that occur in viral and mycoplasma pneumonias.

The bacteriologic diagnosis of pneumonia is not a primary function of the radiologist because it usually requires laboratory confirmation.

Among the radiologic features that occasionally permit the radiologist to suggest a specific cause for pneumonia are lobar opacities with associated diffuse, reticular, nodular interstitial disease, which suggest a nonbacterial pneumonia. An expanded lobe with cavitation is strongly suggestive of *K. pneumonia.*

Aspiration pneumonia should be particularly suspected in patients who develop segmental or lobar opacities and who have known predisposing conditions such as alcoholism, recent anesthesia, head and neck tumors, mental retardation, seizure disorders, and disturbances in esophageal motility. Lipoid pneumonia should be especially considered in the older patient who uses mineral oil.

Primary tuberculosis is an important cause of lobar and segmental opacities, which are frequently associated with hilar adenopathy. This combination may also be seen in children with viral pneumonia, and in older patients it may be an important clue to the diagnosis of obstructive pneumonia caused by endobronchial lung cancer.

Obstructive pneumonia is a particularly important cause of segmental and lobar consolidations in middle-aged smokers. The persistence of a lobar or segmental consolidation following antibiotic therapy for a presumed pneumonia is extremely suggestive of obstructive pneumonia. Suspicion of this abnormality warrants further investigation and the collection of sputum samples for cytologic study. Bronchoscopy and biopsy are frequently required for the definitive diagnosis.

Invasive mucinous adenocarcinoma, which was formerly classified as bronchioalveolar cell carcinoma, causes air space consolidations resembling pneumonia rather than nodules or masses.

ANSWER GUIDE

Legends for introductory figures

Fig. 14.1   A, Homogeneous consolidation in the left upper lobe is the result of *S. pneumoniae.* This organism is the most common cause of community-acquired lobar pneumonia. **B,** Computed tomography scan confirms consolidation with air bronchograms and surrounding ground-glass opacity.

Fig. 14.2   A, Posteroanterior view shows consolidation of the right upper lobe with inferior displacement of the horizontal fissure *(arrows).* **B,** Lateral view further confirms consolidation of the right upper lobe by revealing posterior inferior displacement of the oblique fissure in addition to depression of the minor fissure *(white arrowheads).* Interspersed lucent spaces *(black arrows)* are due to early cavitation. This is a classic appearance for *K. pneumonia.*

ANSWERS

1. b   2. b   3. b   4. d

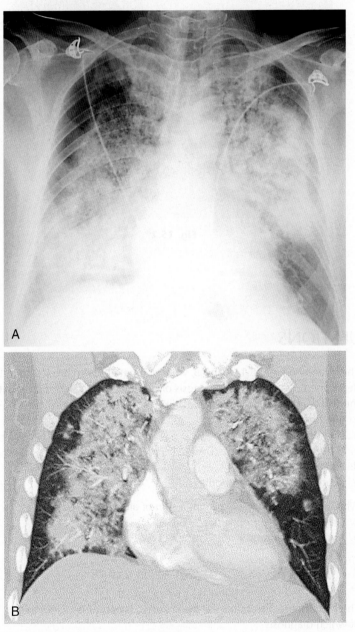

Fig. 15.1

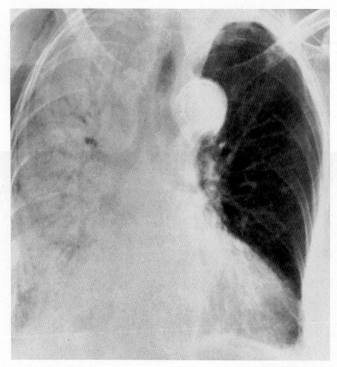

Fig. 15.2

QUESTIONS

1. The images in Fig. 15.1, *A* and *B*, were of a patient who presented in the emergency department with a known diagnosis of granulomatosis with polyangiitis. Which one of the following complications is most likely?
   a. Pneumonia.
   b. Hemorrhage.
   c. Diffuse alveolar damage (DAD).
   d. Pulmonary edema.
   e. Acute interstitial pneumonia (AIP).

2. Which one of the following is not a sign of air space disease?
   a. Diffuse coalescent opacities.
   b. Air bronchograms.
   c. Acinar nodules.
   d. Fine reticular opacities.
   e. Air alveolograms.

3. The asymmetric distribution of the diffuse coalescent opacities in Fig. 15.2 is suggestive of which diagnosis?
   a. Pneumonia.
   b. Goodpasture syndrome.
   c. Chronic renal failure.
   d. Alveolar proteinosis.
   e. Congestive heart failure.

4. A 24- to 48-hour delay in the development of pulmonary edema is commonly observed in which of the following conditions?
   a. Congestive heart failure.
   b. Pulmonary emboli.
   c. Smoke inhalation.
   d. Heroin reaction.
   e. High-altitude pulmonary edema.

Chart 15.1	**DIFFUSE AIR SPACE OPACITIES**

I. Edema
  A. Cardiac failure
  B. Noncardiac (see Chart 15.2)
II. Exudate (pneumonias)
  A. Bacteria[50,117]
  B. Viruses[95,235,382]
  C. Mycoplasma[159,250]
  D. Fungi[93,372,450,534]
  E. *Pneumocystis jiroveci* pneumonia (also known as PCP)[69,96,114]
  F. Parasites (strongyloidiasis)[653]
  G. Aspiration
  H. *Rickettsia* (Rocky Mountain spotted fever)[333,365]
  I. Tuberculosis[405]
  J. Severe acute respiratory syndrome (SARS)[44,70,408,412]
III. Hemorrhage
  A. Anticoagulation therapy
  B. Bleeding diathesis (e.g., leukemia)
  C. Disseminated intravascular coagulation (18- to 72-hour delay)[447]
  D. Blunt trauma[609] (pulmonary contusion, usually is not diffuse)
  E. Vasculitis
    1. Infections (e.g., mucormycosis, aspergillosis, Rocky Mountain spotted fever)
    2. Granulomatosis with polyangiitis (formerly Wegener granulomatosis,[441,606] classic and variant forms)
    3. Goodpasture syndrome[441]
    4. Systemic lupus erythematosus[441]
  F. Idiopathic pulmonary hemosiderosis[163,589]
  G. Infectious mononucleosis[595]
IV. Other
  A. Pulmonary alveolar proteinosis[176,249,457,487]
  B. Acute respiratory distress syndrome (ARDS)[130,277,278,291,421,663]
  C. Acute interstitial pneumonia (AIP)[12,257]
  D. Sarcoidosis (very unusual)[386,457,467]
  E. Mineral oil aspiration (exogenous cholesterol pneumonia)
  F. Eosinophilic lung disease[85,181,274]
  G. Chemical pneumonitis
  H. Drug reactions (see Chart 15.3)

Chart 15.2	**NONCARDIAC PULMONARY EDEMA**

  I. Chronic renal failure
 II. Toxic inhalations
    A. Nitrogen dioxide (silo filler's disease)
    B. Sulfur dioxide[74]
    C. Smoke[285,446]
    D. Beryllium
    E. Cadmium
    F. Silica (very fine particles; silicoproteinosis)[299]
    G. Carbon monoxide[549]
III. Anaphylaxis (e.g., penicillin, transfusion,[62] radiologic contrast medium[205])
 IV. Narcotics (e.g., morphine, methadone, cocaine, heroin)[201,473,671]
  V. Drug reaction (e.g., interleukin-2 therapy,[90,518] β-adrenergic drugs[391])
 VI. Acute airway obstruction[422] (e.g., foreign body)
VII. Near-drowning[448]
VIII. High altitude[254]
 IX. Fluid overload
  X. Cerebral (trauma, stroke, tumor)[467]
 XI. Hypoproteinemia
XII. ARDS (early stages)[277,291]
XIII. Pancreatitis[494]
XIV. Amniotic fluid embolism[537]
 XV. Fat embolism
XVI. Re-expansion following treatment of pneumothorax or large pleural effusion
XVII. Organophosphate insecticide ingestion[339]
XVIII. Hanta virus pulmonary syndrome[291]

Chart 15.3	**PULMONARY DRUG REACTIONS**

  I. Edema
    A. Narcotics[671]
    B. Radiologic contrast[205]
    C. Interleukin-2 therapy[90,518]
    D. β-Adrenergic drugs[391]
 II. Hemorrhage[489]
    A. Anticoagulants
    B. Amphotericin B
    C. Cytarabine
    D. Cyclophosphamide
    E. Penicillamine
III. Diffuse alveolar damage (DAD)[489]
    A. Bleomycin
    B. Busulfan
    C. Carmustine
    D. Cyclophosphamide
    E. Gold
    F. Melphalan
    G. Mitomycin
 IV. Eosinophilic pneumonia[489]
    A. Nitrofurantoin
    B. Nonsteroidal antiinflammatory drugs
    C. Para-aminosalicylic acid
    D. Penicillamine
    E. Sulfasalazine

Chart 15.3	**PULMONARY DRUG REACTIONS—cont'd**

V. Cryptogenic organizing pneumonia (COP)[489]
    A. Amiodorone[426]
    B. Bleomycin
    C. Cyclophosphamide
    D. Gold
    E. Methotrexate[554]
    F. Nitrofurantoin
    G. Penicillamine
    H. Sulfasalazine
VI. Nonspecific interstitial pneumonitis (NSIP)[489]
    A. Amiodarone
    B. Carmustine
    C. Chlorambucil
    D. Methotrexate

Modified from Rossi SE, Erasmus JJ, McAdams HP, et al. Pulmonary drug toxicity: radiologic and pathologic manifestations. *Radiographics.* 2000;20:1245-59. Used with permission.

Discussion

The diffuse air space consolidation[22,601] shown in Fig. 15.1, *A* and *B*, is a classic appearance and consists of the following: coalescent or confluent opacities with ill-defined borders; butterfly-shaped perihilar distribution; ill-defined nodular opacities around the periphery of the process ("acinar pattern")[601,666]; and interspersed small lucencies.[457,460] Air-filled bronchi surrounded by the confluent opacities are seen as dark branching shadows. These were described by Fleischner[162] as the "visible bronchial tree" and are commonly referred to as *air bronchograms*[150] (see Fig 15.2). The small, interspersed lucent spaces represent groups of air-filled alveoli surrounded by airless consolidated lung. The term *air alveologram* was applied to these lucent spaces by Felson[150]; they are the alveolar equivalent of the air bronchogram. The distribution of opacities caused by air space consolidation may be diffuse, lobar, or segmental (see Chapter 14). There is a tendency for air space opacities to be labile—that is, changing in severity over a short period of time on serial examinations.

Diffuse ground-glass opacity is occasionally used to describe less opaque, diffuse, confluent opacities seen on chest radiographs, but is more commonly used in reporting high-resolution computed tomography (HRCT). This differs from consolidation in degree of opacity and implies minimal disease. Ground-glass opacities appear on HRCT as gray areas of confluent attenuation that fail to obliterate normal vascular shadows. Ground-glass opacity demonstrated by HRCT results from minimal filling of the alveolar spaces or from thickening of the alveolar walls and septal interstitium.[133] Reticular opacities, whether or not they are demonstrated on a chest radiograph or computed tomography (CT) scan, are not a finding of air space disease. (Answer to question 2 is *d*.)

CARDIAC PULMONARY EDEMA

Pulmonary alveolar edema (Fig 15.3) is a classic example of a diffuse air space filling process (Chart 15.1). The presence of alveolar edema, however, does not imply the absence of interstitial edema. Cardiac pulmonary alveolar edema is always preceded by interstitial edema, but the extensive alveolar consolidation obscures the fine reticular opacities of the interstitial process. Radiologic documentation of the underlying interstitial process entails examination of areas not significantly involved by the alveolar filling process. When alveolar pulmonary edema is secondary to congestive heart

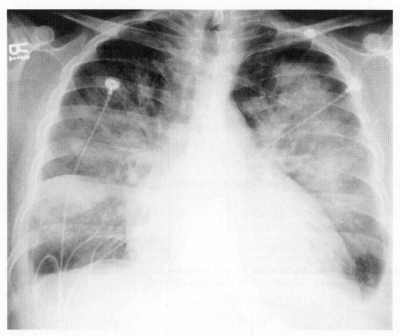

Fig. 15.3   Pulmonary edema is one of the most common causes of diffuse bilateral confluent air space opacities. Associated pleural effusions and cardiac enlargement should confirm the diagnosis of pulmonary alveolar edema resulting from congestive heart failure.

failure, the alveolar edema often has a perihilar distribution, and Kerley B lines may be present in the costophrenic angles.

The latter sign confirms the underlying interstitial process. Other radiologic signs that may be associated with cardiopulmonary edema and can be helpful in suggesting the diagnosis include: (1) prominence of the upper lobe vessels[454]; (2) indistinctness of vessels[291]; (3) peribronchial cuffing[390]; (4) increased width of the vascular pedicle[390]; (5) pleural effusion, frequently with fluid in the fissures; and (6) cardiac enlargement with a left ventricular prominence. Correlation of the radiologic findings with clinical findings usually confirms the diagnosis. An electrocardiogram indicating cardiac enlargement or an old or acute myocardial infarction is also supportive evidence, whereas an S3 heart sound, neck vein distention, hepatomegaly, or peripheral edema usually confirm the diagnosis of congestive failure. Also, auscultation over the lungs usually reveals characteristic basilar rales.

Occasionally, alveolar edema is not distributed uniformly. As a result of gravity, when the patient is upright, the edema fluid has a predominantly lower lobe distribution, but when the patient is supine, the fluid tends to have a more posterior distribution. When the patient favors one side, the fluid tends to gravitate to the dependent side. The resolution of pulmonary edema is often not uniform, so that serial chest radiographs reveal a change in the distribution from diffuse perihilar opacities to a pattern of more uneven multifocal opacities. Other causes for atypical or nonuniform distribution of pulmonary edema are usually of pulmonary origin. The best known of these is severe emphysema, which results in a patchy distribution of the alveolar edema. Presumably, loss of vasculature in the emphysematous areas of the lung results in the development of edema in the more normal areas. Pulmonary embolism is a complication of pulmonary edema that may result in a nonuniform or patchy distribution of the alveolar edema. Two factors may determine the distribution of the air space edema following pulmonary embolism: (1) abrupt interruption of perfusion to an area of lung may prevent the development of typical pulmonary edema; and (2) severe ischemia of the lung may give rise to pulmonary hemorrhage. Clinical suspicion of pulmonary embolism in a patient with congestive heart failure will usually require computed tomography angiography (CTA).

Concomitant infection is another cause of uneven distribution of pulmonary edema. Like the diagnosis of pulmonary embolism, this requires correlation with the clinical history. An elevated temperature, leukocytosis, or purulent sputum should prompt a bacteriologic study to rule out superimposed pneumonia.

Cardiac enlargement in combination with diffuse alveolar opacities that are otherwise characteristic of pulmonary edema is not always a reliable indicator that the patient's primary problem is a cardiac disorder. For instance, chronic renal failure with uremia can cause pulmonary edema (uremic pneumonitis) as well as hypertension and associated heart disease, with the result of cardiac enlargement. Not only does uremia cause true cardiomegaly, which is probably related to chronic hypertension, but it also may cause pericardial effusion. Thus, the pulmonary edema that results from chronic renal failure and uremia is typically associated with enlargement of the cardiac silhouette. Correlation with the clinical history should readily identify uremic pneumonitis.

In contrast to pulmonary alveolar edema and cardiac enlargement, the presence of a normal-sized heart might suggest a noncardiac form of pulmonary edema, but there are situations in which such patients may actually have cardiac pulmonary edema. These include acute cardiac arrhythmias and acute myocardial infarction, which result in pulmonary edema before dilation of the heart. Thus, there are at least two mechanisms for cardiac pulmonary edema with a normal-sized heart.

NONCARDIAC PULMONARY EDEMA

The preceding discussion suggests that the radiologic appearance of noncardiac pulmonary edema is similar to that of cardiac pulmonary edema.[546] In general, the most helpful radiologic feature for distinguishing the two is the presence or absence of cardiac enlargement. Accurate assessment of heart size is often difficult. Technical factors—including supine and anteroposterior positioning, especially when done with portable units—may all contribute to cardiac magnification. Patient condition may also lead to inaccurate cardiac size estimation. Patients with emphysema often have cardiac enlargement, although the chest radiograph is suggestive of a normal or even small heart size. Aggressive intravenous (IV) fluid resuscitation may actually enlarge the heart and cause pulmonary edema. The evaluation of serial radiographs is especially useful for distinguishing a number of the causes of noncardiac edema because the evolution of the edema may be strikingly different. Many of the entities listed in Chart 15.2 may result in acute alveolar edema in the absence of the pulmonary vascular and interstitial changes that precede the edema because of either renal failure or cardiac failure. These entities tend to occur in very acute cases of pulmonary edema and are often best diagnosed by clinical correlation,[5] as is shown in the following discussions of acute toxic inhalations, near-drowning, acute airway obstruction, drug reactions, and ARDS.

Acute Toxic Inhalations

Nitrogen dioxide inhalation (silo filler's disease) is an excellent model for acute toxic pulmonary edema. In the first few days after a grain storage silo is filled, nitrogen dioxide forms. The gas reacts with water in the respiratory tract to produce an irritation of the tracheobronchial tree and alveoli. In the acute phase, this disease has the radiologic appearance of bilateral diffuse alveolar edema. This phase is usually followed within a few days or weeks by complete resolution, although bronchiolitis obliterans may develop weeks to months later as a result of the small airway injury. Chest radiographs of patients with bronchiolitis obliterans often show a fine nodular or reticular pattern. The other chemicals listed in Chart 15.2 produce a similar reaction.

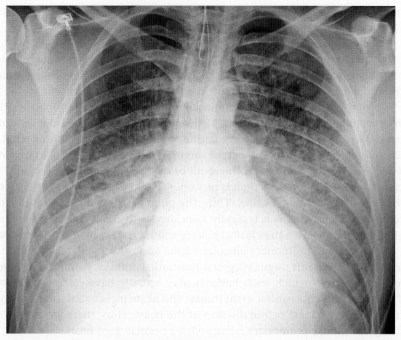

Fig. 15.4   Smoke inhalation produces diffuse bilateral air space opacities with a normal heart size. There is often delayed onset of edema following smoke inhalation. The presence of edema soon after the exposure indicates that the patient is at increased risk for diffuse alveolar damage.

Smoke inhalation is the most common cause of death due to fires. Fire victims may have thermal injuries to the airways and are exposed to toxic gases, soot, and carbon monoxide. Inhalation of these substances may cause airway and alveolar injury with alveolar leak as the cause of pulmonary edema (Fig 15.4). Patients with smoke inhalation must be carefully monitored because the radiologic appearance of pulmonary edema may be delayed by as much as 24 to 48 hours (answer to question 3 is c). The risk of a delayed onset of edema is greatest in patients with low oxygen saturation and elevated carboxyhemoglobin, which reflects carbon monoxide poisoning with potential concomitant lung damage.[445] Early onset of pulmonary edema indicates severe alveolar injury with increased risk of diffuse alveolar damage and ARDS.

Near-Drowning

Near-drowning[448] is another important cause of noncardiac pulmonary edema. The history should confirm the diagnosis; however, aspiration of water provides only a partial explanation for the diffuse alveolar opacities that may develop in near-drowning victims. Again, there may be a delay of 24 to 48 hours before edema develops. Other mechanisms that may contribute to the development of this type of edema include prolonged hypoxia, respiratory obstruction, and fibrin degradation. Fibrin degradation raises the possibility of a subclinical consumptive coagulopathy with microembolization, which may lead to a diffuse pulmonary capillary leak and thus to pulmonary edema. Severe hypoxia may occur in a near-fatal–drowning victim, even when the initial chest radiograph is normal. Patients should therefore be followed for 24 to 48 hours to exclude a significant pulmonary injury.

Acute Airway Obstruction

The diagnosis of acute airway obstruction is usually made on the basis of the clinical history. The obstruction is frequently an aspirated object, such as a large bolus of food or a surgical sponge. The resultant pulmonary edema is usually related to severe hypoxia. This mechanism may be nearly identical to that described for near-drowning.

The collection of alveolar fluid is most likely due to a diffuse alveolar leak caused by severe injury to the alveolar capillary membrane.[422]

Drug Reactions

Adverse reactions to a variety of drugs (Chart 15.3) may cause acute and chronic pulmonary responses.[18,52] These reactions have been described as *chemotherapy lung*,[551] but a large variety of drugs have pulmonary complications. These include antibiotics, narcotics, heart medications, arthritis drugs, radiographic contrast, and a number of chemotherapeutic agents. Acute drug reactions may cause the rapid development of diffuse, confluent air space opacities or patchy, multifocal, confluent opacities (as seen in Chapter 16). These acute reactions are the result of edema, hemorrhage, or DAD, which may resemble ARDS. Subacute and chronic reactions include eosinophilic pneumonia, COP, and NSIP. The more chronic reactions cause air space opacities in the early stages but later progress to cause reticular opacities, indicating a fibrotic reaction. Pleural effusions (see Chart 4.1) may also be associated with some of these reactions. This is especially true of drugs that are known to cause a lupus-like reaction.[489]

Anaphylaxis is an acute response to a variety of substances and is a cause of edema. Acute alveolar edema may occur following administration of IV radiologic contrast, morphine, heroin, and other opiates. Cocaine has been reported as a cause of both cardiac and noncardiac pulmonary edema.[201,473] Although the mechanism for the noncardiac pulmonary edema is unknown, it is generally believed to represent an idiosyncratic reaction with an alveolar capillary injury. Since the opiates cause central nervous system depression, there may also be a relationship to neurogenic edema. Methadone, a slow-acting narcotic, may cause a slower onset of edema than heroin or morphine, and may also resolve more slowly.[201,671] The typical radiographic pattern for narcotic-induced edema is diffuse, bilateral, confluent air space opacification without cardiomegaly and without pleural effusion. In contrast to narcotics, the allergic edema of interleukin-2 commonly causes interstitial edema (as seen in Chapter 18) with septal lines and peribronchial edema.[90,518] This so-called *allergic edema* infrequently becomes more severe with the development of alveolar edema.[291]

Acute DAD causes permeability edema with the radiologic appearance of diffuse confluent opacities that may sometimes appear multifocal. Therefore, in its early stages, DAD may be indistinguishable from hydrostatic pulmonary edema. The acute edema is rapidly followed by cellular necrosis, inflammation, and later fibrosis. Bleomycin, busulfan, and cyclophosphamide are all possible causes of DAD, and the resulting ARDS is the most severe life-threatening drug reaction.

Eosinophilic pneumonia is a true allergic reaction. Diffuse confluent air space opacities with a peripheral distribution are typical. Histologic changes include infiltration of alveolar walls with eosinophils and other inflammatory cells. Peripheral eosinophilia is also a common finding. Eosinophilic pneumonia responds well to withdrawal of the medication but sometimes requires steroid therapy for complete resolution. Nitrofurantoin is a urinary antibiotic that may cause eosinophilic pneumonia.

COP, previously known as BOOP (*b*ronchiolitis *o*bliterans *o*rganizing *p*neumonia), is more likely to produce multiple areas of diffuse confluent opacity. Like eosinophilic pneumonia, the opacities tend to be in the periphery of the lung. CT often shows the areas of consolidation to be more nodular than expected from the radiograph. Even though there is histologic evidence of fibrosis, this reaction usually responds well to withdrawal of the drug and steroid therapy.[489] Amiodarone, bleomycin, methotrexate, and nitrofurantoin are all possible causes of COP.

NSIP is more likely to present with minimal patchy or multifocal basilar opacities that may appear confluent on the chest radiograph. HRCT shows mainly ground-glass opacity with some reticular opacities. This reaction is more likely to progress to interstitial fibrosis with reticular opacities, honeycombing, and traction bronchiectasis.[489] Amiodarone and methotrexate are also causes of NSIP.

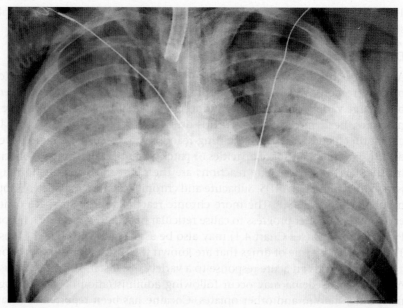

Fig. 15.5 Diffuse pulmonary consolidations in this case are the result of acute respiratory distress syndrome. This appearance is radiologically indistinguishable from diffuse pneumonia and other causes of pulmonary alveolar edema. In the early stages of diffuse alveolar damage, the alveoli are filled by edema resulting from alveolar capillary leak. The pneumomediastinum is the result of barotrauma caused by positive pressure ventilation.

The diagnosis of drug reaction is best suggested by a history of medication with any of the drugs known to produce pulmonary reactions. In patients who are undergoing chemotherapy for cancer, the differential includes the following: (1) opportunistic infection; (2) diffuse hemorrhage; (3) drug reaction; and (4) spread of the primary tumor.[94]

Acute Respiratory Distress Syndrome

ARDS is a complex clinical syndrome that may occur after a variety of severe pulmonary injuries[130] including trauma, shock, sepsis, severe pulmonary infection, transfusion reaction, or cardiopulmonary bypass. These conditions cause an alveolar capillary injury with leakage of edematous fluid into the alveolar spaces. This is so severe that increasing concentrations of inspired oxygen are required to maintain adequate arterial oxygen saturation, while at the same time high ventilator pressures are needed to combat the decreasing lung compliance. The radiologic appearance is that of diffuse coalescent opacities similar to those described for alveolar edema, alveolar hemorrhage, or diffuse air space pneumonia. The sequence of events in patients with ARDS, however, is different from that in patients with typical pulmonary edema. Unlike cardiac pulmonary edema, which clears in response to therapy, the edema in ARDS may persist for days to weeks. As the diffuse coalescent opacities begin to clear, an underlying reticular pattern emerges. Patients who succumb to the illness usually have a complex pulmonary reaction that includes the formation of hyaline membranes, extensive fibrosis, and development of areas of organizing pneumonia. Grossly, the lungs are stiff and firm. The mechanisms for this catastrophic course are not completely understood. It has been suggested that diffuse intravascular clotting and platelet aggregation within the capillary bed (disseminated intravascular coagulation) probably lead to interstitial edema, altered capillary permeability, atelectasis, and hyaline membrane formation. This is pathologically described as DAD and includes injury to the capillary endothelium and alveolar epithelium.[291] Oxygen toxicity may also be a factor in the pathogenesis of many cases of ARDS. In addition, bacterial superinfection is very common. This entity should be suspected on the basis of the clinical presentation and the presence of persistent, diffuse, coalescent opacities (Fig 15.5).

Acute Interstitial Pneumonia

AIP is a fulminant form of interstitial pneumonia that was originally described by Hamman and Rich.[217] It is an idiopathic interstitial pneumonia that is often grouped with usual interstitial pneumonia, desquamative interstitial pneumonia, and NSIP. It has a different clinical course in that it occurs in previously healthy individuals and is rapidly progressive with a poor prognosis. The histologic findings are described as DAD and are similar to findings of ARDS. It has even been described as an idiopathic form of ARDS.

The first phase is an exudative reaction that is followed by a proliferative reaction. The chest radiograph typically shows diffuse air space opacities. HRCT may show additional findings of ground-glass opacities and reticular or linear opacities. The proliferative phase may begin after the first week. Additional CT findings that result from the retracting fibrosis during the proliferative phase include architectural distortion, traction bronchiectasis, and cystic spaces.[12,257]

Re-expansion Pulmonary Edema

Re-expansion pulmonary edema is an infrequent complication that occurs after treatment of pneumothorax or a large pleural effusion. Rapid reinflation of the lung probably causes alveolar capillary injury initiated by ischemia. Re-expansion edema is most likely when the lung has been collapsed for a prolonged period of time. In cases of pneumothorax the history often suggests a delay in treatment of more than 24 hours (Fig 15.6, *A* and *B*).

Other Causes

Other causes of pulmonary edema that must be diagnosed on the basis of the clinical history include high-altitude pulmonary edema,[254] amniotic fluid embolism,[537] and fat embolism. As indicated in the previous discussion of smoke inhalation and near-drowning, there may be a delay in the development of the diffuse coalescing opacities with fat embolism, but it should not exceed the time of the fracture by more than 24 to 48 hours. Repositioning or orthopedic manipulation of a fracture occasionally accounts for fat emboli occurring days to weeks after the initial fracture. In the absence of a history of manipulation, however, the development of pulmonary opacities from days to weeks after a fracture is more suggestive of other diagnoses, such as venous thromboembolism or pneumonia.

PULMONARY HEMORRHAGE

Hemorrhage is an important cause of diffuse coalescent opacities because it may lead to extensive air space consolidation (see Fig 15.1, *A* and *B*). Some of the causes of pulmonary hemorrhage, such as anticoagulant therapy and pulmonary contusion, are easily identified from the clinical history. Hemoptysis is a common clinical finding because a large amount of blood fills the lungs.

Bleeding disorders that may lead to pulmonary hemorrhage include hemophilia, anticoagulation therapy, and hematologic malignancy. The differential of diffuse alveolar consolidation in the leukemic patient is that of: (1) opportunistic infection; (2) drug reaction; (3) diffuse hemorrhage; (4) leukemic infiltration; and (5) pulmonary edema. Severe hemoptysis confirms the diagnosis of diffuse pulmonary hemorrhage in such a clinical setting, but the absence of hemoptysis does not exclude the diagnosis.

Drug reactions that result in pulmonary hemorrhage produce radiologic appearances identical to those of alveolar edema. The chest radiograph may show either diffuse, symmetric, confluent opacities with a perihilar or basal distribution, or the pattern of multifocal opacities. Sometimes, HRCT may show that the distribution is more patchy or multifocal than suspected from the radiograph. Additional HRCT findings include ground-glass opacities that indicate less severe alveolar hemorrhage.

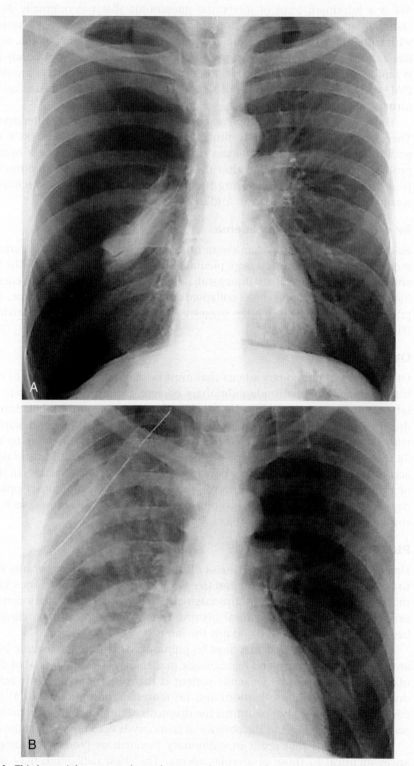

Fig. 15.6 A, This large right pneumothorax has caused near-complete collapse of the right lung. **B,** Following treatment of the pneumothorax with a thoracostomy tube, the patient developed diffuse confluent opacity throughout the right lung. This has been described as re-expansion pulmonary edema.

Anticoagulants, amphotericin B, and some of the cytotoxic drugs are all possible causes of acute pulmonary hemorrhage.[489]

Trauma is not a common cause of diffuse pulmonary hemorrhage, but in the setting of severe trauma, diffuse air space opacities may result from pulmonary contusion (Fig 15.7, *A* and *B*). More frequently, trauma results in asymmetric, localized, or multifocal areas of contusion. The radiologic presentations range from minimal ground-glass opacities on CT to multiple areas of air space opacity or even diffuse air space consolidation. Associated fractures, extrapleural hematoma, and pleural effusion are common associated findings but are not always present. A history of rapid deceleration injury, blunt trauma, or penetrating trauma can confirm the diagnosis of contusion with pulmonary hemorrhage.

Goodpasture syndrome,[522] although not a common entity, must be seriously considered in a patient with hemoptysis, hematuria, and diffuse air space consolidations. The diagnosis is usually confirmed by renal biopsy with specific immunofluorescent stains. Because these patients have antibodies to their glomerular basement membrane, the condition has been renamed *antiglomerular basement membrane disease.*[441]

Idiopathic pulmonary hemosiderosis is another rare pulmonary disease that causes diffuse pulmonary hemorrhage. The radiologic pattern depends on the stage of the disease. In the acute phases, there are bilateral, diffuse coalescent opacities with air bronchograms. As the disease resolves, the clearing may be patchy, leaving the multifocal ill-defined opacities described in Chapter 16. This entity tends to be recurrent with the development of an interstitial pattern that is frequently of a fine reticular nature and occurs as a late complication of the disease. This generally follows many recurrences of the acute alveolar hemorrhage. During the phases of the hemorrhage, the fine reticular pattern is obscured by extensive alveolar consolidation.

Granulomatosis with polyangiitis is a diffuse pulmonary vasculitis that may produce either localized or diffuse pulmonary hemorrhage (see Fig 15.1, *A* and *B*; answer to question 1 is *b*). This diagnosis is easily confirmed when the classic triad of pulmonary, nasopharyngeal, and renal involvement is present. The limited form of granulomatosis with polyangiitis requires lung biopsy for confirmation. Other patterns associated with this entity include multiple ill-defined opacities and multiple lesions that may cavitate (see Chapters 16 and 24). Systemic lupus erythematosus is another collagen vascular disease that sometimes causes diffuse pulmonary hemorrhage.[441]

INFLAMMATORY DISEASES

Acute pulmonary infections are a major consideration in the differential of diffuse coalescent opacities. The entity is commonly distinguished from pulmonary edema on clinical grounds. Patients with diffusely coalescent bilateral pneumonias are usually profoundly ill, with an elevated temperature, elevated white blood cell count, severe dyspnea, and productive sputum.

Pneumonia

Bronchopneumonias are the most common infections producing diffuse coalescent opacities. Gram-negative organisms are particularly notorious for producing such fulminant pneumonias.[235] This pattern is frequently preceded by radiographs showing multifocal ill-defined opacities like those described in Chapter 16. There is a tendency for the patient to have some volume loss because of the bronchial inflammation. The loss of volume may cause one lobe to appear predominantly involved during the course of the illness. In some cases, the radiologic patterns of bronchopneumonia and pulmonary edema are identical, but an asymmetric, patchy, or even unilateral presentation (see Fig 15.2) is more consistent with the diagnosis of bronchopneumonia. (Answer to question 2 is *a*.) It must be remembered that pulmonary edema may also produce a patchy or asymmetric distribution when there is underlying disease such as

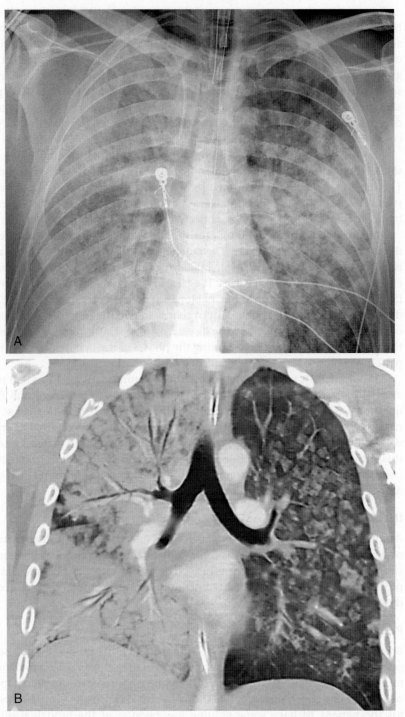

Fig. 15.7 A, Pulmonary contusion should be suspected as the cause of diffuse air space opacities in patients who have sustained major thoracic trauma. In this case, the extensive air space opacities are bilateral but more severe on the right. The patient was in a motor vehicle collision and experienced major rapid deceleration and blunt force trauma. **B,** Coronal computed tomography shows confluent opacities with air bronchograms on the *right* and lobular ground-glass opacities on the *left*.

emphysema or pulmonary embolism. Clinical and laboratory data may be useful in distinguishing bronchopneumonia from pulmonary edema. Bronchopneumonia should result in a febrile response with productive purulent sputum and leukocytosis. Culture of sputum and blood usually confirms the diagnosis and identifies the organisms.[67]

Viral Pneumonia

Viral pneumonias are best known for producing a diffuse interstitial pattern—usually a fine reticular or fine nodular pattern—but fulminant cases may also lead to diffuse air space consolidations. The appearance varies depending on the severity, ranging from ground-glass opacities with areas of consolidation to near-complete alveolar consolidation. This has been reported in detail with descriptions of SARS.[70,322,427] Viral pneumonia may be especially severe in immunologically compromised patients, in particular those with hematologic malignancies, acquired immunodeficiency syndrome (AIDS), or an organ transplant, and especially those who are receiving immunosuppressive therapy. Severe viral pneumonia with air space consolidation is infrequently encountered in the otherwise normal patient.

ARDS is a well-documented complication of a number of viral and mycoplasma infections,[159] and it is a likely explanation for the pattern of diffuse air space opacities in patients with viral pneumonia. Chickenpox pneumonia carries a very high risk for this complication, especially in pregnant patients. ARDS is also a concern with emerging infections including SARS.[44,420] This complication could also be the cause for a high mortality rate in an influenza pandemic.

Aspiration Pneumonia

Aspiration pneumonia is another cause of diffuse coalescent opacities that should be diagnosed by correlating the radiologic appearance with the clinical setting. Aspiration pneumonia may produce diffuse bilaterally coalescent opacities, although these tend to be more localized than in pulmonary edema. Because the aspirated material usually goes to the dependent portions of the lung, the distribution of the radiologic abnormality is directly related to the position of the patient at the time of aspiration. Material aspirated while the patient is in the upright position tends to go to the medial basal segments of the lung and to the right middle lobe, whereas in the supine patient aspirated material tends to collect in the superior segments of the lower lobes and the posterior segments of the upper lobes. Knowledge of the material aspirated and of the patient's position at aspiration often confirms the diagnosis. The clinical setting is very important. For example, the postoperative or comatose patient is very susceptible to aspiration, and alcoholic patients are especially prone to aspiration pneumonia.

Chronic aspiration is often more difficult to confirm and requires careful evaluation of the patient's history. For example, air space consolidation in the right middle lobe in an older patient who is otherwise not particularly ill should prompt suspicion of an exogenous lipoid pneumonia—mineral oil aspiration. This type of aspiration pneumonia should not result in diffuse confluent opacities. Patients with disturbances of esophageal motility, obstructive lesions of the esophagus, and head or neck tumors are all candidates for chronic aspiration. Aspiration may also be the underlying factor in the tendency for these patients to have gram-negative pneumonias. Gram-negative pneumonias are a much more likely cause of diffuse confluent opacities than is uncomplicated chronic aspiration.

Opportunistic Pneumonia

Immunologically compromised patients are susceptible not only to common pyogenic, viral, and fungal pneumonias but also to a more virulent infection. Viral infections that may cause minimal abnormality in a patient with a competent immune system may cause a fatal hemorrhagic pneumonia in a patient with severe immunosuppression.

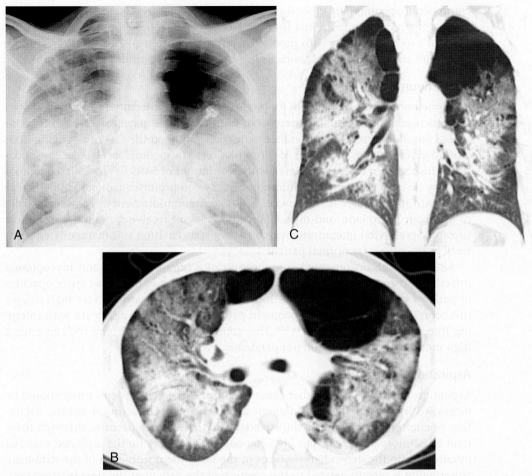

Fig. 15.8   A, Diffuse bilateral confluent opacities in a patient with AIDS are strongly suggestive of pneumocystis pneumonia. **B,** Axial computed tomography (CT) confirms the presence of extensive bilateral alveolar consolidations and ground-glass opacities. The upper lobes are spared because of severe bullous disease. **C,** Coronal CT shows the opacities to have air bronchograms and a distribution resembling pulmonary edema.

Fungi that are nonpathogenic in patients with normal immunity may cause diffuse coalescent opacities in the patient who is immunologically compromised.[423] These uncommon pathogenic fungi include *Aspergillus, Candida, Cryptococcus,* and *Phycomycetes.*[372] Infection by *Phycomycetes* is commonly called *mucormycosis.* Both *Phycomycetes* and *Aspergillus* invade the pulmonary vessels, leading to a diffuse hemorrhagic pneumonia and even pulmonary necrosis or gangrene.

PCP is an AIDS-defining disease and one of the most common infections in patients with AIDS.[196,605] It is not expected to occur until the CD4 cell count has dropped to less than 200 cells/μl.[223,559] The organisms spread through the airways and interstitium with minimal or no visible abnormality on the initial radiograph. During the earliest stages, gallium scans and HRCT are more sensitive for early diagnosis. The earliest chest radiograph appearance is a subtle, fine, reticular pattern, but many cases follow a more fulminant course, with rapid development of diffuse coalescent opacities (Fig 15.8, *A-C*). This results from alveolar wall injury followed by filling of the air spaces with plasma proteins, inflammatory cells, and organisms. The chest radiographic appearance is often that of diffuse symmetric coalescent opacities and resembles noncardiac edema. CT often confirms a mixed pattern of reticular interstitial opacities with thickening of the interlobular septa, ground-glass opacities, and alveolar consolidation. The combination of interlobular septal thickening and ground-glass opacities is common and has been described as the "crazy-paving pattern."[221,490] An atypical upper lobe distribution may be seen in patients who are receiving prophylactic treatment with aerosolized pentamidine.[69,96] Associated pleural effusions are rare in patients with pneumocystis, occurring as infrequently as in 2% of patients, and should be considered evidence of another diagnosis.

Pyogenic pneumonias typically occur in the earlier stages of HIV infection—that is, before the first AIDS-defining disease with a CD4 count between 200 and 500 cells/μl. Bacterial pneumonias may be severe and cause a pattern of diffuse consolidations in approximately 20% of cases, but lobar consolidations are more common with a frequency of 50%. The most common organisms are *Haemophilus influenzae* and *Streptococcus pneumoniae*.[106]

CHRONIC DIFFUSE CONSOLIDATIONS

Diffuse coalescent opacities usually indicate either an acute process, such as pulmonary edema, or the acute phase of a chronic relapsing disease, such as idiopathic pulmonary hemosiderosis. However, although rare, there are a few conditions that cause persistent chronic diffuse pulmonary consolidations. This somewhat rare radiologic presentation may be seen with chronic granulomatous diseases and pulmonary alveolar proteinosis.

Chronic Granulomatous Diseases

Chronic granulomatous diseases rarely cause diffuse coalescent opacities. Fungal infections may produce this pattern in immunologically compromised patients but rarely in the uncompromised host. Although rarely seen in tuberculosis, this pattern may occur when there is extensive pulmonary hemorrhage in conjunction with aspiration of blood to other portions of the lung from a cavitary lesion, or when patients with miliary tuberculosis develop secondary pulmonary edema or ARDS.[405] Once this complication develops, the underlying miliary nodules are obscured by pulmonary edema.

Sarcoidosis is a rare cause of diffuse bilaterally symmetric consolidations that may resemble pulmonary edema. The mechanism for this pattern is considered in detail in Chapter 16. Sarcoidosis more often causes multifocal ill-defined opacities, which may have air bronchograms, than a pattern of diffuse confluent opacities. In contrast to the other entities considered in this chapter, there may be a striking disparity between the severity of the radiologic appearance of sarcoidosis and the clinical well-being of the patient. Although the abnormalities may appear to be very extensive, patients with sarcoidosis are often only mildly dyspneic and may otherwise be asymptomatic.

Alveolar Proteinosis

Alveolar proteinosis[176,487] is an unusual disease that results in diffuse bilateral confluent opacities that often have air bronchograms (Fig 15.9, *A* and *B*). Occasionally, a fine nodular pattern with ill-defined borders may be seen around the periphery of the confluent opacities, but these are not interstitial nodules like the nodules discussed in Chapter 17. They represent acinar nodules and are the smallest unit of air space filling that can be detected radiologically. CT usually confirms extensive air space consolidation, but also reveals ground-glass opacities and thickened interlobular septa,[249] or the crazy-paving pattern.[490] These consolidations may appear acutely and resolve spontaneously or may persist, requiring pulmonary lavage. The time required for their spontaneous resolution is highly variable. Alveolar proteinosis is also observed to be a chronic relapsing disease and one of the few diseases that may produce diffuse air space consolidation while the patient remains relatively asymptomatic. In fact, the radiologic presentation of diffuse bilateral air space consolidations that are either recurrent or chronic in a patient who complains only of mild dyspnea strongly suggests this diagnosis.

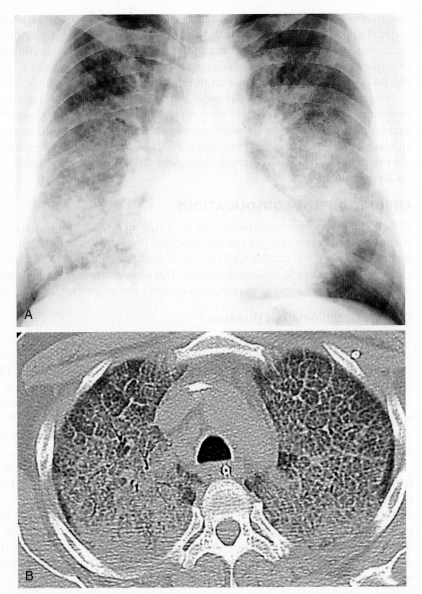

Fig. 15.9 **A,** Diffuse bibasilar confluent opacities fade into the more normal-appearing aerated lung with an intermediate, poorly defined, ground-glass appearance. This radiologic appearance is similar to pulmonary edema, hemorrhage, and diffuse pneumonia, but this patient's opacities were chronic and relapsing. **B,** Axial computed tomography (CT) through the upper lungs confirms extensive ground-glass opacities with associated thickening of the interlobular septa. This combination is described as the *crazy-paving pattern*. These chest radiographic and CT patterns in combination with the history of a chronic and relapsing clinical course are the expected presentation of pulmonary alveolar proteinosis.

Top 5 Diagnoses: Diffuse Air Space Opacities

1. Edema
2. Pneumonia
3. ARDS
4. Pneumocystis
5. Hemorrhage

Summary

Diffuse coalescent opacities with air bronchograms, air alveolograms, and acinar nodules constitute the classic radiologic appearance of alveolar disease.

Pulmonary edema is the most common cause of this pattern. Pulmonary edema may be divided into cardiac and noncardiac categories on the basis of cause. Clinical correlation is extremely important in identifying the cause in pulmonary edema of noncardiac origin.

ARDS is a complex clinical syndrome that results in diffuse coalescing opacities. The diagnosis should be suspected when the patient has acute pulmonary edema following severe injury or shock, particularly after a drug reaction, gram-negative sepsis, transfusion reactions snake bite, or the use of a pump oxygenator in cardiopulmonary bypass surgery.

Diffuse pneumonias are another extremely important cause of diffuse coalescent opacities. They should be easily distinguished from pulmonary edema when seen in an acutely ill and toxic febrile patient. The radiologic appearance is of little value in determining the specific organism. Bacteria, viruses, and fungi may also produce this appearance. Viruses and fungi are more likely in the immunologically compromised host, and a prompt specific diagnosis is essential because failure to initiate immediate therapy may result in death.

Diffuse pulmonary hemorrhage with extensive bilateral confluent opacities is frequently but not invariably associated with hemoptysis. Clinical correlation is essential for determining the cause of diffuse pulmonary hemorrhage (e.g., anticoagulation therapy, hemophilia, leukemia, or trauma). Biopsy is required for a diagnosis of the idiopathic sources of such hemorrhage, including Goodpasture syndrome, pulmonary hemosiderosis, and granulomatosis with polyangiitis.

ANSWER GUIDE

Legends for introductory figures

Fig. 15.1 A, Pulmonary hemorrhage fills the alveoli with blood and often causes bilateral symmetric, coalescent opacities. This patient presented with massive hemoptysis. The bleeding was the result of pulmonary vasculitis from granulomatosis with polyangiitis. **B,** Coronal reconstruction emphasizes the diffuse alveolar consolidation with air bronchograms.

Fig. 15.2 Bronchopneumonia has caused consolidation of the entire right lung. Note the air-filled branching bronchial tree. Air bronchograms are a reliable sign of pulmonary consolidation.

ANSWERS

1. b   2. d   3. a   4. c

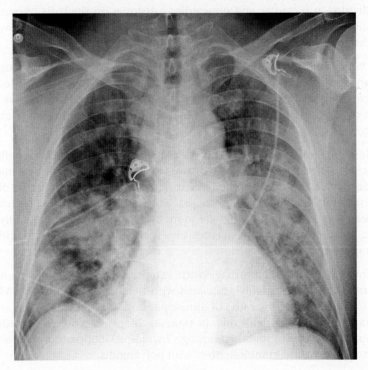

Fig. 16.1

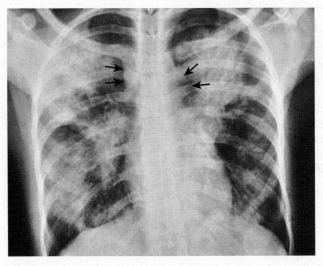

Fig. 16.2

QUESTIONS

1. Which one of the following is the most likely diagnosis in the case seen in Fig. 16.1?
   a. Tuberculosis.
   b. Lung cancer
   c. Melanoma.
   d. Silicosis.
   e. Pneumonia.

2. Referring to Fig. 16.2, the combination of hilar adenopathy and multifocal ill-defined opacities is most consistent with which one of the following?
   a. Granulomatosis with polyangiitis.
   b. Sarcoidosis.
   c. Hypersensitivity pneumonitis.
   d. Langerhans cell histiocytosis.
   e. Choriocarcinoma.

3. The presence of an air bronchogram throughout a large irregular opacity is inconsistent with which one of the following diagnoses?
   a. Silicosis.
   b. Invasive mucinous adenocarcinoma.
   c. Lymphoma.
   d. Granulomatosis with polyangiitis.
   e. Sarcoidosis.

Chart 16.1	**MULTIFOCAL ILL-DEFINED OPACITIES**

I. Infectious diseases
   A. Bacterial pneumonias (*Staphylococcus, Streptococcus, Pseudomonas, Legionella,*[498] *Klebsiella, Haemophilus influenzae,*[428] *Escherichia coli*, other gram-negative bacteria, *Nocardia*[29,145])
   B. Fungal pneumonias (histoplasmosis,[97] blastomycosis,[450] candidiases,[56] actinomycosis,[26,91] coccidioidomycosis, aspergillosis,[591] cryptococcosis[229,346,,499] mucormycosis,[33] sporotrichosis[89])
   C. Tuberculosis[198,388,644]
   D. Viral[95,382,599] and mycoplasma pneumonias[170,250]
   E. Rocky Mountain spotted fever[333,365]
   F. *Pneumocystis jiroveci* pneumonia
   G. Paragonimiasis[416]
   H. Q fever[385]
   I. Atypical mycobacteria in patients with acquired immunodeficiency syndrome (AIDS)[363]
   J. Severe acute respiratory syndrome (SARS)[412]
   K. Septic emboli[312,491]
II. Autoimmune diseases
   A. Sarcoidosis[460]
   B. Granulomatosis with polyangiitis[4,177]
   C. Goodpasture syndrome[441]
   D. Connective tissue diseases (e.g., rheumatoid arthritis, scleroderma, dermatomyositis) complicated by diffuse alveolar damage (DAD)
   E. Systemic lupus erythematosus[441] (lupus pneumonitis or hemorrhage)
III. Neoplasms
   A. Invasive mucinous adenocarcinoma (formerly classified as bronchioloalveolar cell carcinoma)[9,457,597,598]

Continued

Chart 16.1	MULTIFOCAL ILL-DEFINED OPACITIES—cont'd

B. Metastases (e.g., vascular tumors, malignant hemangiomas, choriocarcinoma,[341] adenocarcinoma[526])

C. Kaposi sarcoma in patients with AIDS[209,406,545]

IV. Lymphoproliferative disorders

    A. Non-Hodgkin lymphoma[21,27] (mucosa-associated lymphoid tissue [MALT] lymphoma is most common)[543]

    B. Hodgkin lymphoma (rarely primary in lung)

    C. Lymphomatoid granulomatosis[343,345,543]

    D. Posttransplant lymphoproliferative disorder[119]

    E. Mycosis fungoides[264,362]

    F. Waldenström macroglobulinemia[410,457]

V. Environmental diseases

    A. Hypersensitivity pneumonitis (allergic alveolitis)[86,299,565,570]

    B. Coal worker's pneumoconiosis

    C. Silicosis

VI. Smoking-related diseases

    A. Langerhans cell histiocytosis[1,355]

    B. Desquamative interstitial pneumonitis (DIP)[355,398]

VII. Idiopathic

    A. Amyloid[246,581]

    B. Acute interstitial pneumonitis (AIP)[12]

    C. Cryptogenic organizing pneumonia (COP)[86,329]

    D. Eosinophilic pneumonitis[85,181,344] (idiopathic, drug reaction,[489] or secondary to parasites[175])

VIII. Other disorders

    A. Drug reactions[52,426,434]

    B. Radiation pneumonitis[384,425]

    C. Metastatic pulmonary calcification (secondary to hypercalcemia)[158,228]

    D. Fat emboli

Discussion

Multifocal ill-defined opacities (see Fig 16.1) result from a great variety of diffuse pulmonary diseases (Chart 16.1). This pattern is sometimes referred to as a *patchy alveolar pattern*, but it should be contrasted with the bilaterally symmetric, diffuse, coalescing opacities described as the classic appearance of air space disease in Chapter 15. Many of the entities that cause multifocal ill-defined opacities do result in air space filling, but they also may involve the bronchovascular and septal interstitium. Acute diseases may present as patchy scattered opacities and progress to complete diffuse air space consolidation. Some of the additional signs of air space disease are also encountered in this pattern, including air bronchograms, air alveolograms, and a tendency to be labile.

Because many of the entities considered in the differential are in fact primarily interstitial diseases, complete examination of the chest radiograph may reveal an underlying fine nodular or reticular pattern. Distinction of this multifocal pattern from the fine nodular pattern may also become somewhat of a problem because the definition of the opacities is one of the primary distinguishing characteristics of the two patterns. The description for miliary nodules usually requires that the opacities be sharply defined, in contrast to the less defined opacities currently under consideration. Most entities considered in this differential produce opacities that are larger than 1 to 2 cm in diameter, in contrast to the fine nodular pattern in which the opacities tend to be less than 5 mm in diameter. Additionally, this pattern may result from diseases that cause multiple larger nodules and masses. Some tumors may be locally invasive

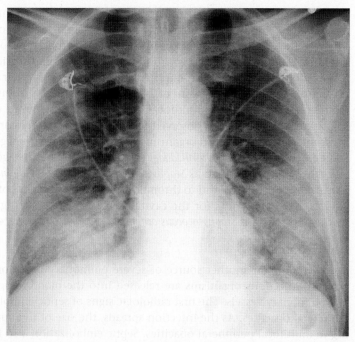

Fig. 16.3 Bilateral multifocal areas of consolidation caused by bronchopneumonia often progress with large areas of multilobar involvement. This patient has bilateral lower lobe consolidations with multiple smaller foci of pneumonia in the upper lobes. As the infection spreads this appearance of multilobar pneumonia may become more uniform and may even resemble pulmonary edema.

and appear ill defined because of their growth pattern, whereas others may develop complications such as hemorrhage. Because the differential for multifocal ill-defined opacities is lengthy, its identification obligates the radiologist to review available serial examinations, carefully evaluate the clinical background of the patient, and recommend additional procedures.

INFECTIOUS DISEASES

Bacterial Bronchopneumonia

Multiple areas of consolidation are the characteristic pattern of bacterial bronchopneumonia (see Fig 16.1; answer to question 1 is *e*). Because this type of infection spreads via the tracheobronchial tree, large areas of air space consolidation are often preceded by lobular opacities[238] that tend to be ill defined because the fluid and inflammatory exudate that produce the opacities spread through the interstitial planes in addition to spilling into the alveolar spaces.[235] In some cases, the lobular pattern may have sharply defined borders where the exudate abuts an interlobular septum. The size of the radiologic opacities depends on the number of contiguous lobules involved. Intervening normal lobules lead to a very heterogeneous appearance. As the infection progresses, the consolidations will begin to coalesce and form a pattern of multilobar consolidation (Fig 16.3) that may even become indistinguishable from the diffuse confluent pattern commonly associated with alveolar edema. This is a common pattern for hospital-acquired pneumonias.

The radiologic patterns of bronchopneumonia are determined by the virulence of the organism and the host's defenses. The primary sites of injury are the terminal and respiratory bronchioles. The disease starts as an acute bronchitis and bronchiolitis. The large bronchi undergo epithelial destruction and infiltration of their walls by polymorphonuclear leukocytes. Epithelial destruction results in ulcerations that are covered with a fibrinopurulent membrane and that contain large quantities of multiplying organisms. As the inflammatory reaction spreads through the walls of the bronchioles to involve the alveolar walls, there is an exudation of fluid and inflammatory cells into the acinus, which results in the pattern of multifocal consolidations. As noted in Chapter 15, patients with bronchopneumonia occasionally have only one lobe predominantly involved, but there are almost always other areas of involvement. An unusually virulent organism or failure of the patient's immune response leads to rapid enlargement of the multifocal opacities and, finally, to diffuse air space consolidations. This has been observed in patients infected by common organisms and those infected with unusual organisms, including those with Legionnaires' disease and those infected by *Legionella micdadei* (Pittsburgh pneumonia agent).[311,436] With more aggressive organisms, such as *Staphylococcus aureus* and *Pseudomonas*, a necrotic bronchitis and bronchiolitis lead to thrombosis of lobular branches of the small pulmonary arteries, which accounts for the cavitation seen in necrotizing pneumonias such as methicillin-resistant *Staphylococcus aureus* (MRSA; see Chapter 24).

Septic Emboli

Septic emboli are another source of severe pulmonary infection that occurs when a bolus of infectious organisms are released into the blood and spread to the peripheral pulmonary vessels. The first radiologic signs of septic emboli are small, ill-defined peripheral opacities. As the infection spreads, the size of the opacities increases, leading to multifocal peripheral opacities. Septic embolization also has a high probability of cavitation, which makes it different from many of the other causes of this pattern. Clinical correlation is essential in the diagnosis of septic embolization. There should be a history of a significant febrile illness. Risk factors for septic embolism include sepsis, osteomyelitis, cellulitis, carbuncles, and right-sided endocarditis. Patients with right-sided endocarditis frequently have a history of intravenous drug abuse and are at increased risk for MRSA infection.

Viral Pneumonia

Viruses produce their effect in the epithelial cells of the respiratory tract, leading to tracheitis, bronchitis, and bronchiolitis.[295] The bronchial and bronchiolar walls become very edematous, congested, and infiltrated with lymphocytes. The bronchial infiltrate may extend into the surrounding peribronchial tissues, which become swollen. This infiltrate spreads into the septal tissues of the lung, leading to a diffuse, interstitial, mononuclear, cellular infiltrate. The changes in the airways may extend to the alveolar ducts, but most severe changes occur proximal to the terminal bronchioles. The adjacent alveolar cells, both type 1 and type 2, become swollen and detached. These surfaces then become covered with hyaline membranes. In fulminant cases, there are additional changes in the alveoli. The alveoli are filled with a mixture of blood, edema, fibrin, and macrophages. In the most severely affected areas, there is focal necrosis of the alveolar walls and thrombosis of the alveolar capillaries, leading to necrosis and hemorrhage.

The radiologic pattern of a viral pneumonia depends on both the virulence of the organism and host defenses.[50] The mildest cases of viral infection are confined to the upper airways and manifest no radiologic abnormality. The earliest radiologic abnormalities are the signs of bronchitis and bronchiolitis, which may include peribronchial thickening and signs of air trapping. When the infection spreads into the septal tissues, a reticular pattern with interlobular septal lines may result, as described in Chapter 18. The more serious cases lead to hemorrhagic edema and areas of air space consolidation. These opacities may be small and appear as a fine nodular pattern similar to that described in Chapter 17, but the nodules tend to be less well defined than the classic miliary pattern. As the process spreads, lobular consolidations develop, as in bacterial bronchopneumonia. In the most severe cases, the lobular consolidations may coalesce into diffuse consolidation, resembling pulmonary edema or bacterial bronchopneumonia.

Influenza viral pneumonia should be suspected in patients with typical influenza symptoms of fever, dry cough, headache, myalgia, and prostration. As the infection spreads to the lower respiratory tract, the patient notices an increased production of sputum that may be associated with dyspnea, pleuritic chest pain, or both. Physical examination reveals rales that may be accompanied by diminished or harsh breath sounds. Because of the bronchial involvement, wheezes are occasionally noted. High-resolution computed tomography (HRCT) may reveal multifocal ground-glass opacities while the chest radiograph appears to be normal. The chest radiographic patterns evolve from a minimal reticular pattern to small, ill-defined nodules to lobular consolidations, and finally to diffuse confluent opacities. Influenza pneumonia may be complicated by adult respiratory distress syndrome or superimposed bacterial pneumonia. At this time, laboratory examination of the sputum and blood becomes paramount to rule out a superimposed bacterial bronchopneumonia. The organisms most likely to present a superimposed bacterial infection are pneumococci, staphylococci, streptococci, and *H. influenzae*. In this clinical setting, the development of a superimposed cavity virtually confirms a superimposed bacterial infection. Other causes of viral pneumonia are less commonly encountered in patients with normal immunity, but have been reported with hanta viruses, Epstein-Barr virus, adenoviruses,[295] and SARS.[412]

Fulminating cases of viral pneumonia are rarely encountered in patients with normal immunity but may occur in patients with suppressed immune systems including those receiving high-dose steroid therapy, patients receiving chemotherapy, patients with AIDS, organ transplant patients, pregnant women, and older adults. Herpes simplex, varicella, rubeola, cytomegaloviruses, and adenoviruses occur mainly in immunocompromised patients.[295]

Varicella pneumonia characteristically occurs from 2 to 5 days after the onset of the typical rash. It is most commonly noted in infants, pregnant women, and adults with altered immunity. Approximately 10% of adult patients may have some degree of pulmonary involvement. In contrast to what is seen in bacterial pneumonias, sputum examination shows a predominance of mononuclear cells and giant cells. As in the consideration of other viral pneumonias, the possibility of superimposed bacterial infection is best excluded by laboratory examination of the sputum and blood. Because the viruses of herpes zoster and varicella are identical, patients with an atypical herpetic syndrome consisting of a rash with pain that follows the nerves of a single dermatome are also at increased risk for development of this type of pneumonia.

Rubeola (measles) pneumonia may be more difficult to diagnose by clinical criteria because the pneumonia occasionally precedes the development of the rash. As with other viral pneumonias, the clinical findings are nonspecific and consist of fever, cough, dyspnea, and minimal sputum production. Increasing sputum production requires exclusion of a superimposed bacterial pneumonia. Timing is important for evaluating a pneumonia associated with measles. The development of primary viral pneumonia in rubeola is synchronous with the first appearance of a rash, whereas secondary bacterial pneumonias are most likely to occur from 1 to 7 days after the onset of the rash. Bacterial infection is strongly suggested in the patient with a typical measles rash whose condition improves over a period of days before pneumonia develops. A third type of pneumonia associated with measles pneumonia is histologically referred to as *giant cell pneumonia*. This may follow overt measles in otherwise normal healthy children, but children with an altered immune system may develop subacute or chronic, but often fatal, pneumonias. Pathologically, giant cell pneumonia is characterized by an interstitial mononuclear infiltrate with giant cells.

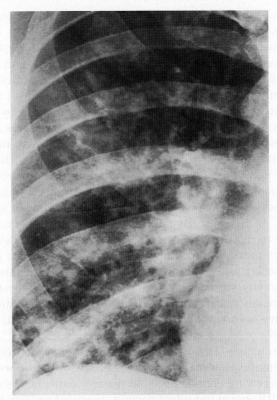

Fig. 16.4 Histoplasmosis is caused by a fungus and is well known to produce a radiologic appearance similar to that of lobular pneumonia.

Cytomegalic inclusion disease[2] has few distinguishing clinical features, has a radiologic presentation suggestive of bronchopneumonia, and is frequently fatal in patients who are immunosuppressed. Histologically, the lung reveals a diffuse mononuclear interstitial pneumonia accompanied by considerable edema in the alveolar walls that may even spill into the alveolar spaces. In addition, the alveolar cells have characteristic intranuclear and intracytoplasmic occlusions. The radiologic opacities are the result of cellular infiltrates in the interstitium, as well as intra-alveolar hemorrhage and edema. Other viruses, including the coxsackie viruses, parainfluenza viruses, adenoviruses, and respiratory syncytial viruses, may result in disseminated multifocal opacities. When the course of the viral infection is mild, confirmation is rarely obtained during the acute phase of the disease, but may be made by viral culture or acute and convalescent serologic studies.

Rickettsial Infection

Rocky Mountain spotted fever is a lesser known cause of pulmonary vasculitis that may lead to the appearance of multiple areas of air space consolidation and even an appearance similar to that of pulmonary edema.[333,365] This rickettsial infection also results in a diffuse vasculitis. It is best diagnosed by the clinical findings of a rash and central nervous system findings. A history of tick bite and an increase in antibody titers strongly support the diagnosis.

Granulomatous Infections

Histoplasmosis[97] (Fig 16.4) is the most likely of the granulomatous infections to produce ill-defined multifocal opacities of varying sizes. This form of histoplasmosis is usually seen after a massive exposure to *Histoplasma capsulatum*. This organism is a soil contaminant found primarily in the Mississippi and Ohio River valleys, and histoplasmosis should be suspected when this pattern is seen in acutely ill patients from these endemic areas. A history of prolonged exposure to contaminated soil is frequently obtained and helps confirm the diagnosis. A marked rise in serologic titers is also confirmatory. The radiologic course is characterized by gradual healing of the process, involving contraction of the opacities; resolution of a large number of opacities; and the development of a pattern of scattered, more circumscribed nodules. This may precede the characteristic appearance of multiple calcifications that develops as a late stage of histoplasmosis.

Blastomycosis[142,450] and coccidioidomycosis[373] are two other fungal infections likely to result in this pattern. These fungi are also soil contaminants with a well-defined geographic distribution. Coccidioidomycosis is primarily confined to the desert Southwest of the United States, although the fungus may be found as a contaminant of materials such as cotton or wool transported from this area. The geographic distribution of blastomycosis is less distinct than that of histoplasmosis or coccidioidomycosis, but it is generally confined to the eastern United States, with numerous cases reported from Tennessee and North Carolina.

Opportunistic fungal diseases,[98] such as candidiasis,[173] cryptococcosis,[502] aspergillosis,[172,591] and mucormycosis, may produce this pattern but are rarely encountered in patients who are immunologically normal. Aspergillosis and mucormycosis[33] are part of a small group of pulmonary infections that tend to invade the pulmonary arteries. These invasive fungal infections produce multifocal areas of consolidation as a result of pulmonary hemorrhage and infarction. Invasive aspergillosis is a cause of masses with ill-defined borders that may have the appearance of a halo on HRCT. Infarction causes cavities that are often filled with a mass of necrotic tissue that causes the appearance of an air crescent sign on both chest radiographs and computed tomography (CT) scans.[524]

Tuberculosis[388] less commonly produces multifocal ill-defined opacities, but should be strongly considered in the case of an apical cavity followed by the development of this pattern. In such an instance, the opacities most probably are the result of bronchial dissemination of the organisms.

Large, poorly defined, mass-like opacities may form by the coalescence of small nodules.[244] The diagnosis is confirmed by sputum stains for acid-fast bacilli or by cultures.

AUTOIMMUNE DISEASES

Sarcoidosis

Sarcoidosis[235,457,460] is a well-documented cause of the radiologic appearance of bilateral nodular or even mass-like foci (Fig 16.5, *A* and *B*). These opacities often have ill-defined borders, sometimes becoming confluent and showing air bronchograms (see Fig 16.2). The clinical manifestation of sarcoidosis is in striking contrast to that of the other inflammatory conditions. Patients with sarcoidosis are afebrile and often virtually asymptomatic, although they may complain of mild dyspnea. This marked disparity of the radiologic and clinical findings virtually eliminates all of the entities considered so far in this chapter. When the pattern of multifocal ill-defined opacities is combined with bilaterally symmetric hilar adenopathy and the typical clinical presentation of the disease, the diagnosis becomes nearly certain. In this diffuse pulmonary disease, the diagnosis is easily confirmed by transbronchial biopsy.

The pathologic explanations for this presentation of sarcoidosis have stimulated considerable discussion in the radiologic literature. Some authors describe this pattern as nodular sarcoidosis, whereas others consider it to be an alveolar sarcoidosis. The radiologic features supporting the appearance of alveolar sarcoidosis are primarily those of confluent opacities with ill-defined borders, which may contain air bronchograms. It should be noted that sarcoidosis rarely causes bilaterally symmetric confluent

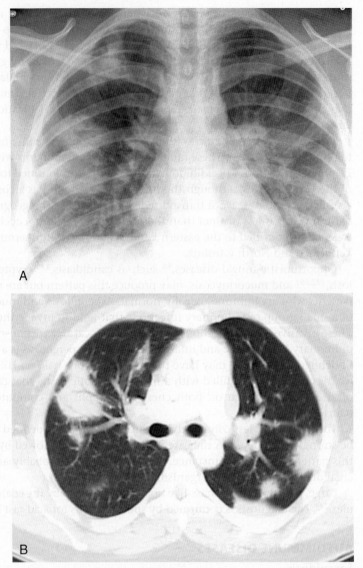

Fig. 16.5 **A,** Multifocal opacities often resemble nodules and masses. **B,** The presence of air bronch-ograms and less well-defined borders on this computed tomography scan make metastatic nodules a less likely diagnosis. This is a multinodular manifestation of sarcoidosis.

opacities with a bilateral perihilar (butterfly) distribution, as seen in alveolar edema, pulmonary hemorrhage, or alveolar proteinosis. Consequently, sarcoidosis is not a serious consideration in the differential of the pattern considered in Chapter 15. Heitzman[235] reported histologic evidence that patients with this "alveolar pattern" may have massive accumulations of interstitial granulomas, which by compression of air spaces could mimic an alveolar filling process. This is essentially a form of compres-sive atelectasis. The histologic observation of a massive accumulation of interstitial granulomas can easily be confirmed by examination of a number of cases with this radiologic pattern. Therefore, this mechanism almost certainly accounts for some cases with this pattern.

One feature of the consolidation of sarcoidosis that is not readily explained by the foregoing observation is their very labile character. Frequently, the opacities accumu-late and disappear dramatically, either spontaneously or in response to steroid treat-ment. It seems unlikely that a massive accumulation of well-organized granulomas could resolve in a matter of days or even a few weeks. Another explanation for this radiologic pattern of fluffy opacities with ill-defined borders and air bronchograms is based on the frequent presence of peribronchial granulomas that cause bronchial obstructions. Peribronchial granulomas are frequently observed on bronchoscopy and HRCT.[335] Distal to these bronchial obstructions there is, in fact, alveolar filling, not by sarcoid granulomas but by macrophages and proteinaceous material. Histologically, this pattern is basically an obstructive pneumonia. The clinical variability of alveolar sarcoidosis is probably accounted for by these two major histologic explanations. For instance, the confluent heavy accumulation of sarcoid granulomas with resultant compressive atelectasis would not be expected to resolve in a short time, whereas the smaller accumulations of granulomas in the peribronchial spaces with distal obstruction could account for cases that follow a much more labile course and respond dramatically to steroid therapy. It should be emphasized that obstructive pneumonia in sarcoidosis is secondary to the obstruction of small distal bronchi and bronchioles. It is very rare for sarcoid granulomas to obstruct large bronchi and produce lobar atelectasis.

Granulomatosis

Granulomatosis with polyangiitis and its variants are probably the best-known sources of pulmonary vasculitis.[146,343,345] Clinical correlation is extremely important because the classic form is associated with severe paranasal sinus and kidney involvement. A history of multifocal ill-defined opacities on the chest radiograph, hemoptysis, and hematuria strongly suggests granulomatosis with polyangiitis or one of its variants. The opacities appearing on the chest radiograph are areas of edema, hemorrhage, or even lung tissue necrosis. Ischemic necrosis results in cavitary opacities in approximately 25% of patients with granulomatosis with polyangiitis. These opacities are more likely to be the result of the vasculitis with ischemia than to the granulomas. Perivascular granulomas, in fact, may be very small and may contribute minimally to the radiologic opacities. Granulomatosis with polyangiitis frequently requires careful histologic evaluation to differentiate it from other diseases that have been referred to as the *pulmonary renal syndromes,* including Goodpasture syndrome and idiopathic pulmonary hemosiderosis.

NEOPLASMS

Neoplasms are not generally regarded as a common cause of multifocal ill-defined opacities in the lung. However, there are a few neoplasms that do produce this pattern and are somewhat characteristic in their radiologic appearance when compared with other pulmonary tumors.

Invasive mucinous adenocarcinoma[457,587,597,598] (Fig 16.6) is the primary lung tumor most likely to produce the radiographic appearance of multifocal ill-defined opacities, which often have air bronchograms.[647] The biologic behavior of this tumor is significantly different from that of most other primary lung tumors because it tends to spread along the alveolar walls while leaving them intact. At the same time the tumor spreads along the walls, there is a tendency for it to produce significant amounts of mucus, which may contribute to the ill-defined opacities. The preservation of the underlying lung architecture permits the tumor to spread around open bronchi and gives rise to air bronchograms. This radiologic pattern of multifocal ill-defined opacities resembles bronchopneumonia and requires careful clinical correlation. The HRCT patterns of invasive mucinous adenocarcinoma are usually a mixture of ground-glass opacities and air space consolidations with air bronchograms.[575]

Metastases rarely present as multifocal opacities with ill-defined borders. The ill-defined borders likely result from the superimposition of a large number of masses and nodules or from the invasive growth of masses into the surrounding lung. Poorly marginated metastases may also result from surrounding opacities, including atelectasis or bleeding that obscures the margin of the masses. It has been suggested that

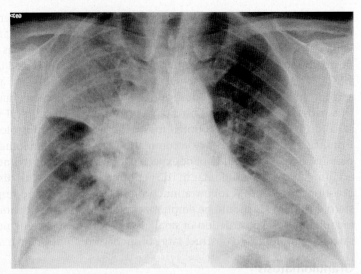

Fig. 16.6 Invasive mucinous adenocarcinoma fills the air spaces with mucus and tumor cells. Bronchogenic dissemination accounts for the appearance of multifocal air space opacities that may progress to cause extensive consolidations.

choriocarcinoma is frequently complicated by bleeding around the periphery of the tumor, giving the radiologic appearance of ill-defined opacities. However, Libshitz et al.[341] have presented more than 100 cases showing that this occurrence is exceptional.

LYMPHOPROLIFERATIVE DISORDERS

Lymphoma[21,328,457,460] is the most common of the pulmonary lymphoproliferative disorders, with non-Hodgkin lymphoma being the most common (Fig 16.7, *A* and *B*). The MALT subtype of B cell lymphoma is the most common primary lymphoma of the lung, but primary lymphoma of the lung is rare at 1% of all lung malignant tumors.[543] When lymphoma involves the lung parenchyma, primarily or secondarily, it spreads via the perivascular and peribronchial tissues and even by way of the interlobular septa. Histologically, its spread is considered to be an interstitial process. However, it is also well known that lymphomatous involvement of the lung may present with consolidative opacities that have ill-defined borders and air bronchograms.[337] There are at least three feasible explanations for this radiographic appearance of lymphoma: (1) the massive accumulation of tumor cells may destroy the alveolar walls and break into the alveolar spaces; (2) there may essentially be a compressive atelectasis or collapse of the alveolar spaces by the massive accumulation of lymphoma cells in the interstitium; and (3) because of the peribronchial infiltration, there may be an obstructive pneumonitis with secondary filling of the distal air spaces by fluid and inflammatory cells rather than by lymphoma cells.

Lymphomatoid granulomatosis was described by Liebow[343] and Liebow et al[345] as an angioinvasive, lymphoproliferative B cell disorder. It involves the lungs but may also involve the skin and central nervous system. Chest radiographic findings include multifocal consolidations, nodules, and masses. Minimal adenopathy has been found in a small number of cases and probably represents reactive hyperplasia.[543] The presence of lymphadenopathy should probably be regarded as a warning to question the diagnosis and suspect progression to lymphoma.

ENVIRONMENTAL DISEASES

The environmental diseases most frequently associated with the pattern of multifocal ill-defined opacities include acute hypersensitivity pneumonitis, silicosis, coal workers' pneumoconiosis,[299,429,565,570] and some of the smoking-related diseases.

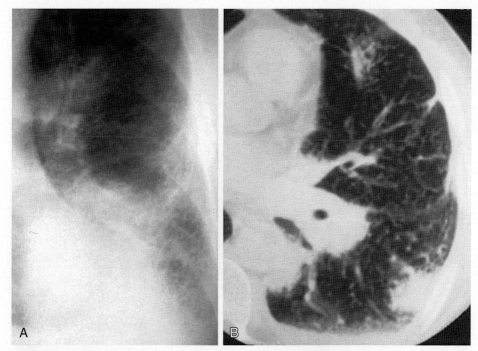

Fig. 16.7 A, Pulmonary lymphoma is a cause of poorly circumscribed masses that may resemble consolidations. This case shows a large opacity in the left lower lobe, a peripheral subpleural opacity, and an opacity above the left hilum. There is also a subtle, diffuse, fine reticular pattern. **B,** Computed tomography section of the same case of lymphoma shows multiple ill-defined opacities. There is an air bronchogram through the most anterior opacity, which has the appearance of a consolidation. There is also diffuse thickening of the interlobular septae. These findings are all the result of lymphomatous masses and interstitial infiltration.

Hypersensitivity pneumonitis is an allergic reaction at the alveolar capillary wall level to mold and other organic irritants. Initially it is an acute reaction consisting of edema with an inflammatory infiltrate in the interstitium. This inflammatory infiltrate may gradually be replaced by a granulomatous reaction with some histologic similarities to sarcoid granulomas. The multiple confluent opacities with air bronchograms tend to represent the acute phase of the disease, and a nodular or even a reticular pattern may be seen in the later stages. Confirmation of the diagnosis is best obtained by establishing a history of exposure followed by skin testing, serologic studies, and correlation with HRCT. Exposure histories are varied; they include molds and fungi from sources such as moldy hay in farmer's lung, bird fancier's disease, bagassosis from mold in sugar cane, mushroom worker's lung, and hot tube lung. Hot tube lung may differ from the other causes of hypersensitivity pneumonitis in that it is a reaction to *Mycobacterium avium* complex (MAC)[227] rather than to molds.

Silicosis and coal workers' pneumoconiosis are inhalational diseases that frequently result in multiple opacities. The border characteristics of these opacities are quite different from those considered in the remainder of this discussion. These borders tend to be more irregular rather than truly ill defined. The irregularities are the result of strands of fibrotic reaction around the conglomerate masses. In addition, the opacities tend to be much more homogeneous because they represent large masses of fibrotic reaction. There should be no normal intervening alveoli to give a soft heterogeneous appearance. Furthermore, there should be no evidence of air bronchograms. (Answer to question 3 is *a.*) These opacities tend to be in the periphery of the lung with an upper lobe predominance. However, they are frequently not pleural-based; rather, they appear to parallel the chest wall. The opacities are usually bilateral but may be asymmetric. As they enlarge, they are often mass-like and described as *progressive massive fibrosis* (Fig 16.8).

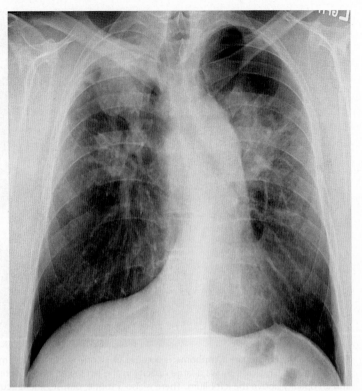

Fig. 16.8 Upper lobe opacities in this case of coal workers' pneumoconiosis are similar to those of other cases in this chapter. The associated coarse reticular opacities are the result of interstitial scars. Progressive fibrosis causes the larger opacities to have irregular rather than ill-defined borders. This is often described as progressive massive fibrosis.

A history of exposure in mining or sandblasting is usually confirmatory. Coal workers' pneumoconiosis is radiologically indistinguishable from silicosis. Comparison with old examinations is essential to ensure stability and eliminate the possibility of a new super-imposed process, such as tuberculosis or neoplasm.

SMOKING-RELATED DISEASES

Langerhans cell histiocytosis (LCH) is a smoking-related[1,355] inflammatory condition that may present with a variety of patterns, including nodules ranging in size from 1 to 10 mm.[1] The nodular opacities are caused by a granulomatous infiltrate with histiocytes, eosinophils, plasma cells, lymphocytes, and Langerhans cells. The nodular phase of the disease is generally believed to represent an early stage of the disease, which precedes the development of reticular opacities, small cavities, or multiple cysts. There is typically an upper lobe predominance in the nodular, reticular, and cystic phases of the disease. HRCT should confirm the presence of nodular and reticular opacities with an upper lobe distribution and is very sensitive for the detection of small peripheral cavities and cystic spaces[42,319] (Fig 16.9, *A* and *B*). LCH is an afebrile illness with much milder symptoms than all of the infectious diseases hitherto considered.

DIP causes filling of the alveoli with macrophages and minimal interstitial fibrosis. In contrast with LCH, it produces ground-glass opacities with a peripheral basilar distribution.[20] The chest radiograph may reveal subtle opacities in the periphery of the lung bases that are difficult to characterize and are best evaluated with HRCT.

IDIOPATHIC DISEASES

Cryptogenic organizing pneumonia (COP),[329] formerly known as *bronchiolitis obliterans with organizing pneumonia* (BOOP), is a subacute or chronic inflammatory process involving

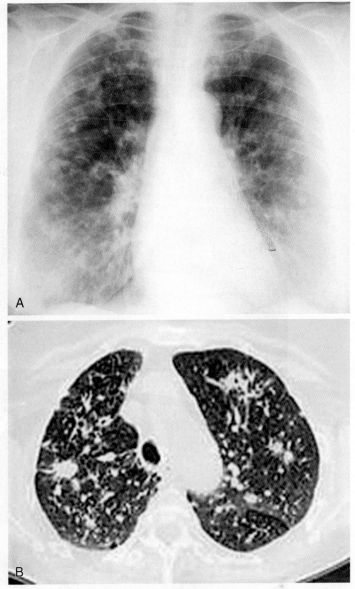

Fig. 16.9 **A,** Langerhans cell histiocytosis is a cause of multifocal, poorly defined nodular opacities with a tendency toward an upper lobe predominance, as illustrated by this case. **B,** High-resolution computed tomography section through the upper chest reveals multiple, poorly defined nodular opacities with interspersed, coarse, reticular opacities.

the small airways and alveoli. COP has extensive alveolar exudate and fibrosis that may resemble or overlap the changes of usual interstitial pneumonia (UIP), but COP can usually be distinguished from UIP. COP has multifocal air space opacities with normal lung volume, whereas UIP has irregular reticular opacities with reduced lung volume. The radiologic presentation resembles that of bronchopneumonia (Fig 16.10, *A* and *B*); patients with the disease are often unsuccessfully treated with antibiotics on the basis of a presumed diagnosis of pneumonia. Corticosteroid therapy has been reported to produce clearing of the radiologic abnormalities, but there is a high relapse rate following steroid withdrawal.

Eosinophilic pneumonias[85,181,344] with peripheral eosinophilia or eosinophilic infiltrates of the lung are often of unknown cause but may occur as a drug reaction or as a response to parasites. Radiologically, these infiltrates appear as patchy areas of air space consolidation that tend to be in the periphery of the lung[86] (Fig 16.11). When these

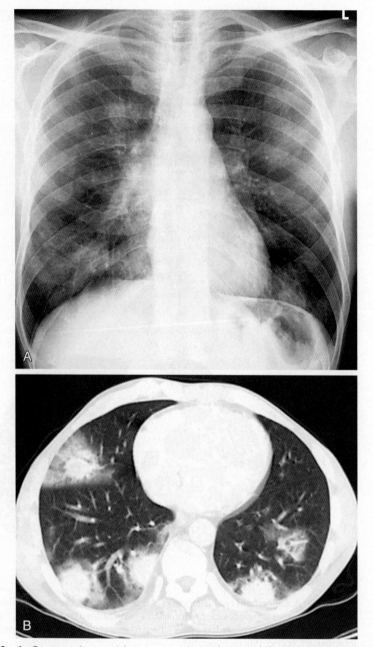

Fig. 16.10   A, Cryptogenic organizing pneumonia produces multifocal ill-defined opacities that resemble bronchopneumonia. **B,** Computed tomography scan reveals multifocal air space consolidations with a halo of peripheral ground-glass opacities and a lower lobe predominance.

eosinophilic infiltrates become extensive, the radiologic picture has been compared with a photonegative picture of pulmonary edema because of the striking peripheral distribution of the opacities.[181] These opacities have very ill-defined borders, tend to be coalescent, and frequently have air bronchograms.

There are two important groups of eosinophilic pneumonias. The first group consists of the idiopathic varieties of eosinophilic pneumonia that are generally divided into those associated with peripheral eosinophilia, referred to as *Loeffler syndrome,* and those that are comprised primarily of eosinophilic infiltrates in the lungs without peripheral eosinophilia, referred to as *chronic eosinophilic pneumonia.* Besides tending to be peripheral, the infiltrates have the additional characteristic of being recurrent and are frequently described as fleeting.[175]

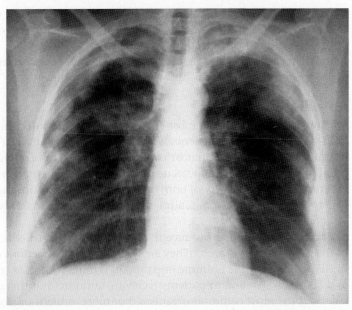

Fig. 16.11 Eosinophilic pneumonia typically produces multifocal ill-defined opacities that tend to be in the periphery of the lung. This is often described as the photonegative of pulmonary edema. Note the peripheral opacities with a clear area between the opacities and central pulmonary arteries.

The second group of pulmonary infiltrates associated with eosinophilia includes those with a known causal agent. A variety of parasitic conditions are associated with pulmonary infiltration and are likewise well known for the association of eosinophilia. These include ascariasis, *Strongyloides* infection, hookworm disease (ancylostomiasis), *Dirofilaria immitis* and *Toxocara canis* infections (visceral larva migrans), schistosomiasis, paragonimiasis, and, occasionally, amebiasis.[175]

Correlation of the clinical, laboratory, and radiologic findings often makes a precise diagnosis of parasitic disease a straightforward matter. For example, *T. canis* infection results from infestation by the larva of the dog or cat roundworm and has a worldwide distribution. The disease is most commonly encountered in children. The symptoms are nonspecific, but there is usually the physical finding of hepatosplenomegaly. There is also marked leukocytosis. In addition, a liver biopsy usually reveals eosinophilic granulomas containing the larvae.

The diagnosis of ascariasis is similarly made by laboratory identification of the organism. Larvae may be detected in sputum or gastric aspirates, whereas the adult forms of ova may be found in stool. The disease is usually associated with a marked leukocytosis and eosinophilia. As mentioned earlier, the chest radiographic appearance is that of nonspecific multifocal areas of homogeneous consolidation that are frequently transient and therefore virtually identical to the opacities described as Loeffler syndrome. Strongyloidiasis, like ascariasis, produces mild clinical symptoms at the same time that the radiograph demonstrates peripheral ill-defined areas of homogeneous consolidation. The diagnosis is made by finding larva in the sputum or in the stool. Exceptions to this clinical course occur in the compromised host. A fatal form of strongyloidiasis has been reported in patients who are immunologically compromised, particularly by corticosteroids.[175]

Amebiasis is different from the other parasitic diseases in both its clinical and radiologic presentations. Patients with amebiasis frequently have symptoms of amebic dysentery and complain of right-sided abdominal pain, which is related to the high incidence of liver involvement. There is often elevation of the right hemidiaphragm because of liver involvement and, as in other cases of subphrenic abscess, there is frequently right-sided pleural effusion. Furthermore, the areas of homogeneous consolidation are not evenly distributed throughout the periphery of the lung, as in other cases of eosinophilic infiltration, but tend to be in the bases of the lungs, particularly in the right lower lobe and right middle lobe. Because the opacities correspond to areas of abscess formation, they occasionally develop cavities.[175]

AIDS-RELATED DISEASES

Pneumocystis is one of the most common pulmonary infections in patients infected with human immunodeficiency virus (HIV). It most often presents with a pattern of uniform bilateral reticular or confluent opacities that often resemble noncardiac pulmonary edema. The appearance of scattered or patchy opacities requires consideration of a greater variety of both infections and neoplasms including bacterial, fungal, and mycobacterial pneumonias, and neoplasms such as lymphoma and Kaposi sarcoma.[538]

Bacterial pneumonias produce the same patterns in patients with HIV infection as in the general population.[106] They are the most likely infections during the early stages of HIV infection while immune impairment is mild, with CD4 cell counts between 200 and 500 cells/μl,[36] and in patients receiving antiretroviral therapy. *Streptococcus pneumoniae* is the most common organism, but more virulent organisms such as *Staphylococcus* should be suspected when the pneumonias are complicated by cavitation.

Tuberculosis in patients who have early HIV infection (CD4 counts between 200 and 500 cells/μl) produces the same patterns seen in patients with normal immunity.[223,531] At this early stage, tuberculosis usually causes apical disease with cavitation. The bronchial dissemination of organisms from an apical cavity may lead to multifocal opacities that resemble bacterial bronchopneumonia. Following the development of AIDS after the CD4 count is lower than 200 cells/μl, patients are at increased risk for miliary tuberculosis[515] with a fine nodular pattern (see Chapter 17), or multifocal air space opacities with hilar or mediastinal adenopathy resembling primary infection.[203]

Fungal infections are less frequent. However, candidiasis, cryptococcosis, histoplasmosis, and coccidioidomycosis have all been reported to produce patterns similar to tuberculosis in patients with AIDS.[93,98,555]

MAC infection most frequently causes diffuse, bilateral, reticular, and nodular opacities in patients with AIDS.[363] In contrast, the patients with normal immunity who are at greatest risk for MAC infection are those with chronic pulmonary disease. In this latter group of patients, MAC may be radiographically indistinguishable from tuberculosis. The reticular pattern of MAC should be coarser and more disorganized than *Pneumocystis* pneumonia (PCP); however, when PCP is chronic, it may result in a similar appearance. When MAC causes air space opacities, the air space opacities are segmental or multifocal, and the multifocal opacities are likely to resemble poorly circumscribed masses. The air space opacities are also often associated with pleural effusions or adenopathy, which may also be seen in tuberculosis but are not expected in pneumocystis pneumonia. Disseminated MAC is a terminal infection that occurs after the CD4 count has declined below 50 cells/μl.

Lymphoma may cause multiple poorly defined masses or multiple nodules. Lymphoma in patients with HIV is usually β-cell non-Hodgkin lymphoma[94] and differs from patients with normal immunity in that AIDS-related lymphomas are more often extranodal.[328,539] Lymphoma is probably the most likely diagnosis of lobulated pulmonary masses in patients with AIDS. These masses often show a very aggressive growth pattern and may double in size within 4 to 6 weeks.

Kaposi sarcoma is the most common AIDS-related neoplasm,[94] but has decreased in frequency for unexplained reasons. It is a highly vascular tumor that involves any mucocutaneous surface and produces characteristic red plaques. It is usually a skin lesion, but it also involves the trachea, bronchi, and lungs. The radiographic appearance of pulmonary opacities may result from atelectasis, hemorrhage, or hemorrhagic masses. Multiple nodules or masses are the most common pattern. More confluent, patchy, air space opacities may resemble PCP. Associated adenopathy or pleural effusions are reported to occur in 90% of patients with Kaposi sarcoma and may help distinguish Kaposi sarcoma from PCP, but their occurrence would not permit the exclusion of mycobacterial infection. Sequential thallium and gallium scanning has been advocated as a technique for distinguishing PCP, Kaposi sarcoma, and lymphoma. *Pneumocystis* is thallium negative but gallium positive on 3-hour delayed images. Lymphomas are thallium and gallium positive, and Kaposi sarcoma is thallium positive but gallium negative.[332] Bronchoscopy may establish the diagnosis of Kaposi sarcoma. Fine-needle aspiration biopsy has also been advocated for the diagnosis of focal and multifocal lesions.[524] Lymphoma is an aggressive and often fatal neoplasm, in contrast to Kaposi sarcoma, which is an indolent, slow-growing tumor that is rarely fatal.

Top 5 Diagnoses: Multifocal Ill-Defined Opacities

1. Pneumonia
2. Sarcoidosis
3. Invasive mucinous adenocarcinoma
4. Granulomatous pneumonias
5. Septic emboli

Summary

Small multifocal ill-defined opacities are distinguished from miliary nodules by evaluation of their borders. Miliary nodules should be sharply defined.

Multifocal ill-defined opacities most commonly result from processes that involve both the interstitium and air spaces. Careful evaluation of the chest radiograph frequently reveals the classic signs for both components of the disease.

Bacterial bronchopneumonias typically present with this pattern, which is a common appearance of hospital-acquired pneumonias.

Histoplasmosis is one of the most common fungi to produce the pattern.

Unusual pulmonary infections, including aspergillosis, mucormycosis, cryptococcosis, and nocardiosis, may lead to the pattern in the patient who is immunocompromised.

Sarcoidosis causes this pattern when there are extensive accumulations of granulomas or when small granulomas occlude bronchioles with a resultant obstructive pneumonia.

Eosinophilic pneumonias should be suspected when the opacities are peripherally located and are recurrent or fleeting.

The large opacities seen in granulomatosis with polyangiitis frequently represent areas of necrosis or of hemorrhage and edema resulting from ischemia. Remember, this is a disease of the vessels.

Invasive mucinous adenocarcinoma is the only primary lung tumor that is expected to produce this pattern.

Lymphoma and other lymphoproliferative disorders of the lung are rare, but this is their most likely appearance. MALT lymphomas are the most common type of primary pulmonary lymphoma.

Kaposi sarcoma in patients with AIDS is an important cause of this pattern. These patients usually have advanced cutaneous Kaposi sarcoma. The pulmonary involvement must be distinguished from lymphoma and opportunistic infection. For unexplained reasons, the incidence of Kaposi sarcoma is declining.

Metastases rarely lead to this pattern but some may be invasive, hemorrhagic, or numerous masses may be superimposed.

Silicosis and coal workers' pneumoconiosis may cause large, bilateral, irregular, upper lobe masses (conglomerate masses). They are fibrotic and should therefore not produce air bronchograms. Peripherally, their margins often parallel the lateral pleura.

Drug reactions frequently result in this pattern. They are best diagnosed by clinical correlation. Biopsy is frequently required in the patient who is immunocompromised to rule out opportunistic infection.

ANSWER GUIDE

Legends for introductory figures

Fig. 16.1   Multifocal ill-defined opacities are a common pattern for bronchial spread of infection and are a common appearance of hospital-acquired pneumonias.

Fig. 16.2   The multifocal ill-defined opacities in this case are very nonspecific, but the observation of enlargement of the nodes in the aortic pulmonary window *(left arrows)* and paratracheal lymph nodes *(right arrows)* combines two patterns and thus narrows the differential. Either sarcoidosis or lymphoma could account for this combination. The fact that the patient is relatively asymptomatic supports the correct diagnosis of sarcoidosis.

ANSWERS

1. e   2. b   3. a

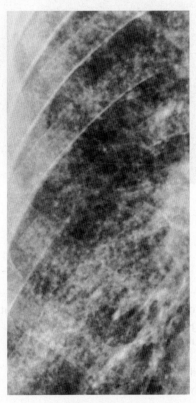

Fig. 17.1

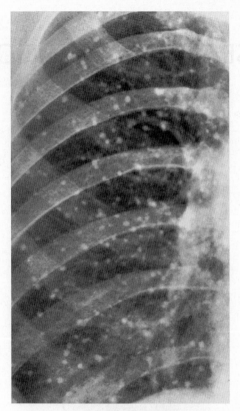

Fig. 17.2

QUESTIONS

1. Based on the radiologic appearance of the case illustrated in Fig. 17.1, which one of the following diagnoses is the most urgent one?
   a. Miliary tuberculosis.
   b. Silicosis.
   c. Langerhans cell histiocytosis.
   d. Hypersensitivity pneumonitis.
   e. Sarcoidosis.

2. Regarding Fig. 17.2, which of the following is the most likely diagnosis?
   a. Sarcoidosis.
   b. Metastatic carcinoma.
   c. Langerhans cell histiocytosis.
   d. Hypersensitivity pneumonitis.
   e. Histoplasmosis.

Mark the following questions **True** *or* **False:**

3. _____ Sarcoidosis and silicosis may present with the pattern seen in Fig. 17.1 in combination with hilar adenopathy.

4. _____ Bronchoscopy with biopsy is contraindicated in the evaluation of patients in whom the pattern is believed to be secondary to tuberculosis.

Chart 17.1	DIFFUSE FINE NODULAR OPACITIES

I. Infections
   A. Tuberculosis[41,235,288]
   B. Fungus infections (histoplasmosis,[97] blastomycosis,[450,561] coccidioidomycosis[373]), Aspergillosis (rare),[46] cryptococcosis (rare)[200,252,321]
   C. Bacterial infections (bronchopneumonia—unusual early presentation), nocardiosis[208]
   D. Viral pneumonia (e.g., varicella)[382,451,599]
II. Environmental diseases
   A. Silicosis and coal workers' pneumoconiosis[80,86,429]
   B. Berylliosis[80,175]
   C. Siderosis[80,175]
   D. Hypersensitivity pneumonitis or allergic alveolitis (farmer's lung)[353,497,570]
   E. Hard metal pneumoconiosis[299]
III. Langerhans cell histiocytosis[1,585]
III. Sarcoidosis[86,103,407]
VIII. Metastatic tumor[175]
   A. Thyroid carcinoma
   B. Melanoma[76]
   C. Other adenocarcinomas (e.g., gastrointestinal tumors)
IX. Other
   A. Alveolar microlithiasis (rare)[467]
   B. Gaucher disease[645]
   C. Granulomatosis with polyangiitis (rare)
   D. Immunotherapy (bacillus Calmette-Guérin)[272]

Discussion

Detection of very small nodules is a serious challenge for the radiologist. Nodules measuring 1 to 3 mm (see Fig. 17.1) are marginally detectable on the chest radiograph and may require high-resolution computed tomography (HRCT) for confirmation (Fig. 17.3, *A* and *B*). Examination of gross specimens often reveals many more nodules of a much smaller size than can be resolved as separate opacities on the chest radiograph. Heitzman suggested that miliary nodules are probably seen on the radiograph because of the effect of summation—that is, a "stacked coin effect."[235] These very small nodules are sometimes more easily appreciated on the posteroanterior view in the costophrenic angle and on the lateral view in the retrosternal clear space. Furthermore, small nodular opacities may occasionally be confused with very small pulmonary vessels seen on end. This mistake is usually avoided by identifying an associated, branching vascular pattern around the nodule. Also, miliary nodules are typically much more diffuse than the fine nodular appearance created by normal vessels.

The sharpness of the borders of the nodules is an important criterion for narrowing the differential. Small opacities may be caused by small, sharply defined interstitial nodules or by minimal involvement of the distal air spaces, which results in ill-defined opacities with an acinar pattern.[175,601] This distinction is the key to limiting the differential. If the pattern includes small, fluffy, or ill-defined opacities, then alveolar edema, exudate, or hemorrhage should be considered. The presence of ill-defined borders should prompt examination of the radiograph for other signs of air space filling disease (see Chapter 15). In contrast, the pattern of very small but sharply defined or discrete opacities should reassure the radiologist that the nodules are more likely interstitial and are thus associated with one of the entities listed in Chart 17.1.

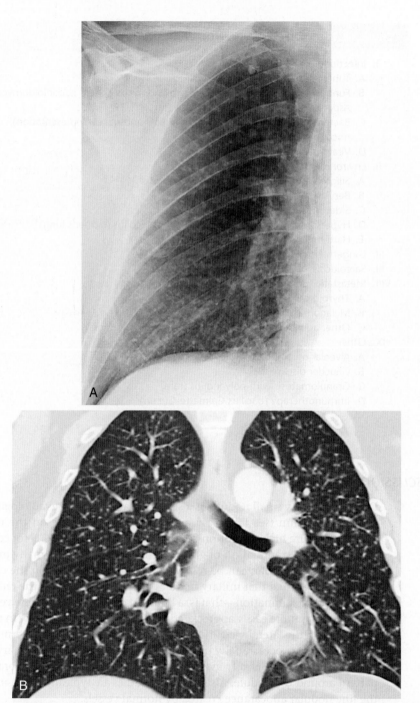

Fig. 17.3   A, Posteroanterior chest radiograph of a patient treated for acute myeloid leukemia with a bone marrow transplant demonstrates increased opacities that are suggestive of diffuse small nodules. **B,** High-resolution computed tomography confirms a random distribution of small nodules suggesting miliary tuberculosis, and transbronchial biopsy confirmed the diagnosis.

Miliary nodules are usually 1 or 2 mm in diameter and not more than 3 mm,[221,601] but size should rarely influence the differential diagnosis because all of the entities listed in Chart 17.1 may produce larger nodules (i.e., up to 3 to 4 mm). It is true, however, that the size of the nodules does occasionally influence the radiologist to favor some members of the differential list over others. For example, the small nodules of Langerhans cell histiocytosis are rarely as small as 1 or 2 mm. Although the very small nodular pattern does not eliminate Langerhans cell histiocytosis from the differential, it makes other diagnoses, such as sarcoidosis, more likely. Very small nodules mixed with larger nodules should not be described as miliary and are more likely to be a clue to suspect metastatic tumor. Because these small nodules usually have no distinguishing features, the radiologist must search for associated radiologic and clinical findings to narrow the differential.

INFECTIOUS DISEASES

Miliary tuberculosis (see Fig. 17.1) results from hematogenous dissemination and almost invariably leads to a dramatic febrile response with night sweats and chills. Exceptions to this clinical presentation are probably the result of altered immune response and are most commonly encountered in older adults, patients receiving steroids or chemotherapy, and patients in the late stages of AIDS with a very low CD 4 count. It must be emphasized that bacteriologic confirmation of miliary tuberculosis is not always easily obtained. Despite the disseminated disease, the miliary nodules are interstitial. Sputum cultures may continue to be negative in the face of miliary tuberculosis because the organisms are primarily in the interstitium rather than in the air spaces. More invasive procedures, such as bronchoscopy with transbronchial biopsy, may be required to confirm the diagnosis (answer to question 4 is *False*). Miliary tuberculosis has a high mortality rate, which requires prompt diagnosis and treatment (answer to question 1 is *a*).

Any of the fungal infections listed in Chart 17.1 may mimic the radiologic appearance of miliary tuberculosis, but this pattern is most commonly the result of histoplasmosis, coccidioidomycosis, or North American blastomycosis. The clinical response to these fungal infections may be more varied than to tuberculosis. For example, some patients have a profound systemic response leading to death, others have a mild, influenza-like syndrome, and a few are minimally symptomatic. In the last instance, the radiologic abnormality may be more impressive than the clinical course. A history of exposure to a specific fungus is occasionally obtained. For example, history of a trip to the desert virtually confirms the diagnosis of coccidioidomycosis, whereas exposure to soil contaminated with bird or chicken droppings in the Ohio River Valley strongly suggests histoplasmosis. Such histories also suggest that the nodules are not always the result of hematogenous dissemination, such as in miliary tuberculosis, but may also be due to an inhaled organism. This difference in cause helps explain some of the clinical and radiologic differences in the two conditions. The acute epidemic form of histoplasmosis produces the radiologic appearance of larger, ill-defined nodules, similar to that of bronchopneumonia (see Chapter 16). As the patient recovers, the nodules may regress in size and become more sharply defined and may even begin to calcify (Fig. 17.4). Therefore, the fine nodular pattern may represent acute hematogenous dissemination of the fungi or the healed phase of the disease. Some patients with histoplasmosis who develop this diffuse nodular pattern are later observed to develop diffuse, small, calcified nodules (answer to question 2 is *e*). Numerous calcified nodules are virtually diagnostic of histoplasmosis, especially when associated with hilar lymph node or splenic calcifications.

Bacterial infections generally do not produce this fine nodular pattern of pulmonary involvement. However, there are occasional reports of early bacterial pneumonias leading to this pattern. *Nocardia*, previously regarded as a fungus, is now considered to be a gram-positive bacterium that rarely causes infection in normal patients but is an opportunistic infection in patients who are immunosuppressed. *Nocardia* may produce a variety of pulmonary patterns, including miliary nodules.[208,467]

Viral pneumonia, especially varicella or chickenpox pneumonia, may result in fine nodules.[382] The nodules represent localized collections of inflammatory cells. When the course of the illness is severe, the pattern may be transient and rapidly

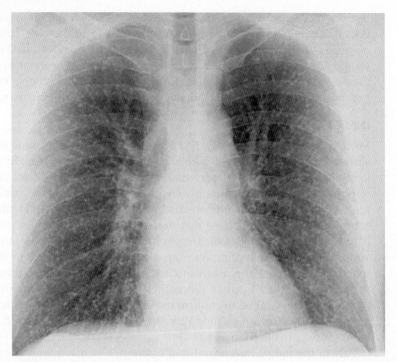

Fig. 17.4   The small nodules seen in this case of histoplasmosis are more circumscribed than expected with miliary spread of infection and likely indicate that the patient has recovered from a transbronchial infection.

followed by larger, multifocal, ill-defined opacities or even diffuse coalescent opacities and is complicated by adult respiratory distress syndrome. Such a course is frequently encountered in patients who are immunosuppressed. As with histoplasmosis, the small nodules caused by varicella pneumonia may heal with the development of multiple, calcified nodules. However, confirmation of this cause of the calcified nodules may be virtually impossible unless the diagnosis of varicella pneumonia is established in the acute phase of illness. Clinical correlation makes diagnosis of the acute illness relatively simple because most patients have the characteristic skin lesions of chickenpox. Chickenpox pneumonia is much more common in adults than in children.

ENVIRONMENTAL DISEASES

Silicosis and coal workers' pneumoconiosis[80,429] are the occupational diseases most commonly associated with the pattern of diffuse fine interstitial nodules. The predicted distribution of fine nodules based on lung volume would favor a basilar predominance, but this is not the case in silicosis. The fine nodules caused by silicosis are predominantly in the upper lobes (Fig. 17.5, *A* and *B*).[214,299] Histologically, these nodules are localized areas of fibrosis, and the summation of shadows probably contributes to the nodular appearance. In many cases of silicosis, the chest radiograph shows a fine reticular and nodular pattern, which suggests that crossing reticulations may contribute to the nodular appearance. Because this a chronic, long-standing process, the nodules may very slowly increase in size and may also calcify. Exposure to free silica occurs in a variety of occupations including sandblasting, quarrying, and coal mining.

There is some controversy as to whether coal workers' pneumoconiosis and silicosis are two separate entities. Radiologic and histologic evidence indicates that the interstitial reaction that results in reticulations, nodules, and conglomerate masses is a stronger reaction to silica than to anthracotic pigments. In most cases, a history of exposure is easily obtained. It is also important to compare the current chest radiograph with old examinations to confirm the stability of the process. Patients with a history of coal

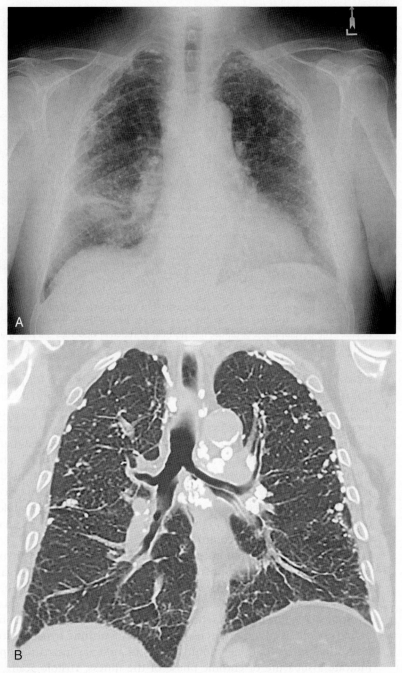

Fig. 17.5 A, Silicosis has caused numerous small nodules that are more conspicuous in this case because of calcification. They have an upper lobe predominance, with the more peripheral nodules appearing to blend in. The patient had a long history of working as a tombstone engraver. **B,** Coronal computed tomography image confirms the peripheral upper lobe predominance of the nodules. Calcified hilar and mediastinal lymph nodes are also consistent with silicosis. This combination could also result from histoplasmosis.

mining are at increased risk for the development of superimposed tuberculosis or silicotuberculosis. A change in the radiographic pattern or the rapid development of diffuse fine, interstitial nodules, in combination with a febrile response and night sweats, is strongly suggestive of tuberculosis rather than simple pneumoconiosis.

Other occupational exposures known to produce diffuse, fine, nodular patterns are berylliosis,[80] hypersensitivity pneumonitis,[501,570] hard metal pneumoconiosis, and

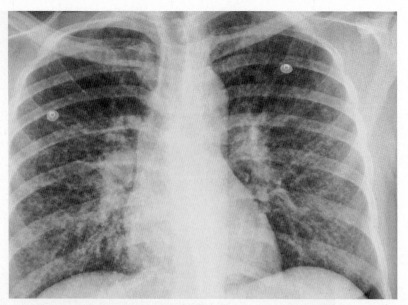

Fig. 17.6 Diffuse fine nodules are a classic but uncommon appearance for lung involvement by sarcoidosis. The expected adenopathy may regress before there is radiologic evidence of interstitial disease. The development of diffuse fine nodular or reticular opacities is a sign that the patient is at risk for the development of advanced pulmonary scarring.

siderosis.[80,299] Asbestosis, on the other hand, is best known for producing reticular or linear opacities, as described in Chapter 18, rather than fine nodular opacities. The diagnosis of berylliosis is usually suggested by a history of exposure. However, the incidence of berylliosis has become rare, primarily because the number of occupations in which there is potential exposure to beryllium has decreased dramatically. Historically, beryllium was used as a coating for fluorescent light bulbs, and this was one of the most common sources of exposure to the metal. It is still used in the aerospace industry, particularly in aircraft brake linings. Confirming the diagnosis of berylliosis is sometimes difficult because the histologic examination of the nodules reveals a granulomatous reaction identical to that seen in sarcoidosis. Chemical analysis of wet tissue is frequently required for confirmation.

Hypersensitivity pneumonitis (allergic alveolitis) is an allergy involving the alveolar wall that results from exposure to a variety of noninvasive fungi, organic materials, and chemicals.[299,353,501,570] Hypersensitivity pneumonitis causes a number of patterns, and fine nodular opacities are common. The HRCT patterns may be mixed, with ground-glass, air space, fine nodules, reticular opacities, and mosaic perfusion. The observation of fine nodules is an important feature for distinguishing hypersensitivity pneumonitis from usual interstitial pneumonitis. The fine nodular interstitial opacities frequently indicate a subacute or chronic phase of the illness. Histologically, the nodules correspond with the presence of sarcoid-like granulomas. Sources of exposure include moldy hay (farmer's lung), saw dust, humidifiers, bird droppings, cork, chemicals such as isocyanates, and use of hot tubs.

SARCOIDOSIS

Sarcoidosis is an autoimmune disease that causes an inflammatory response with granulomas that spread through the bronchovascular bundles and lymphatics[103] (Fig. 17.6). Small granulomas may cause very fine nodular opacities that resemble those of miliary tuberculosis. Sarcoidosis may be distinguished from a number of other entities considered in this differential because of their relatively mild symptoms, despite radiologic findings that suggest a severe pathologic condition. Patients with sarcoidosis may complain of very mild dyspnea and virtually no other symptoms. The combined presence

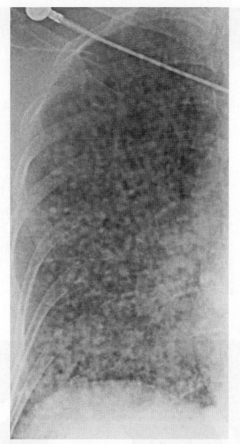

Fig. 17.7 Papillary carcinoma of the thyroid is a well-known cause of diffuse small nodular metastases. Because patients with this tumor often have a relatively long survival, the profusion may be great and the nodules may be larger than the nodules of granulomatous infections.

of hilar adenopathy and a fine nodular pattern is an important feature to suggest sarcoidosis, but the adenopathy often regresses as the lung disease advances. Therefore, an old examination that demonstrates bilaterally symmetric hilar adenopathy is virtually diagnostic of sarcoidosis. Silicosis is another entity considered in this differential of fine nodules and hilar adenopathy, but silicosis should be confirmed with an exposure history. (Answer to question 3 is *True*.) Additionally, eggshell calcifications of lymph nodes are considered a classic sign of silicosis, but they have also been observed in sarcoidosis.

Langerhans cell histiocytosis[1,585] is a smoking-related disease that is best known as a cause of upper lobe cysts, but in its earliest stages it causes interstitial nodules that also have an upper lobe predominance. The nodules may be very small with the appearance of miliary nodules but become larger as the disease progresses.

METASTATIC DISEASE

The development of a fine nodular pattern in a patient with a known distant primary tumor, such as a thyroid tumor (Fig. 17.7),[467] is strongly suggestive of disseminated metastatic disease. These patients often have signs of severe systemic illness, including weight loss, but careful clinical correlation is required because many patients with malignant tumors receive chemotherapy with potent immunosuppressive agents. A febrile response strongly suggests opportunistic infection, and prompt biopsy of the lung is advisable for establishing the diagnosis of a treatable infectious disease. Other primary tumors that have been observed to lead to this pattern include melanoma (Fig. 17.8, *A* and *B*), breast cancer, and gastrointestinal tumors, including pancreatic cancer.

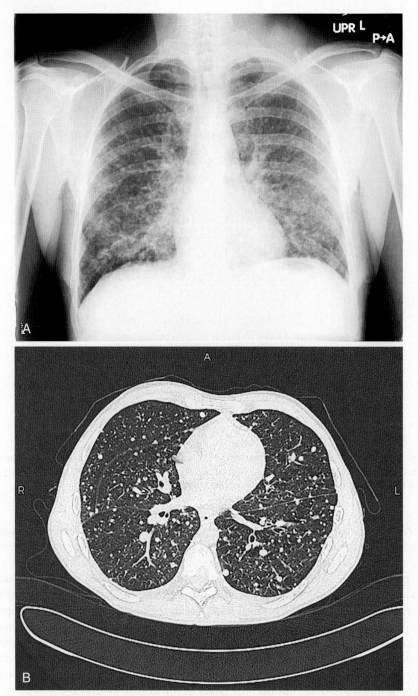

Fig. 17.8 A, Melanoma frequently metastasizes to the chest with a variety of manifestations including numerous small nodules. These nodules often vary in size and are larger than miliary nodules. **B,** Computed tomography image confirms that the nodules are well circumscribed, vary in size, and have a basilar distribution. This is very characteristic of metastatic nodules.

Top 5 Diagnoses: Diffuse Fine Nodular Opacities

1. Miliary tuberculosis
2. Fungal infections
3. Sarcoidosis
4. Pneumoconiosis (coal workers' pneumoconiosis, silicosis)
5. Metastases

Summary

Miliary tuberculosis is the classic example of a disease producing a fine nodular interstitial pattern on radiographic examination of the chest.

The most common fungal infections that produce a fine nodular interstitial pattern are histoplasmosis, coccidioidomycosis, and blastomycosis.

Silicosis and coal workers' pneumoconiosis are the most common inhalational diseases to produce the pattern. Asbestosis, in contrast, produces a reticular interstitial pattern.

Sarcoidosis and Langerhans cell histiocytosis may produce a fine nodular interstitial pattern, although the patient may have only minimal symptoms of shortness of breath or easy fatigability. Associated bilateral hilar adenopathy or even previous examinations revealing hilar adenopathy are strongly suggestive of sarcoidosis.

Patients who are immunosuppressed are susceptible to infection by less common organisms (e.g., *Nocardia, Cryptococcus,* and *Aspergillus*), but we must not minimize the frequency of infection by common organisms in these patients (e.g., viral pneumonia, tuberculosis, coccidioidomycosis, histoplasmosis, and blastomycosis).

ANSWER GUIDE

Legend for introductory figures

Fig. 17.1 Diffuse fine nodular opacities are the classic radiologic appearance of miliary tuberculosis. This patient was treated with steroids for rheumatoid arthritis and within 1 month developed the diffuse nodules. Transbronchial biopsy confirmed the diagnosis.
Fig. 17.2 Histoplasmosis is the most common cause of disseminated calcified nodules. Chickenpox pneumonia may also heal and leave residual nodules that may calcify.

ANSWERS

1. a   2. e   3. True   4. False

18 | FINE RETICULAR OPACITIES

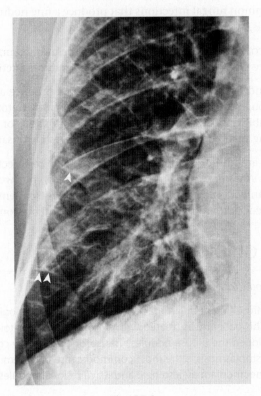

Fig. 18.1

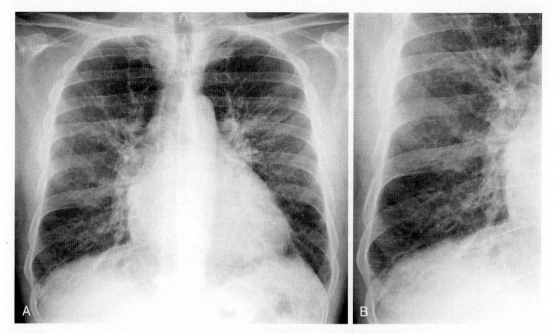

Fig. 18.2

QUESTIONS

1. Kerley B lines (Fig. 18.1) represent which one of the following?
   a. Thick interlobular septa.
   b. Dilated lymphatic vessels.
   c. Dilated venules.
   d. Thick alveolar walls.
   e. Fibrosis.

2. Which one of the following statements is not true?
   a. Kerley B lines are perpendicular to the pleura.
   b. Kerley A lines are deep in the lung parenchyma.
   c. Kerley lines are diagnostic of pulmonary edema.
   d. Kerley lines indicate interstitial disease.
   e. Dilated lymphatics are one cause of Kerley lines.

3. Which one of the following diagnoses is most likely in the case illustrated in Fig. 18.2?
   a. Pulmonary edema.
   b. Lymphangitic carcinomatosis.
   c. Lymphoma.
   d. Sarcoidosis.
   e. Idiopathic pulmonary fibrosis.

4. Which one of the following causes of fine reticular opacities is least likely to be associated with pleural effusion?
   a. Lymphangitic carcinomatosis.
   b. Lymphoma.
   c. Scleroderma.
   d. Rheumatoid disease.
   e. Pulmonary edema.

| Chart 18.1 | **DIFFUSE FINE RETICULAR OPACITIES** |

I. Acute
  A. Edema
    1. Congestive heart failure[75]
    2. Uremia[175]
    3. Fluid overload
  B. Infection
    1. Viral pneumonia[235,475,547]
    2. Mycoplasma pneumonia[170]
    3. Infectious mononucleosis
    4. Malaria[68] (*Plasmodium falciparum*)
    5. *Pneumocystis jiroveci* pneumonia
II. Chronic
  A. Chronic edema
    1. Atherosclerotic heart disease
    2. Mitral stenosis[75]
    3. Left atrial tumor (myxoma)
    4. Pulmonary veno-occlusive disease[529]
    5. Sclerosing mediastinitis
  B. Granulomatous disease
    1. Sarcoidosis[86]
    2. Langerhans cell histiocytosis[1,86,440]
  C. Collagen vascular disease[241,497,541]
    1. Rheumatoid lung[576]
    2. Scleroderma lung[19]
    3. Dermatomyositis and polymyositis[259]
    4. Sjögren syndrome[307]
  D. Lymphangitic carcinomatosis[235,258,269,279]
  E. Lymphocytic disorders
    1. Lymphoma and leukemia
    2. Waldenström macroglobulinemia[410,643]
    3. Lymphocytic interstitial pneumonia[49,374,543]
  F. Environmental disease[182,299,429]
    1. Asbestosis[37,80,99,100] and talcosis[144]
    2. Silicosis
    3. Hard metals[166,299]
    4. Hypersensitivity pneumonitis[58,128,353,501,565]
  C. Drug reactions (see Chart 18.1)[18,52,434,489,562]
  D. Idiopathic
    1. Idiopathic pulmonary fibrosis[104,364,398,440,553,569]
    2. Desquamative interstitial pneumonia[355]
    3. Tuberous sclerosis[24]
    4. Lymphangioleiomyomatosis[24,401,510]
    5. Idiopathic pulmonary hemosiderosis
    6. Amyloidosis[246]
    7. Interstitial calcification (chronic renal failure)[158]
    8. Alveolar proteinosis (late complication)
    9. Gaucher disease[645]
    10. Nonspecific interstitial pneumonitis[305,354]

Chart 18.2	**FINE RETICULAR OPACITIES AND PLEURAL EFFUSION**

I. Acute
  A. Pulmonary edema
  B. Infection (viral or mycoplasma pneumonia)
  C. Malaria[68] (rare)
II. Chronic
  D. Congestive heart failure
  E. Rheumatoid disease
  F. Lymphangitic spread of tumor
  G. Lymphoma and leukemia
  H. Lymphangioleiomyomatosis

Chart 18.3	**FINE RETICULAR OPACITIES AND HILAR ADENOPATHY**

I. Viral pneumonia (rare combination)
II. Sarcoidosis
III. Lymphoma and leukemia
IV. Metastases (lymphangitic carcinomatosis)
V. Silicosis

Chart 18.4	**CAUSES OF INTERLOBULAR SEPTAL THICKENING**

I. Acute
  A. Edema
  B. Viral pneumonia
  C. *Mycoplasma pneumoniae*
  D. *Pneumocystis jiroveci* pneumonia (formerly known as *Pneumocystis carinii* pneumonia [PCP])
II. Chronic
  A. Lymphangitic carcinomatosis
  B. Lymphoma
  C. Kaposi sarcoma
  D. Sarcoidosis

Discussion

The diffuse, fine reticular pattern (see Fig. 18.1) is one of the most reliable patterns for identifying diffuse interstitial disease. Because this pattern is linear, the lines must be distinguished from the normal pattern of blood vessels. In the early stages of an interstitial disease, this may be impossible by chest radiography, and high-resolution computed tomography (HRCT) may be required to confirm minimal interstitial disease. Interstitial diseases may spread throughout the bronchovascular or the septal interstitium while fibrotic diseases destroy the normal lung tissues, but both processes cause fine reticular opacities.

Kerley lines are the most reliable radiologic observation for making the distinction of bronchovascular versus septal interstitial disease.[150,175,235] Kerley B lines are short lines that are perpendicular to the pleura and continuous with it. The latter feature distinguishes the Kerley B lines from small vessels. Kerley B lines are usually observed in the costophrenic angles on the posteroanterior view and, occasionally, on the lateral view in the retrosternal clear space. They were first thought to represent only enlarged lymphatics but, based on pathologic correlations, these lines represent more generalized, enlarged interlobular septa. (Answer to question 1 is *a*.) Although it is true that the engorgement of septal lymphatic vessels would contribute to Kerley B lines, this has probably been overemphasized. In lymphangitic carcinomatosis, metastatic tumor spreads through dilated lymphatics in the interlobular septa and causes fine reticular opacities. In the other entities listed in Chart 18.1, dilation of lymphatics is not a sufficient explanation for the presence of Kerley B lines. Furthermore, in congestive heart failure, edema of the loose connective tissue of the interlobular septa accounts for Kerley lines, rather than engorged lymphatics.

Kerley A lines are also important and reliable signs of interstitial disease. These lines are linear opacities that appear to cross the normal vascular markings. Heitzman[235] showed that they correspond anatomically to thick interlobular septa. They differ from Kerley B lines only by their location, representing thick interlobular septa that are deep in the lung parenchyma. Kerley A lines may be suspected from the chest radiograph and account for the fine reticular interstitial pattern, but HRCT is often required to confirm the pattern by showing thickened interlobular septa, which outline the secondary pulmonary lobules.[221,614,617] (Answer to question 2 is *c*; pulmonary edema is only one cause of Kerley lines.)

Fibrosis of the interstitium may involve the septal and bronchovascular interstitium but revises and destroys the normal lung architecture as it progresses. The radiologic result is a pattern of irregular fine linear and curvilinear opacities that appear more disorganized. Thickened interlobular septa are not an expected result of fibrosis.

PULMONARY EDEMA

Pulmonary interstitial edema is the most common cause of fine reticular opacities. (Answer to question 3 is *a*). Edema first spreads through the bronchovascular interstitium and later through the septal interstitium, but Kerley B lines are an infrequent observation in patients with congestive heart failure. Kerley lines are most often seen in patients with chronic or recurrent heart failure. The next step in the evaluation of this pattern is to check for other signs that might suggest congestive heart failure. These include an enlarged heart with left ventricular or left atrial enlargement, prominence of upper lobe vessels, constriction of lower lobe vessels (cephalization of flow), peribronchial cuffing, increased width of the vascular pedicle, and signs of pleural effusion, including thickening of the interlobar fissures[75,390] (Figs 18.2 and 18.3). Prominence of the left atrium without left ventricular enlargement, in combination with fine reticular opacities and prominence of upper lobe vessels, strongly suggests mitral valve disease.[659] A clinical history of rheumatic fever and a murmur indicating mitral stenosis should be sufficient to confirm the diagnosis. Cardiac ultrasound examination is a reliable noninvasive method for confirming such a diagnosis and for excluding the rare atrial myxoma, which may also produce the classic chest radiographic findings of mitral stenosis.

Fluid overload is another common cause of interstitial edema. Fluid overload may be iatrogenic, but it is also commonly encountered in patients suffering from chronic renal failure.[175] Correlation with the clinical setting is particularly important in renal transplant patients because they are susceptible to interstitial edema and infections. Therefore, a febrile response should suggest an interstitial pneumonia rather than interstitial edema. In addition, any cause of severe hypoproteinemia, including cirrhosis and nephrosis, may lead to interstitial edema.

All these causes of interstitial edema, except mitral stenosis and pulmonary venoocclusive disease, are acute or recurrent processes; the pattern tends to be transient and changes rapidly. A changing course can be ascertained by examining old examinations and obtaining serial examinations.

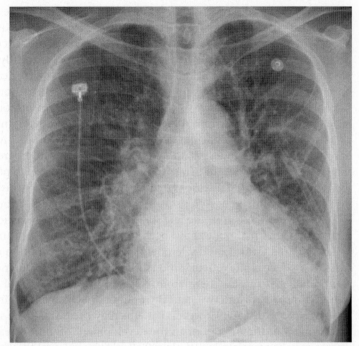

Fig. 18.3　The increased size and loss of definition of the pulmonary vessels, especially with more prominent upper lobe vessels (cephalization of pulmonary vasculature), results from edema in the bronchovascular interstitium. This helps confirm congestive heart failure as the cause of the more peripheral fine reticular opacities.

ACUTE INFECTIOUS INTERSTITIAL PNEUMONIAS

After pulmonary edema has been eliminated, viral, pneumocystis, and mycoplasma pneumonias are the major causes of acute, fine, reticular opacities (see Fig. 18.1). The acuteness of the interstitial pattern is best documented with serial radiographs. These patterns usually change over a few days. Both viral and mycoplasma pneumonias characteristically produce a febrile response and a nonproductive cough. They are commonly associated with a flu-like syndrome. The reticular opacities may appear coarse on occasion, but this is the result of a heavy accumulation of inflammatory cells in the interstitium and should not be confused with honeycombing (see Chapter 19 for a discussion of honeycomb lung).

CHRONIC INTERSTITIAL INFLAMMATORY DISEASE

Distinguishing acute from chronic interstitial opacities requires careful clinical correlation and serial examinations; a single chest radiograph is rarely adequate. Serial examinations not only document the chronicity of the disease but may also reveal information about changing patterns. This is particularly important in the diagnosis of diseases that may change from a nodular to a fine reticular pattern. Langerhans cell histiocytosis and sarcoidosis are two diseases well known for this type of radiologic evolution—nodules to lines. Both diseases may be very similar in their radiologic appearances, except for the presence of hilar adenopathy, which is not commonly seen in Langerhans cell histiocytosis and is therefore diagnostic of sarcoidosis. The first manifestations in the classic pattern of the progression of sarcoidosis are bilaterally symmetric hilar and paratracheal adenopathy. A small percentage of patients have radiologically detectable fine nodules (described in Chapter 17) at the time of their initial visit. The nodules are small noncaseating granulomas. If the nodules become very extensive, they appear to line up along the bronchovascular bundles and interlobular septa. This arrangement of the nodules produces fine reticular opacities and may occur at the time of the adenopathy, but it more typically occurs in the later stages of the disease, that is, after the adenopathy has regressed. The granulomas may regress spontaneously or in response to steroids. In some cases, the diffuse reticular opacities resolve, but in a small number of patients the granulomas are gradually replaced by fibrosis. This replacement may not be radiologically detectable. In other cases, the fine reticular opacities increase and may eventually lead to a coarse reticular or honeycomb pattern.

Langerhans cell histiocytosis progresses from a pattern of nodular to fine reticular opacities. The changing appearance suggests that histiocytes and eosinophils, which give rise to the nodular opacities, are being replaced by fibrosis.[1] As in sarcoidosis, if the fibrotic reaction continues, the fine reticular opacities will progress to a multicystic or honeycomb appearance. In Langerhans cell histiocytosis, an upper lobe distribution of the reticular interstitial disease is frequently observed, in contrast to the entities listed in Chart 18.2, which characteristically have a lower lobe distribution. Hilar adenopathy is not typically seen in the late stage of Langerhans cell histiocytosis, but enlarged hilar and mediastinal nodes have been reported in up to one-third of cases.[355,619]

Rheumatoid arthritis and scleroderma are the most common collagen vascular diseases to produce a fine reticular interstitial pattern, but reticular opacities may also be seen in polymyositis and dermatomyositis.[241,259,592] The clinical presentation of these entities is usually distinctive, and the pulmonary changes are almost always seen in a late stage of the disease. However, patients may occasionally be seen with rheumatoid involvement of the lung prior to the development of joint disease. Rheumatoid lung disease may be associated with pleural effusions or pleural thickening, either of which helps distinguish it from scleroderma (answer to question 4 is *c*). Pleural reactions secondary to sarcoidosis are rare. Rheumatoid lung disease has a tendency to involve the lung bases with the same distribution seen with idiopathic pulmonary fibrosis. As the fibrosis of rheumatoid progresses, the linear opacities will become more diffuse. This is in contrast to scleroderma, which is usually but not necessarily confined to the bases, even after it has progressed from a fine reticular to a coarse honeycomb pattern. In addition to the fine reticular pattern, multiple areas of air space consolidation may be observed in patients with scleroderma. These consolidations represent edema in the acute or early phases of the disease and therefore often precede fine reticular opacities. Since many patients with significant pulmonary involvement from scleroderma have a serious esophageal motility disturbance with a dilated atonic esophagus, aspiration is another possible factor contributing to the development of air space opacities in scleroderma. It is necessary to document any acute changes in the patterns of pulmonary disease in patients with scleroderma or rheumatoid arthritis to detect an acute opportunistic pneumonia. This is most important for patients with rheumatoid arthritis who are being treated with steroids and are thus susceptible to opportunistic infections or reactivation of previous tuberculosis.

NEOPLASMS

Fine reticular opacities with Kerley A and B lines are the classic radiologic findings of lymphangitic carcinomatosis. This is usually a bilateral process with a predominantly basilar distribution. In the early stages, lymphangitic carcinomatosis may be very subtle. HRCT is very sensitive for the detection of the early spread of tumor through the bronchovascular and septal interstitium (Fig. 18.4, *A* and *B*). The procedure has also been reported to be useful for distinguishing carcinomatosis from benign diseases such as sarcoidosis, idiopathic pulmonary fibrosis (IPF), and drug reactions.[42,560] The radiologic appearance of reticular opacities correlates well with the typical histologic appearance of tumor that has spread through the bronchovascular bundles and interlobular septa. As the tumor becomes more extensive, the radiologic pattern may change from a reticular to a reticulonodular or even a fine nodular pattern (see Chapter 17). Kang et al.[284] have emphasized that HRCT often demonstrates nodular thickening

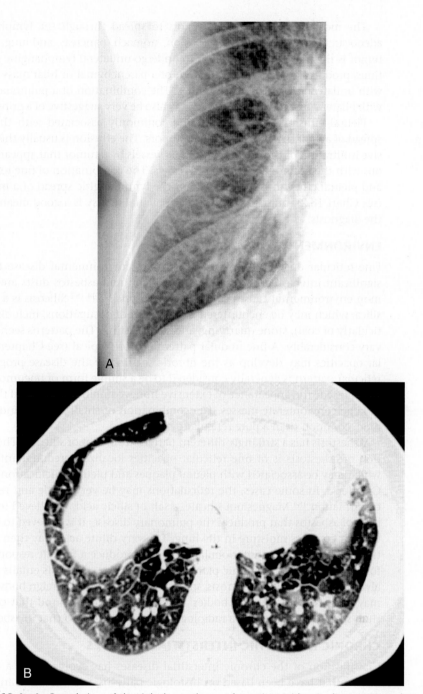

Fig. 18.4   A, Coned view of the right lower thorax of a patient with prior breast cancer shows peripheral reticular opacities with Kerley B lines in the costophrenic angle. **B,** High-resolution computed tomography section through the bases of the lungs confirms thickened interlobular septa outlining the secondary pulmonary lobules. This is the result of lymphangitic carcinomatosis.

of the interlobular septa, but this appearance is not specific. Nodular thickening of the interlobular septa would not be expected to result from edema, but may result from lymphangitic carcinomatosis, Kaposi sarcoma, lymphoma, sarcoidosis, tuberculosis, and histoplasmosis. As lymphangitic spread of the tumor becomes more extensive, it may even give the appearance of basilar consolidation and thus mimic the appearance of an air space consolidation (see Chapter 15).

The most common primary tumors to spread through the lymphatic vessels are adenocarcinomas from the breast, colon, stomach, pancreas, and lung. A primary lung tumor is the most common tumor to undergo unilateral lymphangitic spread. It sometimes produces a characteristic pattern of a parenchymal or hilar mass in combination with unilateral, fine reticular opacities. The combination of a pulmonary or hilar mass with bilateral fine reticular opacities may also be very suggestive of a primary lung tumor.

Pleural effusion is another finding commonly associated with the lymphangitic spread of any of the aforementioned tumors. The effusion is usually the result of extensive infiltration of the pleural lymphatic vessels by a tumor that appears to be continuous with the pulmonary lymphatic vessels. The combination of fine reticular opacities and pleural effusion is not specific for the lymphangitic spread of a malignant tumor (see Chart 18.2), but thoracentesis with pleural biopsy is a good means of confirming the diagnosis.

ENVIRONMENTAL DISEASES

Fine reticular opacities may occur with any environmental disease that produces a significant interstitial fibrotic reaction. Silicon and asbestos dusts are the most common environmental causes of interstitial fibrosis.[37,144,182] Silicosis is a reaction to free silica, which may be encountered in a number of occupations, including mining (particularly of coal), stone quarrying, and sandblasting. The patterns seen in silicosis may vary considerably. A fine nodular pattern is more typical (see Chapter 17), but reticular opacities may develop as the fibrotic scarring of the disease progresses. The fine reticular pattern is generally considered to be a simple form of pneumoconiosis, which may precede the appearance of extensive honeycombing fibrosis and the development of large conglomerate masses. The combination of small nodules and reticulations is more common than a pure reticular pattern.

Asbestosis has a strikingly different pattern from that of silicosis. The classic description of asbestosis is of fine reticular opacities localized predominantly in the bases, which may be associated with pleural plaques and pleural calcification, as described in Chapter 5. In some cases, the reticulations may be very subtle and require HRCT for confirmation.[184] Magnesium silicate, a salt of silicic acid, is believed to be the component of asbestos that produces the pulmonary disease; it is believed to form silicic acid when it contacts moisture in the lung. The very dilute acid may then diffuse through the alveolar walls and interlobular septa and produce a fibrotic response that initially follows the normal anatomic planes. Histologically, asbestosis entails reactions in the alveolar walls, involving fibrosis, inflammatory cells, and foreign body giant cells that may even contain asbestos bodies. Talc is another compound that contains magnesium silicate and produces a radiologic picture identical to that in asbestosis.[144]

CHRONIC IDIOPATHIC INTERSTITIAL DISEASES

Classification of the chronic interstitial diseases has evolved with a number of synonyms that have been based on histologic patterns and variations in clinical course. A widely accepted clinical classification includes acute interstitial pneumonitis (AIP), cryptogenic organizing pneumonia (COP), nonspecific interstitial pneumonia (NSIP), desquamative interstitial pneumonia (DIP), respiratory bronchiolitis–associated interstitial lung disease (RB-ILD), IPF, and lymphocytic interstitial pneumonia (LIP).[86,354,398]

AIP[12] (discussed in Chapter 15) has a predominant pattern of diffuse air space consolidation and may represent an idiopathic form of adult respiratory distress syndrome. This presentation of interstitial pneumonitis with rapidly developing fibrosis was first described in 1944 by Hamman and Rich.[217] A significant number of patients with a variety of idiopathic interstitial diseases have been diagnosed with Hamman-Rich syndrome, but the clinical description of these patients best matches the cases currently classified as AIP.

COP, also known as bronchiolitis obliterans with organizing pneumonia,[86] has a pattern of peripheral basilar air space opacities that most often resemble a multifocal pneumonia that has failed to respond to antibiotic therapy. The predominant histologic feature is organizing pneumonia, with bronchiolitis obliterans appearing as a secondary feature. In contrast with AIP, the opacities resulting from COP are more chronic and multifocal. Reticular opacities may be seen as a late finding. The latter appearance requires differentiation from usual interstitial pneumonia (UIP).

DIP[355] is a smoking-related disease that is histologically characterized by the filling of the alveolar spaces with macrophages and inflammatory changes in the alveolar walls. Even with this predominant alveolar reaction, the radiographic appearance of air space opacities is infrequent. Peripheral basilar opacities that may be reticular are the most common chest radiographic finding, but HRCT is often required for characterization. Ground-glass opacities are the most common feature on HRCT, with reticular opacities developing as the disease progresses. HRCT may also reveal cystic changes, which are not expected from the radiographic appearance. The changes of DIP often regress in response to smoking cessation and steroid treatment, but DIP is a progressive disease that may end with honeycombing fibrosis.

RB-ILD[221,355] has histologic similarities to DIP with macrophages around the respiratory bronchioles, but also has peribronchiolar inflammation and fibrosis. The radiographic findings are usually minimal, but RB-ILD may cause fine reticular opacities that likely result from the peribronchiolar changes. HRCT may show centrilobular nodules resembling hypersensitivity pneumonitis, ground-glass opacities, and bronchial wall thickening. Like DIP, this is a smoking-related disease that is reversible and responds to smoking cessation, especially when combined with steroid therapy.

NSIP[305,354] is a more recently recognized subtype of interstitial pneumonitis that causes a mild or moderate chronic, interstitial inflammatory, cellular infiltrate with minimal or no fibrosis. NSIP causes peripheral basilar opacities that may appear to be fine reticular or linear, but are often difficult to characterize by radiography. Ground-glass opacities are the predominant HRCT finding with minimal reticular changes that indicate fibrosis. NSIP is distinguished from UIP based on histologic differences, predominant radiographic and HRCT patterns, and prognosis. Because fibrosis is a minimal part of the histologic pattern of NSIP, it is considered reversible and therefore has a better prognosis than UIP.

IPF is the most common of the idiopathic interstitial pneumonias.[398] IPF is the end-stage scarring of the lung that is the result of the idiopathic form of UIP.[354,440] UIP is the histologic pattern of IPF and is characterized by a pattern of nonuniform and variable interstitial changes that include zones of interstitial fibrosis, inflammation, fibroblastic activity, honeycombing fibrosis, and normal lung. This histologic appearance often resembles a number of specific diseases including rheumatoid, scleroderma, asbestosis, and hypersensitivity pneumonitis, which should be eliminated based on the patient's history and associated findings. Because IPF is a disease that is histologically characterized by fibrosis, reticular opacities are the primary radiologic pattern. These opacities are usually peripheral and basilar. HRCT[571] may be required to confirm the dominant pattern and distribution of the opacities. Because of superimposition, the reticular opacities may appear uniform on the chest radiograph, whereas HRCT (Fig. 18.5) reveals a heterogeneous distribution with zones of normal lung interspersed with reticular opacities and honeycombing fibrosis. Ground-glass opacities are less prominent in IPF than in NSIP and correspond with zones of minimal disease. Because IPF is a primary pulmonary disease, additional findings such as adenopathy may not be expected; however, Bergin et al.[42] have reported that computed tomography (CT) detects small mediastinal nodes measuring from 10 to 15 mm in a high percentage of patients. These nodes are not usually detectable on chest radiographs. Most importantly, IPF is a progressive fibrotic disease that ends

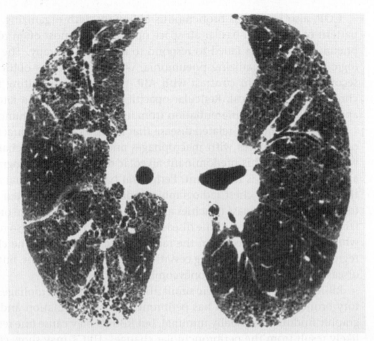

Fig. 18.5 High-resolution computed tomography (HRCT) scan of a patient with idiopathic pulmonary fibrosis (IPF) was taken at a level just below the carina and shows irregular reticular opacities in the periphery of the lungs. Notice the involvement of the posterior aspect of the lower lobes and the lateral aspect of the right middle lobe. There are large areas of intervening normal lung. This heterogeneous appearance is a common finding of IPF on HRCT that may not be obvious on the chest radiograph.

with irreversible fibrosis and a characteristic radiographic and HRCT appearance of diffuse honeycombing.

LIP is a lymphocytic cellular infiltrate that spreads through alveolar walls and interlobular septa.[543] It involves an infiltration of the pulmonary interstitium with mature lymphocytes and, histologically, may closely resemble a lymphocytic lymphoma. In contrast with the previously mentioned idiopathic interstitial diseases, LIP is not fibrotic and does not progress to honeycombing. The radiographic opacities are typically in the bases and may appear reticular or confluent on the chest radiograph. HRCT most often shows ground-glass opacities, but also shows reticular opacities and, like DIP, may show cystic changes. Because LIP is a lymphoproliferative disorder, it is imperative that patients with LIP be carefully evaluated to rule out a malignant process. Associated adenopathy is evidence to question the diagnosis of LIP and should therefore influence the histologist to consider the diagnosis of a well-differentiated lymphocytic lymphoma. There is a strong clinical association of LIP with Sjögren syndrome and other collagen vascular diseases. LIP has also been observed as an additional complication of the acquired immunodeficiency syndrome that occurs primarily in children.[374,417]

OTHER CHRONIC INTERSTITIAL DISEASES

Tuberous sclerosis may result in a smooth muscle proliferation in the lung and therefore may result in diffuse, fine reticular opacities.[175] It is best diagnosed on clinical grounds because patients with the disease usually have other associated signs.

Lymphangioleiomyomatosis (LAM) is a rare cause of fine reticular opacities that may result from smooth muscle proliferation in the lung but are more likely the result of superimposed thin-walled cysts. HRCT shows extensive cystic changes with very thin walls that are often not visible on the chest radiograph.[175,401] The clinical setting may be very specific. It typically occurs in young women and is accompanied by recurrent pleural effusions and pneumothoraces. Examination of pleural fluid reveals a chylous effusion. This complex of radiologic and clinical findings is so specific that biopsy is unnecessary.

Idiopathic pulmonary hemosiderosis is a rare disease that produces diffuse air space consolidations (see Chapter 15); however, after multiple episodes of bleeding, fine reticular opacities may develop. This is most prominent in the bases and is the result of an accumulation of iron-laden macrophages in the interstitium, which may gradually be replaced by fibrosis. The pattern can be observed only between episodes of acute bleeding and occurs as a late complication of the disease.[589]

Amyloidosis[246] is also a rare cause of diffuse, fine reticular opacities. This is possibly the rarest of the pulmonary manifestations of amyloidosis.[604] Amyloidosis should be suspected in patients with multiple myeloma and a slowly progressive interstitial pattern, but care must be taken in this setting to rule out opportunistic infections and drug reactions.

Top 5 Diagnoses: Fine Reticular Opacities

1. Edema
2. Interstitial pneumonia (viruses, mycoplasma, pneumocystis)
3. Lymphangitic carcinomatosis
4. Collagen vascular disease
5. IPF

Summary

A fine reticular or linear pattern with Kerley A and B lines is specific for interstitial disease.

One of the earliest steps in evaluating a fine reticular pattern is to determine whether the process is acute or chronic.

The most common acute cause of the pattern is interstitial edema, which should be divided into cardiac and noncardiac edema on the basis of cause.

Other radiologic signs of cardiac pulmonary edema include cardiomegaly, prominence of upper lobe vessels, constriction of lower lobe vessels, loss of definition of vessels, pleural effusion, perihilar haze, and air space consolidations.

Viral, *Mycoplasma,* and *Pneumocystis* are the other major causes of acute interstitial opacities.

Chronic pulmonary edema is usually associated with mitral stenosis and, rarely, with left atrial myxoma. These may be distinguished by cardiac ultrasound examination.

Clinical correlation is essential for evaluating chronic causes of fine reticular opacities. Biopsy is usually not necessary in rheumatoid arthritis, scleroderma, silicosis, asbestosis, tuberous sclerosis, and lymphangioleiomyomatosis.

The most important reason for lung biopsy in patients with a known primary malignancy or lymphoma and in patients who exhibit fine reticular opacities is to exclude an opportunistic pneumonia.

It is important not to assume that a chronic, fine reticular pattern is due to fibrosis. Even when biopsy confirms the diagnosis of a disease that may ultimately lead to fibrosis, such as sarcoidosis, the pattern may be due to an extensive inflammatory reaction rather than fibrosis.

Some of the diagnoses considered in Chart 18.1 must be confirmed by biopsy. These include DIP, LIP, Langerhans cell histiocytosis, and sarcoidosis.

IPF is the most common of the idiopathic interstitial lung diseases. HRCT may confirm the diagnosis, but biopsy is often required.

ANSWER GUIDE

Legends for introductory figures

Fig. 18.1   Kerley B lines *(arrowheads)* are the result of thickened interlobular septa that are perpendicular to the pleura. They are often best seen in the costophrenic angles. In this case, they are the result of mycoplasma pneumonia. (Case courtesy of Dr. Peter Dempsey.)

Fig. 18.2   **A,** Combination of fine reticular opacities in the bases, cardiac enlargement, small pleural effusions, and congestion of upper lobe vessels is the classic appearance of interstitial pulmonary edema secondary to congestive heart failure. **B,** The coned view of the right lower thorax confirms thickening of the interlobular septa.

Answers

1. a   2. c   3. a   4. c

COARSE RETICULAR OPACITIES (HONEYCOMB LUNG)

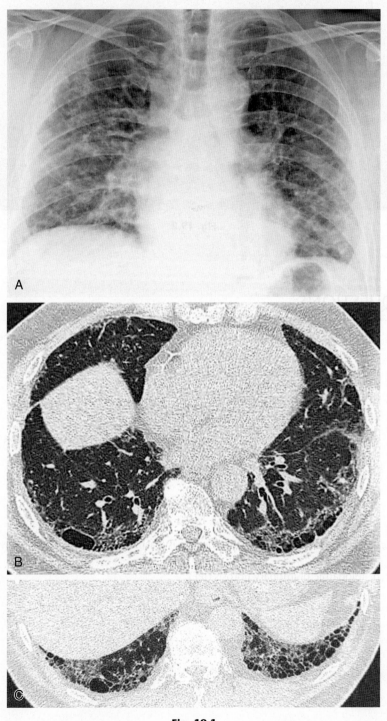

Fig. 19.1

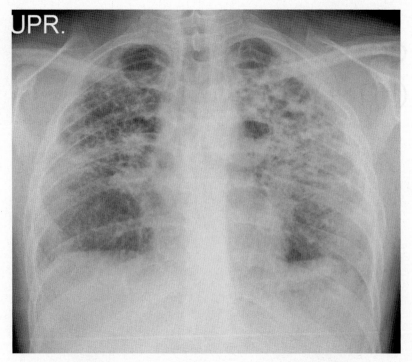

Fig. 19.2

QUESTIONS

1. Refer to Fig. 19.1, *A-C.* The term *honeycomb lung* indicates which one of these processes?
   a. Emphysema.
   b. Cystic bronchiectasis.
   c. Paraseptal emphysema.
   d. End-stage interstitial fibrosis.
   e. Multiple cavities.

2. Which one of the following diagnoses is the least likely in the case shown in Fig. 19.2?
   a. Lymphangitic metastases.
   b. Sarcoidosis.
   c. Asbestosis.
   d. Usual interstitial pneumonia (UIP).
   e. Rheumatoid lung.

3. Basilar distribution of interstitial disease is least likely in which of the following entities?
   a. Asbestosis.
   b. Idiopathic pulmonary fibrosis (IPF).
   c. Scleroderma.
   d. Sarcoidosis.
   e. Rheumatoid lung.

Chart 19.1	**COARSE RETICULAR OPACITIES WITH LUCENT SPACES—HONEYCOMB LUNG**

I. Usual interstitial pneumonitis
  A. Collagen vascular diseases[296]
    1. Rheumatoid lung[59,241,532]
    2. Scleroderma[19]
    3. Dermatomyositis and polymyositis[259,523]
    4. Mixed connective tissue disease[309]
    5. Ankylosing spondylitis[48,646]
  B. Environmental diseases
    1. Asbestosis[37,80]
    2. Chemical pneumonitis[299]
    3. Hard metal pneumoconiosis[299]
  C. Idiopathic pulmonary fibrosis (IPF)[86,104,440,553,569]
II. Inflammatory diseases
  A. Sarcoidosis
  B. Langerhans cell histiocytosis (LCH)[1]
  C. Hypersensitivity pneumonitis (chronic)[58,128,497,501,570]
  D. Desquamative interstitial pneumonitis (DIP; rarely causes honeycombing)[355]
III. Mimicking opacities with lucent spaces
  A. Cystic bronchiectasis
  B. Superimposed cysts (LCH; lymphangioleiomyomatosis [LAM])[424]

Chart 19.2	**RADIOLOGIC STAGING OF SARCOIDOSIS**

I. Stage I—hilar and mediastinal adenopathy
II. Stage II—hilar and mediastinal adenopathy with lung disease
III. Stage III—lung disease without adenopathy
IV. Stage IV—honeycombing fibrosis

Discussion

Honeycomb lung is characterized by coarse reticular interstitial opacities with intervening lucent spaces.[462] The typical appearance of honeycomb lung is shown in Figs. 19.1, *A-C*, and 19.2. Diseases that produce honeycomb lung tend to affect both lungs and are usually extensive, although the degree of involvement is frequently not uniform. The lucent spaces are described as cysts and should not be confused with those seen in emphysema or cavities. Emphysema involves tissue destruction without fibrosis, whereas honeycombing involves tissue destruction by retracting fibrosis. Paraseptal emphysema involves the subpleural portions of the lung and, when it is extensive, may resemble honeycombing. The bullae of paraseptal emphysema are often in a single subpleural layer, in contrast to the cysts of honeycombing which are in multiple layers. Cavities may be multifocal and extensive but are not contiguous diffuse spaces. High-resolution computed tomography (HRCT) should reliably differentiate the cystic spaces caused by honeycombing from emphysema or cavities.[289] HRCT also provides a map of the distribution of the honeycombing and often allows the radiologist to determine a specific cause.[440]

Recognizing the honeycomb pattern is helpful in narrowing the differential diagnosis for reticular interstitial opacities (Chart 19.1). As previously suggested, the honeycomb appearance indicates end-stage scarring of the lung with revision of the pulmonary architecture by fibrosis. (Answer to question 1 is *d*.) Serial examinations may reveal progression from fine reticular opacities to honeycombing. This is often the case in the pneumoconioses, collagen vascular diseases, or idiopathic pulmonary fibrosis (IPF). Additionally, identification of the cystic spaces of honeycomb lung permits exclusion of other causes of reticular opacities such as acute pulmonary edema, viral pneumonia, mycoplasma pneumonia, lymphangitic spread of carcinoma, lymphoma, and lymphocytic interstitial pneumonia (answer to question 2 is *a*). Honeycomb lung also has grave prognostic implications because the cystic spaces are due to end-stage irreversible scarring.

Cystic bronchiectasis (Fig 19.3) sometimes produces a radiologic appearance of coarse irregular opacities with intervening cystic spaces that resemble honeycombing fibrosis. Bacterial, viral, and tuberculous pneumonias may all cause bronchial wall necrosis with late scarring and bronchiectasis, but this necrosis rarely causes diffuse bilateral bronchiectasis that would be confused with honeycombing fibrosis. However, the late stages of cystic fibrosis do cause diffuse disease with extensive scarring.[521] The scarring of cystic fibrosis is caused by recurrent pneumonias that complicate the chronic problems of thick mucus and impaired bronchial clearance. The radiologic appearance differs from the primary interstitial diseases that cause lung fibrosis by the presence of perihilar bronchial thickening. Additionally, because cystic fibrosis is an obstructive bronchial disease, there is often increased lung volume, in contrast with restrictive scarring from the fibrotic interstitial diseases that reduce lung volume.

USUAL INTERSTITIAL PNEUMONITIS

Collagen Vascular Diseases

Rheumatoid arthritis is the collagen vascular disease that is most likely to result in end-stage scarring of the lung.[59] The characteristic radiologic appearance of rheumatoid interstitial disease changes with the stage of the disease. In the earliest stages, there is congestion of the alveolar capillaries, edema of the alveolar walls, and lymphocytic infiltration. There may even be an alveolar fibrinous exudate. This leads to the radiologic appearance of patchy areas of air space consolidation (multifocal ill-defined opacities). The patchy alveolar opacities usually resolve and are followed by the development of fine interstitial opacities that histologically consist of histiocytes and lymphocytes. At this intermediate stage, the radiologic appearance is that of fine reticular or reticulonodular opacities. As the disease progresses, the cellular infiltrate is gradually replaced by fibrosis that destroys the alveolar walls and distal bronchioles, leading to the cystic spaces of honeycomb lung (Fig 19.4). There is a definite tendency for this interstitial reaction to be localized in the bases of the lungs. Because rheumatoid interstitial disease is a restrictive lung disease, there may be evidence of pulmonary volume loss with elevation of both leaves of the diaphragm; this may occur even when the patient attempts to inspire deeply. Clinically, the patient usually has the characteristic joint involvement of rheumatoid arthritis. However, rheumatoid lung disease may rarely occur before the development of the characteristic joint disease. The pulmonary symptoms may be nonspecific and include cough, dyspnea, and even cyanosis. The dyspnea often exceeds what might be expected from the physical signs and radiologic findings.

Scleroderma (progressive systemic sclerosis) is another collagen vascular disease that produces interstitial fibrosis and honeycomb lung. As in rheumatoid arthritis, there is a tendency for the interstitial fibrosis to have a basal distribution; also, the early phases of scleroderma may produce patchy air space consolidations, which may be recurrent, followed by the development of fine reticular interstitial opacities. Histologically,

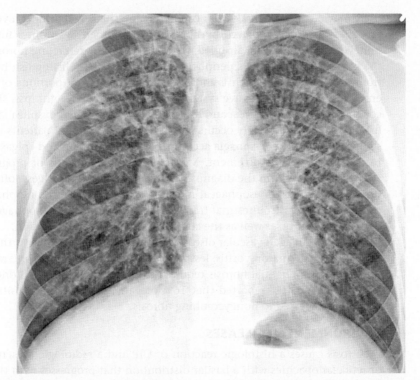

Fig. 19.3 Diffuse cystic bronchiectasis causes coarse reticular scarring with multiple cystic spaces, which must be distinguished from honeycombing fibrosis. Associated bronchial thickening around the hilum and increased lung volume distinguish this appearance from that of honeycombing fibrosis. Also note the relative scarring of the lung periphery in this patient with cystic fibrosis.

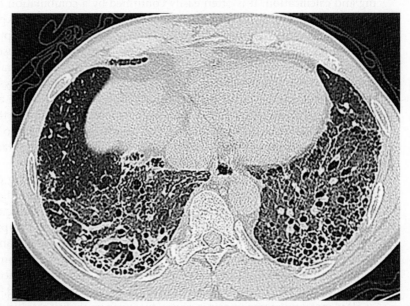

Fig. 19.4 Rheumatoid lung disease may end with advanced honeycombing fibrosis. High-resolution computed tomography of the rheumatoid lung demonstrates honeycombing fibrosis with a basilar peripheral distribution that is indistinguishable from that of idiopathic pulmonary fibrosis.

there may be prominent alveolar capillaries and thickened cellular alveolar walls. This process is gradually replaced by fibrosis, which progresses from a fine reticular to a honeycomb pattern. The air-filled cystic spaces left by retracting fibrosis tend to be in the bases of the lung. This peripheral distribution helps distinguish honeycomb lung from bronchiectasis, which is more severe in the central portions of the lung. General symptoms of progressive systemic sclerosis include weight loss, slight productive cough, progressive dyspnea, and low-grade fever. However, dyspnea is rarely found at first admission and usually occurs late in the disease. Half of patients with pulmonary symptoms also have dysphagia accompanied by substernal and epigastric pain related to the esophageal involvement. More specific clinical signs of progressive systemic sclerosis often confirm the diagnosis. These include skin changes, soft-tissue calcifications, disturbances of esophageal motility, and dilation of the esophagus. Radiologically, an upper gastrointestinal tract series may demonstrate esophageal dilation and decreased motility, as well as the characteristic small bowel dilation.

The other collagen vascular diseases, including systemic lupus erythematosus, polymyositis, and dermatomyositis, less frequently involve the lungs and rarely progress to the degree of interstitial fibrosis required for development of the honeycomb appearance. Ikezoe et al.[259] reported that 16% of patients with polymyositis and dermatomyositis progressed to honeycombing fibrosis.

ENVIRONMENTAL DISEASES

Asbestosis causes a histologic reaction of UIP and a radiologic presentation of linear or reticular opacities with a basilar distribution that progresses with the development of coarse reticular opacities. The reticular opacities are the result of fibrosis, which progresses to revision of the pulmonary architecture with cystic spaces resulting in honeycombing fibrosis. The basilar distribution of the coarse linear opacities causes an appearance that has been described as a "shaggy heart." The diagnosis of asbestosis may also be confirmed by the identification of associated plaques of pleural thickening and calcification. It is often easily confirmed by a combination of the previously mentioned radiologic findings and a clinical history of asbestos exposure. The most common sources of asbestos exposure include asbestos mills, shipyards, plumbing, pipe fitting, insulation, and automobile brake lining work. Because the dangers of asbestos exposure have been recognized, many of these occupational exposures have been eliminated or reduced. Unfortunately, exposure has not always been limited to the industrial worker; asbestosis can also occur in members of the asbestos worker's family. In particular, spouses may have been exposed to asbestos in the worker's dust-contaminated clothing. Other silicates that are chemically similar to asbestos, including talc, have an identical risk for the exposed patient. In fact, the radiologic findings of talcosis and asbestosis are often identical.[144]

Chemical inhalation does not rapidly lead to end-stage scarring of the lungs, but patients who have had massive or recurrent exposures to nitrogen dioxide (silo filler's disease), sulfur dioxide, chlorine, phosgene, cadmium, or the pesticide paraquat may experience extensive parenchymal scarring with revision of the pulmonary architecture and resultant honeycombing fibrosis. Bronchiolitis obliterans with proximal bronchiectasis may also complicate the inhalation of gases such as ammonia and contribute to the appearance of coarse linear opacities with cystic spaces. HRCT should distinguish the chronic bronchial changes from true honeycombing.[299]

Hard metal pneumoconiosis is caused by exposure to dust resulting from the manufacture or use of very hard metal alloys that contain tungsten, carbon, and cobalt with titanium, tantalum, nickel, and chromium. This causes a giant cell interstitial reaction that is replaced by fibrosis. Advanced cases develop basilar fibrosis with honeycombing. HRCT may show ground-glass opacities, fine reticular opacities, traction bronchiectasis, and honeycombing fibrosis.[299]

IDIOPATHIC PULMONARY FIBROSIS

IPF is possibly the most common cause of honeycomb lung, but the radiographic and even the histologic findings are not always specific. The initial injury is at the alveolar capillary wall, with episodes of active alveolitis that may cause a pattern of basilar ground-glass or air space opacities, followed by a progressive development of peripheral basilar reticular opacities. The disease ends in severe scarring with revision of the pulmonary architecture. The radiologic appearance consists of coarse, disorganized, reticular opacities with cystic spaces. Honeycombing occurs in approximately 50% of cases of IPF by chest radiography and is an expected finding on HRCT (see Fig 19.1, *A* and *B*). This extensive fibrosis also leads to severe volume loss that is radiographically apparent in as many as 45% of cases. Because IPF is a slowly progressive disease, it must be emphasized that the histologist may appreciate revision of the pulmonary architecture and report honeycombing by biopsy at a time when the radiograph appears to have only minimal abnormality. HRCT permits an early diagnosis by showing a nonuniform, patchy, peripheral distribution that is diagnostic of IPF and correlates with the histologic hallmarks of UIP. Although this is an idiopathic condition, there is increasing evidence that it occurs in current and former smokers with a prevalence ranging from 40% to 80%.[20,355] The clinical course is gradual decline with a survival of 2 to 4 years.

INFLAMMATORY DISEASES

Sarcoidosis[103,462] is not a common cause of honeycomb lung, but as many as 20% of patients who develop pulmonary sarcoidosis with interstitial nodules or fine reticular interstitial opacities will have progression of their interstitial disease with replacement of the granulomas by fibrosis (Fig 19.5, *A* and *B*; see Fig 19.2). This has the effect of revising the pulmonary architecture through retracting fibrosis in a manner similar to that seen in the collagen vascular, inhalational, and idiopathic group of diseases discussed in this chapter. In contrast with the collagen vascular diseases and idiopathic pulmonary fibrosis, which have a lower lobe distribution, sarcoidosis has a middle and upper zone distribution (answer to question 3 is *d*). Some of the cystic spaces resulting from sarcoidosis may be quite extensive and may even suggest the presence of cavities. However, pathologic documentation of necrotic cavities in sarcoidosis is rare. Most patients who develop large cystic spaces in the end stage of sarcoidosis have retracting fibrosis with traction bronchiectasis and exaggerated revision of the normal pulmonary architecture.[103] Serial chest radiographs are particularly helpful in evaluating these patients. Such late end-stage findings are usually preceded by some of the classic findings, including hilar adenopathy and an interstitial nodular or fine reticular interstitial opacities (see Chapters 11, 17, and 18). The classic description of sarcoid involvement of the lung involves regression of the hilar adenopathy as the interstitial disease progresses. However, the coexistence of hilar adenopathy and extensive interstitial disease still favors the diagnosis of sarcoidosis. The aforementioned progression of sarcoidosis is often used to classify sarcoidosis (Chart 19.2). Honeycombing indicates advanced stage IV disease.

LCH is an infrequent but possible cause of honeycombing fibrosis. Initially, there is infiltration of the lung with histiocytes and eosinophils with the radiologic appearance of small nodules. As the disease progresses, the nodular appearance may be completely replaced by fine reticular opacities and upper lobe cysts. HRCT has shown that the walls of the cystic lesions may contribute to the chest radiographic appearance of reticular opacities, and the appearance of the cystic spaces may mimic honeycombing. Later, as the histiocytic and eosinophilic cellular response is replaced by fibrosis, the fibrosis retracts and may produce the coarse reticular opacities and cystic spaces with the appearance of honeycombing. Pneumothorax occurs in as many as 25% of patients, presumably owing to the rupture of subpleural cystic spaces. LCH has a

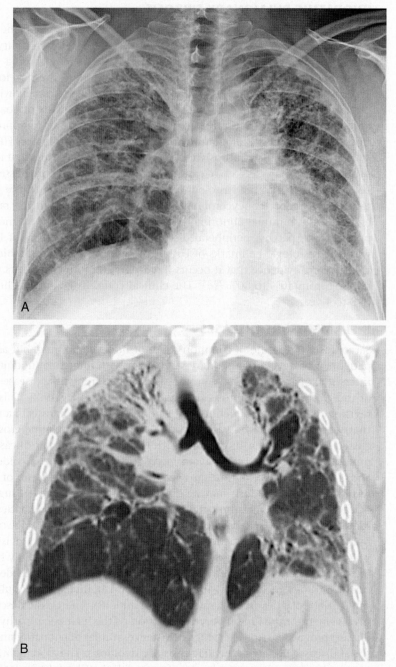

Fig. 19.5   A, Interstitial granulomas may be replaced by fibrosis in the late stages of sarcoidosis. Cystic spaces must not be confused with cavities. Even very large spaces are the result of destruction of lung by retracting fibrosis and are therefore a manifestation of honeycombing. In contrast with idiopathic pulmonary fibrosis, the distribution of honeycombing from sarcoidosis is more upper lobe and central following the bronchovascular interstitium. **B,** Coronal computed tomography emphasizes the large cystic spaces and upper lobe distribution. The asymmetric involvement of one lung is not unusual. In this case, there is more diffuse involvement of the left lung.

predominant upper lobe distribution, which distinguishes it from a number of the other entities considered in this differential, and the costophrenic angles are the last part of the lungs to be affected. Hilar enlargement in patients with LCH may result from pulmonary artery hypertension[143] or lymph node enlargement. Adenopathy has been observed in as many as one-third of cases of LCH and requires careful evaluation to distinguish LCH from sarcoidosis.[355]

Histiocytosis X includes Letterer-Siwe disease, Hand-Schüller-Christian disease, and LCH.[1] These three conditions are histologically related, with histiocytes being the dominant cell type in each, but they are clinically quite different. Letterer-Siwe and Hand-Schüller-Christian disease occur in infants and children and follow a more severe, often fatal course. In contrast, pulmonary LCH tends to occur most frequently in people between the ages of 15 and 40 years and has a comparatively mild course. Patients with pulmonary LCH have a history of cigarette smoking, reported in 80% to 100% of cases. The radiographic changes have been observed to improve or even resolve in patients who stop smoking.[1]

Hypersensitivity pneumonitis[497,501,570] is an inflammatory response to a variety of environmental antigens.[128] The pathologic reaction includes pulmonary lymphocytosis and granulomatous interstitial pneumonitis. With chronic exposure the granulomas are replaced by fibrosis, which leads to honeycombing fibrosis. The distribution of the fibrosis usually differs from IPF with a mid to upper lung zone predominance compared with the basilar peripheral distribution of fibrosis resulting from all of the causes of UIP. Identification and removal of the antigenic agent are important in preventing progression to honeycombing fibrosis.[154] Prevention of exposure may be difficult in occupations such as farming, where noninvasive fungi such as thermophilic actinomycetes grow in moldy hay. Farmer's lung is one of the more likely examples of hypersensitivity pneumonitis to progress to honeycombing fibrosis.

DIP is a smoking-related idiopathic interstitial disease that rarely ends with honeycombing fibrosis. Histologically, DIP is characterized by filling of the air spaces by alveolar macrophages. Areas of patchy ground-glass opacity as seen with HRCT are the most common presentation of DIP, with minimal air space opacities or fine reticular opacities on chest radiographs. Advanced cases with fibrosis may have a basilar distribution with traction bronchiectasis and honeycombing fibrosis on HRCT. Severe lung volume loss is less frequent in DIP (23%) than in IPF (45%). Perhaps the prognostic difference in DIP and IPF is the most important one. DIP responds to steroid therapy and improves with smoking cessation, compared with IPF, which does not respond to steroids and has a mean survival of 2 to 4 years.[355]

Top 5 Diagnoses: Coarse Reticular Opacities (Honeycomb Lung)

1. IPF
2. Rheumatoid lung
3. Scleroderma
4. Sarcoidosis
5. Asbestosis

Summary

The term *honeycomb lung* indicates interstitial fibrosis.

The radiologic appearance of honeycombing fibrosis may be mimicked by severe cystic bronchiectasis, particularly in patients with cystic fibrosis or tuberculous bronchiectasis and severe cystic disease, as seen in lymphangioleiomyomatosis.

Honeycombing fibrosis results in revision of the pulmonary architecture with cystic spaces that are not consistent with the diagnosis of pulmonary interstitial edema, acute viral pneumonia, or lymphangitic carcinomatosis. Therefore a number of common causes of interstitial disease can essentially be ruled out by correct identification of the pattern.

Distribution of the disease is extremely important in considering the differential. For example, an exclusively peripheral location of the cystic spaces in honeycombing fibrosis makes the exclusion of cystic bronchiectasis more definitive.

A basilar distribution is suggestive of asbestosis, scleroderma, rheumatoid lung, DIP, or IPF.

An upper lobe distribution of cystic-appearing spaces is suggestive of LCH, sarcoidosis, ankylosing spondylitis or bronchiectasis secondary to cystic fibrosis, or cavitary granulomatous diseases, including tuberculosis and histoplasmosis.

Clinical correlation frequently confirms the diagnosis of diseases such as rheumatoid arthritis, scleroderma, or hypersensitivity pneumonitis.

ANSWER GUIDE

Legends for introductory figures

Fig. 19.1 A, Diffuse coarse reticular opacities are most often the result of honeycombing fibrosis. Because of summation and superimposition of the opacities, they often appear uniform and diffuse on the chest radiograph. This may lead to overestimation of the severity of the lung destruction. **B,** In this case, high-resolution computed tomography reveals extensive honeycombing fibrosis with a peripheral basilar distribution with more areas of preserved normal lung than expected from the chest radiograph. This is the characteristic pattern of idiopathic pulmonary fibrosis. **C,** The lowest portions of the lung bases are often the most severely involved, as seen in this case.

Fig. 19.2 The combination of coarse reticular opacities and intervening lucent spaces is the expected appearance of honeycomb lung. The spaces accentuate the coarse reticular pattern. Severe involvement of the upper lobes is a feature that should suggest sarcoidosis.

ANSWERS

1. d   2. a   3. d

20 | SOLITARY PULMONARY NODULE

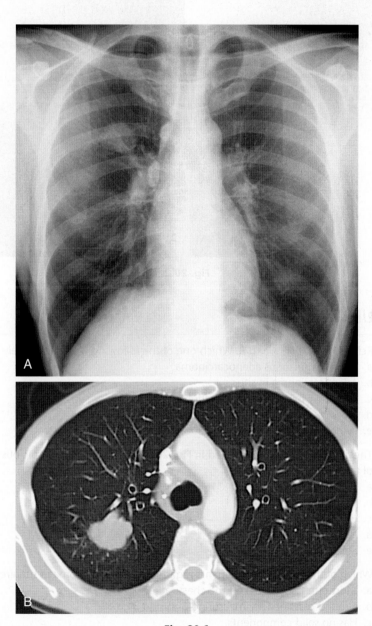

Fig. 20.1

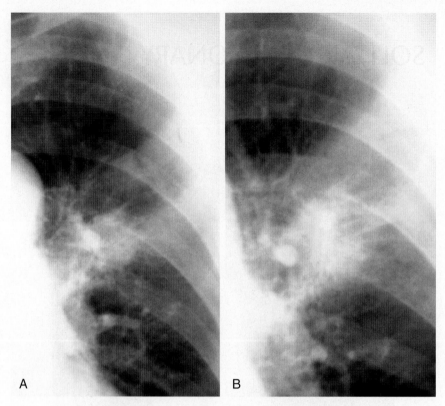

A   B

Fig. 20.2

QUESTIONS

1. Refer to Fig. 20.1, *A* and *B*. Which one of the following is the most likely diagnosis?
   a. Invasive mucinous adenocarcinoma.
   b. Adenocarcinoma in situ.
   c. Minimally invasive adenocarcinoma.
   d. Invasive adenocarcinoma.
   e. Lymphoma.

2. The changing pattern illustrated in Fig. 20.2, *A* and *B*, is most suspicious for which one of the following?
   a. Carcinoid.
   b. Granuloma.
   c. Hamartoma.
   d. Lung cancer.
   e. Solitary metastasis.

3. Which of the following statements regarding adenocarcinoma in situ are true?
   a. Most often not visible on the chest radiograph.
   b. Ground-glass opacity measuring 5 mm to 3 cm.
   c. Has no solid components.
   d. CT may show pulmonary vessels in the nodule.
   e. All of the above.

4. Which one of the following statements regarding carcinoid tumors is true?
   a. Commonly suspected because of carcinoid syndrome.
   b. Benign bronchial tumor.

    c. Malignant neuroendocrine tumor.

    d. Most commonly presents as a peripheral nodule.

    e. Constitutes 15% to 20% of primary lung cancers.

5. Which one of the following features of a peripheral nodule would be most diagnostic?

    a. Spiculated borders.

    b. Air bronchograms.

    c. Central calcification.

    d. Central cavitation.

    e. Eccentric calcification.

Chart 20.1	SOLITARY PULMONARY NODULE OR MASS

I. Neoplasms
  A. Malignant
    1. Primary lung cancer (see Chart 20.4)[234,477,479,598]
    2. Metastasis (e.g., kidney, colon, ovary, testis, Wilms tumor sarcoma)[197,325]
    3. Carcinoid (typical and atypical)
    4. Lymphoma[21,135]
    5. Primary sarcoma of lung
    6. Plasmacytoma (primary or secondary)
  B. Benign[135,469]
    1. Hamartoma
    2. Chondroma
    3. Arteriovenous malformation[456]
    4. Lipoma (usually a pleural lesion)
    5. Amyloidosis[246,430]
    6. Leiomyoma
    7. Hemangioma
    8. Intrapulmonary lymph node
    9. Endometrioma
    10. Fibroma
    11. Neural tumor (schwannoma and neurofibroma)
    12. Paraganglioma (chemodectoma)
II. Inflammatory diseases
  A. Granuloma[590]
    1. Tuberculosis[388]
    2. Histoplasmosis[97,109]
    3. Coccidioidomycosis
    4. Cryptococcosis (torulosis)[200,229,346,380]
    5. Nocardiosis
    6. Talc
    7. *Dirofilaria immitis* (dog heartworm)
    8. Gumma
    9. Atypical measles infection
    10. Sarcoidosis[432]
    11. Q fever[385]
  B. Abscess
  C. Hydatid cyst (fluid-filled)
  D. Bronchiectatic cyst (fluid-filled)
  E. Fungus ball
  F. Organizing pneumonia, cryptogenic organizing pneumonia (COP), atypical measles pneumonia,[661] cytomegalic inclusion virus[455]
  G. Inflammatory pseudotumor (e.g., fibroxanthoma, histiocytoma, plasma cell granuloma,[190,409] sclerosing hemangioma)[10]

continued

Chart 20.1   SOLITARY PULMONARY NODULE OR MASS—cont'd

   H. Bronchocele[334] and mucoid impaction[392]
   I. Round pneumonia[129,608]
III. Vascular diseases
   A. Infarct (organizing)[25,218]
   B. Pulmonary vein varix or anomaly[38]
   C. Rheumatoid nodule
   D. Granulomatosis with polyangiitis (formerly Wegener granulomatosis)
   E. Pulmonary artery aneurysm (Behçet syndrome)[11,414]
IV. Developmental abnormalities
   A. Bronchogenic cyst (fluid-filled)[463]
   B. Pulmonary sequestration
V. Inhalational diseases
   A. Silicosis (conglomerate mass)[636]
   B. Mucoid impaction (allergic aspergillosis)
   C. Paraffinoma (lipoid granuloma)
   D. Aspirated foreign body
VI. Other
   A. Hematoma
   B. Extramedullary hematopoiesis
   C. Emphysematous bulla (fluid-filled)
   D. Thrombolytic therapy
   E. Mimicking opacities[467]
      1. Fluid in interlobar fissure
      2. Mediastinal mass
      3. Pleural mass (mesothelioma)
      4. Chest wall opacities (e.g., nipple, rib lesion, skin tumor)
      5. Artifacts
      6. Atelectasis with bullous emphysema[188]
   F. Posttransplant lymphoproliferative disorder[119,224]
   G. Rounded atelectasis[35,60,64,122]

Chart 20.2   MOST LIKELY CAUSES OF SOLITARY PULMONARY NODULE

I. Neoplasms
   A. Malignant
      1. Primary lung tumor (see Chart 20.4)[222,234]
      2. Metastasis[325]
   B. Benign (less common)[135]
      1. Hamartoma
      2. Arteriovenous malformation
II. Infections
   A. Histoplasmosis[97,199]
   B. Tuberculosis[298]
   C. Coccidioidomycosis
   D. Organizing pneumonia
III. Vascular disease
   A. Infarct
IV. Mimicking opacities
   A. Artifacts (e.g., button, snap)[467,469]
   B. Nipple shadow
   C. Skin and subcutaneous lesions (e.g., mole, neurofibroma, lipoma)
   D. Pleural lesions (loculated effusion or pleural mass)
   E. Chest wall lesions[150,535]

| Chart 20.3 | **SOLITARY PULMONARY NODULE IN CHILDHOOD** |

I. Neoplasms
  A. Malignant
    1. Metastasis (neuroblastoma, Wilms tumor, Ewing sarcoma, osteosarcoma)
    2. Primary carcinoma (exceedingly rare)
    3. Blastoma[219]
  B. Benign
    1. Arteriovenous malformation
    2. Hamartoma
    3. Hemangioma
II. Inflammatory diseases
  A. Granuloma
  B. Organizing pneumonia (especially atypical measles pneumonia)[661]
III. Developmental conditions
  A. Bronchopulmonary sequestration
  B. Bronchogenic cyst

Modified from Young LW, Smith DI, Glasgow LA. Pneumonia of atypical measles. *Am J Roentgenol.* 1970;110:439-448.

| Chart 20.4 | **CLASSIFICATION AND FREQUENCY OF PRIMARY LUNG CANCER** |

I. Adenocarcinoma: 38%
II. Squamous cell carcinoma: 20%
III. Small cell carcinoma: 14%
IV. Large cell carcinoma: 3%
V. Large cell neuroendocrine carcinoma (LCNE): 3%
VI. Carcinoid typical and atypical: 1%
VII. Adenosquamous carcinoma: ≥0.6%
VIII. Sarcomatoid carcinoma: 0.3%

Modified from Travis WD. Pathology of lung cancer. *Clinics Chest Med.* 2011;32:669–692.

| Chart 20.5 | **CLASSIFICATION OF ADENOCARCINOMAS** |

I. Preinvasive
  A. Atypical adenomatous hyperplasia
  B. Adenocarcinoma in situ (formerly part of bronchioloalveolar cell carcinoma [BAC])
II. Minimally invasive adenocarcinoma (formerly part of BAC)
  A. Nonmucinous
  B. Mucinous
  C. Mixed
III. Invasive adenocarcinoma
  A. Lepidic (formerly part of BAC)
  B. Acinar
  C. Papillary
  D. Micropapillary
  E. Solid predominant with mucin
IV. Variants of invasive adenocarcinoma
  A. Invasive mucinous adenocarcinoma (formerly part of BAC)
  B. Colloid (former mucinous cystadenocarcinoma)
  C. Fetal
  D. Enteric

Modified from Tang ER, Schreiner AM, Pua BB: Advances in lung adenocarcinoma classification: a summary of the new international multidisciplinary classification system (IASLC/ATS/ERS). *J Thorac Dis.* 2014;6(Suppl 5):S489-S501.

Discussion

Primary lung cancer is the most critical cause of a solitary pulmonary nodule, but the list of possible causes is long (Chart 20.1). Fortunately, the list of common causes is much shorter (Chart 20.2). Healed granulomas from tuberculosis and fungal infections are the most common cause of a pulmonary nodule. These are benign and indicate prior infection but their diagnosis is important because they must be distinguished from malignant nodules.[613] The radiology report should emphasize the most serious of the possible diagnoses, offer a short differential diagnosis, and help the referring provider develop a plan to confirm the correct diagnosis.

NEOPLASMS

Lung Cancer

Perception is the first challenge confronting the radiologist in the task of lung cancer detection.[23,202,400] Good radiographic technique is essential for the detection of a pulmonary nodule. Woodring's review[651] of the pitfalls in the diagnosis of lung cancer reminds us that detection of small pulmonary nodules requires good technique and careful review of the radiograph. The standard chest examination includes a frontal radiograph, taken with the patient facing the detector and the radiograph beam passing posterior to anterior, and a lateral radiograph, which is taken with the patient's left side against the detector (left lateral). Both images should be taken at maximum inspiration. There is no perfect technique for all cases. The ideal frontal chest radiograph provides good detail of the central structures (e.g., trachea, carina, thoracic spine, intervertebral disk). This permits visualization of the normal vasculature posterior to the heart and thus makes detection of nodules posterior to the heart and posterior to the domes of the diaphragm possible. Adequate penetration of these opaque areas must be done while preserving good visualization of the peripheral vascular markings. This cannot be accomplished with low peak kilovoltage (kVp) techniques.[83,505] For example, a posteroanterior (PA) chest radiograph taken at 60 kVp will be too light for adequate evaluation of the mediastinum. With the low-kVp technique, the lungs will be black if the mediastinum and left lower lobe are adequately penetrated. This has led to the development of higher kVp techniques for standard chest radiography. It is generally agreed that the optimal kVp is in the range of 120 to 150 kVp. This is a major limiting feature of portable chest radiography, which makes it inadequate for the exclusion of pulmonary nodules. The only major disadvantage of the high-kVp technique is the reduced visibility of calcium.

Viewing time for the detection of a nodule on a chest radiograph by an experienced radiologist may be surprisingly short, but it requires a trained, systematic visual search. Kundel et al.[320] demonstrated that obvious cancers are often detected with flash viewing of the image and that subtle cancers may be detected with as short a viewing time as 4 seconds. It was even suggested that prolonged viewing of longer than 10 seconds does not improve the number of true-positive results but increases false-positive results. Detection of less conspicuous nodules is improved by knowledge of the anatomic areas in which lesions are likely to be obscured. Comparisons are vital. For example, the right and left pulmonary arteries should be symmetrically opaque. Asymmetric opacity at the junction of the costal cartilage and the rib must be carefully scrutinized. Nodules in the medial portions of the lung may be obscured by large vessels or the heart and may thus be more easily detected on the lateral than on the PA view (Fig 20.3, *A* and *B*). Obvious abnormalities that may even be insignificant sometimes capture the viewer's attention and interfere with the detection of a subtle lung cancer. After detecting an abnormality, observers should make a conscious effort to complete the review of the examination and avoid the phenomenon of satisfaction of search as a cause of missed

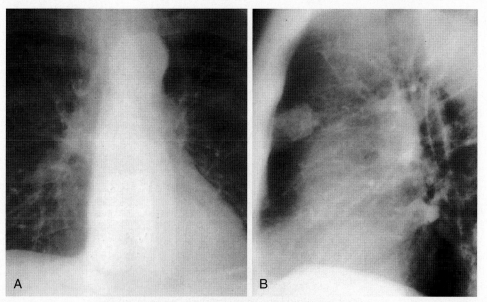

Fig. 20.3   A, This lung cancer projects over the right pulmonary artery and causes only a minimal change in opacity of the right hilum. This would have been missed if the examination had not included a lateral view. **B,** The corresponding lateral view shows an obvious mass in the retrosternal clear space. The lateral view is an essential part of the chest examination and often accounts for the detection of lung cancers that are superimposed over the hilum or mediastinum.

abnormalities.[644] Comparisons with previous examinations also enhance the visual search and may make subtle or minimal opacities more detectable.

Conspicuity of a solitary pulmonary nodule is determined by its size, location, margins, growth patterns, and tissue density.[290] These characteristics of a nodule determine detectability on both the radiograph and computed tomography (CT) scan. Because of its increased sensitivity, CT has even expanded our understanding and definition of nodules by including the categories of ground-glass and mixed ground-glass nodules with partly solid nodules.

Size often determines the conspicuity of a nodule or mass. By definition, a nodule measures up to 3 cm, and above 3 cm it is considered to be a mass. Kundel et al.[320] reported that nodules less than 1 cm in size are not usually detected by chest radiography. Heelan et al.[232] suggested that the threshold nodule size for reliable detection of peripheral lung cancer on the chest radiograph is larger than 1 cm; they reported prospective detection from screening radiographs as ranging from 0.7 to 9.4 cm, with an average size of 2.4 cm. The detection threshold by CT is better, with a threshold of 3 mm, but the average nodule size detected by CT is 1 to 1.5 cm.

Location is also a major variable that affects detection of a solitary pulmonary nodule. Superimposition of normal structures is one of the major problems affecting radiologic detection of lung cancers. This has been described as *anatomic noise*[505] and accounts for some of the well-known blind spots on the chest radiograph. Nodules are often obscured by an overlying rib, costal cartilage calcification, clavicle, scapula, pulmonary vessel, aorta, great vessel, or heart shadow (Fig 20.4, *A* and *B*). A nodule in the apex of the lung may be obscured by the shadow of a rib or the clavicle; the dome of the diaphragm may obscure a posterior lower lobe nodule. The retrocardiac area is a region that is usually obscured on the PA view and is better evaluated on the lateral view. Some nodules in the base of the lung are better visualized on an abdominal examination than a chest radiograph.

The margins of a nodule are determined by the interface of the nodule with the surrounding lung. This frequently influences visibility of the nodule and may also

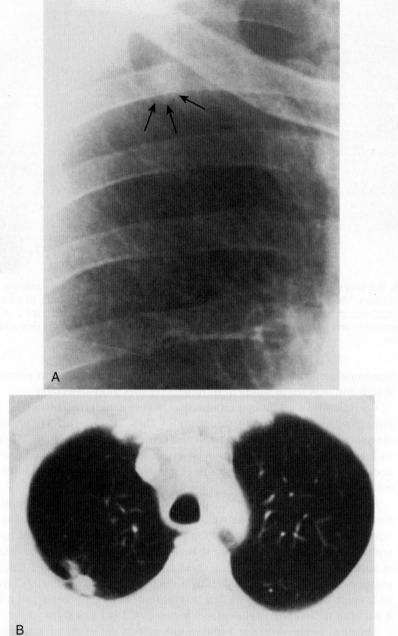

Fig. 20.4   A, This peripheral lung cancer is minimally visible because of its size and position over a posterior rib. Note the rounded inferior border *(arrows).* **B,** Computed tomography confirms an irregular mass that extends to the pleura.

provide clues to the correct diagnosis. The margins may be smooth, lobulated, ill defined, or spiculated. Spiculated margins are a common pattern of lung cancers (Fig 20.5). Heitzman's[234] pathologic correlations of the irregular spiculated margins indicate that some of the spiculations are related to the spread of the tumor into the pulmonary parenchyma, whereas others represent fibrotic strands that presumably are part of a desmoplastic reaction to the tumor. Heitzman also emphasized that similar margin characteristics may be seen in organizing infections and infarcts. Irregular spiculated margins are therefore not regarded as pathognomonic of cancer, but they

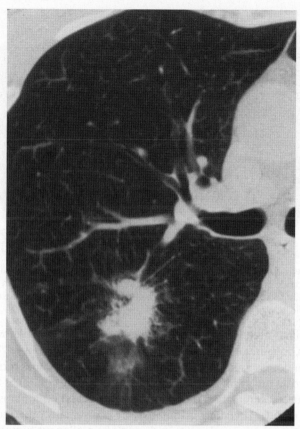

Fig. 20.5 Spiculated masses have a high probability of malignancy. High-resolution computed tomography provides excellent characterization of the margins of this adenocarcinoma. The spiculations may represent desmoplastic fibrosis or interstitial invasion by the tumor. Because inflammatory lesions and infarcts may cause spiculated masses, biopsy is required for diagnosis.

are nevertheless strongly suggestive of malignancy. The value of this sign is greatly enhanced by serial examinations because the organizing processes tend to become smaller and less spiculated as the inflammatory reaction around the resolving infection or infarct fades. This is in marked contrast to the changing margin characteristics that are anticipated in a primary lung cancer. As a primary carcinoma of the lung grows, it continues to invade the surrounding lymphatics and blood vessels of the lung parenchyma. The mass not only enlarges but becomes more spiculated and possibly even ill defined (see Fig 20.2, *A* and *B*). Although the margin characteristics may not be diagnostic on a single chest radiograph, they may be virtually diagnostic on serial examinations.[477] In contrast, a nodule with very smooth margins is not as common in patients with primary lung cancer, but this appearance should not be used to exclude the diagnosis. Slow-growing adenocarcinomas (see Fig 20.1, *A* and *B*), squamous cell carcinomas, and carcinoids may all present as well-circumscribed solitary nodules. Benign slow-growing tumors[135] such as hamartomas are expected to have a sharp interface with the surrounding lung with well-defined margins, and granulomas become more sharply defined as the surrounding inflammatory reactions are replaced by fibrosis.

The growth of lung cancer has been extensively studied using the measure of doubling time. Serial chest radiographs, which document growth of a nodule, are strong evidence that the nodule is malignant (see Fig 20.2, *A* and *B*). (Answer to question 2 is *d.*) Nodules that enlarge very slowly are more likely to be benign.[135] For example, a nodule that doubles its diameter every 18 months suggests a benign tumor, such as

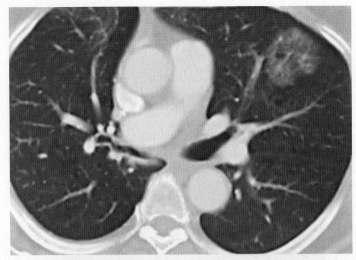

Fig. 20.6 This computed tomography demonstrates a focal area of ground-glass opacity in the left upper lobe. This was minimally detectable on the chest radiograph. The opacity did not resolve with antibiotic treatment and was initially diagnosed as bronchioloalveolar cell carcinoma. A ground-glass opacity measuring under 3 cm is most consistent with the classification of adenocarcinoma in situ.

a hamartoma. Additional diagnostic considerations for slow-growing nodules include carcinoids, inflammatory pseudotumors, and even granulomas.[199] It may be surprising to list granulomas as nodules that may grow, but granulomas form as an immunologic response to an organism. If this immunologic response continues to be active, there will be continued accumulation of inflammatory cells and even fibrosis around the periphery of the nodule. Therefore, granulomas are occasionally observed to slowly increase in size. Slow growth makes absolute exclusion of a malignant tumor difficult because low-grade adenocarcinomas and metastases such as renal cell carcinoma may enlarge very slowly. Despite the lack of specificity, growth of nodules may be carefully followed by CT.[242] When no change is detected after 2 years, it is generally recommended that the lesion be considered benign.[16] Henschke et al.[243] recommend follow-up CT of nodules 5 mm or smaller at 12 and 24 months, but ground-glass nodules may require more than a 24-month follow-up. Growth on an interval scan is considered an indication for biopsy. Alternate strategies have used contrast-enhanced CT scans or fludeoxyglucose–positron emission tomography (FDG-PET) scans.[136] Because both active granulomas and tumors may be positive with either approach, a positive scan is an indication for biopsy.

Tissue density evaluation of suspected lung cancers on the chest radiograph is limited to tumors that appear as solid homogenous opacities and those that are heterogeneous with air bronchograms. The latter group may have an appearance that requires consideration of focal air space opacity versus a nodule. A heterogeneous appearance with air bronchograms is a common pattern for pneumonia but is also the expected pattern of invasive mucinous adenocarcinomas, formerly bronchioloalveolar cell carcinoma (BAC). CT attenuation analysis of a nodule permits the radiologist to classify nodules more precisely as ground-glass, mixed ground-glass with a partly solid component, and solid nodules.[16,268,294] These patterns correlate with the recent classification of adenocarcinomas (Chart 20.5).[577] A ground-glass nodule through which pulmonary vessels are identified measuring 5 mm to 3 cm is the appearance of adenocarcinoma in situ (Fig 20.6; answer to question 3 is *e*), and a partly solid ground-glass nodule measuring less than 3 cm with a solid component measuring less than 5 mm is the expected appearance of minimally invasive adenocarcinoma (MIA). As the size of the solid component in a partly solid nodule increases, the diagnosis of invasive adenocarcinoma becomes more likely, and a solid nodule is the most common presentation of invasive adenocarcinoma (see Fig 20.1). (Answer to question 1 is *d*.)[577,597,598]

The texture of both solid and ground-glass nodules is usually homogeneous, but deviations from this homogeneous character are common and often add diagnostic information. Intervening lucencies may result from air bronchograms, spared parenchyma, necrosis with cavitation, and pseudocavitation. Multiple small lucencies throughout the opacity are more in keeping with an inflammatory process such as a resolving pneumonia. However, caution is warranted in these cases because lymphomas and invasive adenocarcinomas may mimic organizing pneumonias. Demonstration of air bronchograms through an opacity might be considered to be a diagnostic feature in favor of an inflammatory process, but invasive mucinous adenocarcinoma and lymphoma[21,457,460] spread around the bronchi leaving open, air-containing bronchi throughout the tumor. The air bronchogram is therefore not a reliable feature for distinguishing tumor from pneumonia. Opacities with air bronchograms that persist over a period of weeks, particularly after antibiotic therapy, raise the possibility of neoplasm and are an indication for further evaluation that may include sputum cytology or biopsy. CT often reveals small areas of low attenuation in both ground-glass and solid nodules, which may represent spared parenchyma, ectatic bronchi, or focal emphysema and are described as a pseudocavity.[221] Pseudocavities may be seen in pneumonias but are a common observation in adenocarcinomas.

The limitations of the chest radiograph for detection of a solitary pulmonary nodule are well documented.[22,437,505] Even with optimal techniques, careful review of the radiographs, and application of a thorough knowledge of the anatomic structures that may obscure small pulmonary nodules, there are limitations to the sensitivity and specificity of the chest radiograph for detection of a solitary pulmonary nodule. The error rate for the detection of early lung cancer has been reported to vary between 20% and 50%.[651] Studies specifically designed for screening patients at high risk for lung cancer suggest that the error rate may be even higher. Muhm et al.[400] designed a study for screening cigarette smokers older than 45 years with chest radiographs taken at 4-month intervals. The examinations were evaluated twice. The study included more than 4000 patients and detected 92 lung cancers; of these 92, 50 cancers presented as peripheral pulmonary nodules. The researchers reported that in retrospect, 90% of the peripheral cancers were detectable on earlier examinations. Although 27 of the tumors had been visible for 1 year or less, 14 were identified between 12 and 24 months, and 4 had been visible for more than 2 years. Based on these data, the chest radiograph has not been recommended as a screening procedure for lung cancer detection, but lung cancers continue to be diagnosed because of a suspected abnormality on a chest radiograph. CT is the procedure of choice for confirmation and evaluation of a pulmonary nodule that is suspected on a chest radiograph (Fig 20.7, *A* and *B*). It provides precise localization of the nodule and is reliable for detection of other radiologic features of the nodule, including calcification, cavitation, and spiculated borders.[665,669] CT may be done without intravenous contrast when the scan is performed for the detection of calcification, but contrast is often useful for the evaluation of noncalcified nodules. Swensen et al.[572] showed that evaluation of noncalcified nodules with enhanced CT is useful for the distinction of tumor versus granuloma. Tumors were shown to enhance with iodinated contrast, whereas granulomas did not enhance.

Perception challenges are not limited to the radiograph. There have also been studies that indicate a need for caution regarding problems with perception of lung cancer on CT scans. Some of the same perception problems that are applicable to interpretation of the chest radiograph may also apply to the interpretation of chest CT scans. Gurney[211] reported on a series of patients with lung cancers not detected on CT in which five peripheral tumors were below the CT threshold, measuring less than 3 mm in diameter. White et al.[630] reported on 14 patients with primary lung cancer overlooked on CT. They emphasized that problems in detection included nodules in the lower lobes, small focal air space opacities, thickening of the pleura, and endobronchial

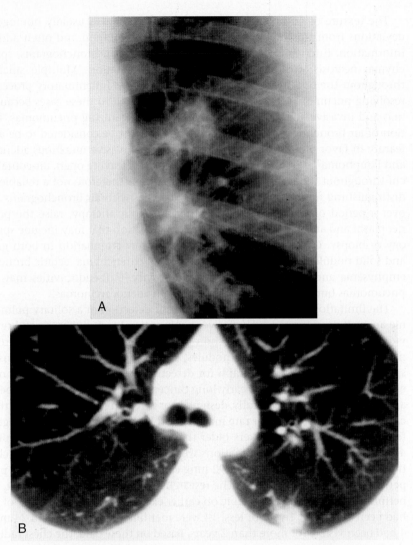

Fig. 20.7 **A,** This opacity with poorly defined margins projects above the left hilum and is suggestive of a hilar mass. **B,** Computed tomography (CT) confirms the presence of a mass in the periphery of the superior segment of the left lower lobe, rather than the left hilum, as suggested by the plain film. CT is essential for confirmation and precise localization of suspected lung cancers.

lesions. This study emphasizes that not all lung cancers present as a solitary pulmonary nodule and it shows the difficulty of correctly recognizing the other patterns of lung cancer.

CT screening for lung cancer is based on the documented sensitivity of CT as opposed to radiography.[399] Coincidental detection of lung cancers on chest CT performed for other indications is not rare, and these cancers are often not detectable on the radiograph even when the observer knows the location of the tumor. The sensitivity of CT led Henschke et al.[242] to conduct a study of CT as a screening procedure for lung cancer. The study enrolled 1000 smokers older than 60 years, which was followed with a second study of 1897 patients.[243] In the first study they detected noncalcified nodules in 233 participants, compared with 68 detected on chest radiographs. Of the CT-detected nodules, 27 were malignant, compared with 7 cancers detected on the radiographs. In addition, 23 of the 27 malignant nodules were stage I, suggesting that CT could be an effective method for the detection of early stage I lung cancer. It was noted that 210 patients with a false-positive CT scan had benign opacities that were managed with follow-up CT scanning and required few invasive procedures. In their second study, Henschke et al.[243] concluded that noncalcified nodules smaller than 5.0 mm should have a 1-year follow-up scan. In a similar study, Swenson et al.[573] showed CT to be sensitive for the detection of lung cancer but reported a high rate of benign nodule detection.

The national lung cancer screening trial was designed and conducted by investigators from multiple institutions to determine the impact of CT screening on mortality of lung cancer. The study ran from 2002 to 2011 and enrolled 54,454 individuals who were at high risk for the development of lung cancer. The positive rate of low-dose CT was 24.2% compared with 6.9% on chest radiography. There was a 20% reduction of the mortality rate from lung cancer with low-dose CT screening.[3] This improvement in the mortality rate is the result of detecting small stage I adenocarcinomas.

Staging of Lung Cancer

The prognosis and treatment of non–small cell lung cancer is directly related to the histologic type and stage at the time of diagnosis. Staging of non–small cell tumors according to the tumor node metastasis system (TNM) provides an estimation of the extent of tumor spread before any therapy is initiated.[397] Staging strategies are based on the correlation of clinical findings via radiologic evaluation by chest radiography, CT, magnetic resonance imaging (MRI), and positron emission tomography (PET) with biopsy results. The findings on chest radiography, CT, and MRI are important but do not have all the information for accurate lung cancer staging.[616] The radiologic abnormalities are evaluated primarily by size criteria. For example, hilar and mediastinal nodes may be measured in either the short or long axis, but are most often measured in the short axis. Nodes measuring more than 10 mm in the short axis are usually defined as abnormal, but using this measurement has a sensitivity and specificity of only 65%. Recognizing this limitation, radiologists may find CT staging most useful for identifying those patients with very advanced disease and for determining the need for preoperative biopsy of lymph nodes. PET-CT provides improved specificity by combing the CT anatomic findings with metabolic activity of lymph nodes and has the added advantage of detecting distant metastases.

Lung cancer presenting as a solitary pulmonary nodule with no evidence of spread to regional nodes and no evidence of distant metastases is a stage I tumor.[397] Stage I tumors should be considered for surgical resection and have the best prognosis. Even within the stage I group, tumor size does affect prognosis and has been emphasized in the updated staging systems.[452] Patients with stage II or stage IIIA tumors have evidence of local spread of tumor that may be extensive. These patients require careful staging to ensure an optimal treatment plan, which may include radical surgery, radiation therapy, and chemotherapy. Stage IIIB tumors are rarely resectable, and stage IV tumors present with distant metastases. Patients with stage IIIB or stage IV tumors are frequently candidates for palliative therapy. The 12-month survival of stage IV tumors is less than 20% and their 5-year survival approaches 0%.

Carcinoid Tumors

Carcinoid tumors are neuroendocrine tumors that usually arise in the gastrointestinal tract, but approximately 20% develop in the bronchi. In contrast with small cell lung cancers, which are also neuroendocrine tumors, these tumors follow an indolent course. Carcinoid tumors account for about 1% of lung cancers. The typical carcinoid may be present for a long time before the patient develops symptoms, but the tumor is malignant and first spreads to regional lymph nodes. Atypical carcinoid is a more aggressive histologic cell type. Since pulmonary carcinoid tumors develop in the airways, they usually cause segmental or lobar atelectasis, but when they arise in more peripheral bronchi, they will present as a solitary pulmonary nodule, which may contain calcification[668] (Fig 20.8, *A-C*). Carcinoid syndrome, which includes skin flushing, bronchoconstriction,

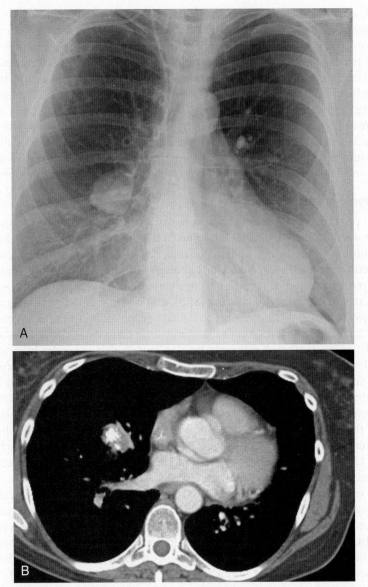

Fig. 20.8 **A,** This well-circumscribed right middle lobe mass was biopsied and confirmed to be a typical carcinoid. **B,** Axial computed tomography showed the nodule to be homogeneous with an inferior calcification.

diarrhea, and right heart failure, occurs in patients with liver metastases; these are usually seen in patients with gastrointestinal carcinoid and are rare in patients with respiratory carcinoid.[39] (Answer to question 4 is *c*.)

Solitary Metastasis

Solitary pulmonary metastasis is the most likely diagnosis in a patient with a well-circumscribed nodule and a history of extrapulmonary malignant neoplasm, but it must be distinguished from a primary lung cancer. Quint et al.[449] reported that patients with the following neoplasms—head and neck, bladder, breast, cervix, esophagus, prostate, stomach, bile duct, or ovarian carcinomas—are more likely to have a primary bronchogenic carcinoma. In this same study, smokers had a 35-fold greater chance of having a primary lung cancer as the cause of a solitary pulmonary nodule rather than a metastasis. Patients with melanoma, sarcoma, or testicular carcinoma were more likely to have a solitary metastasis than a bronchogenic carcinoma.

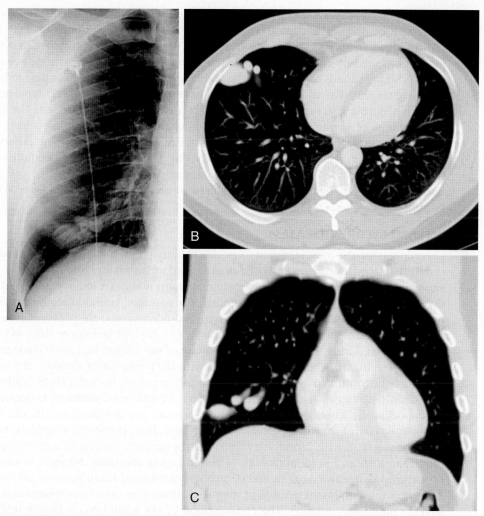

Fig. 20.9   A, This right lower lobe nodular opacity has a lobulated appearance suggestive of feeding vessels. **B,** Axial computed tomography (CT) shows large vessels extending toward the hilum. **C,** Coronal CT confirms the characteristic appearance of an arteriovenous malformation. These may be multiple in patients with Rendu-Osler-Weber disease.

Hamartoma

Hamartomas are benign tumors that contain multiple cell types growing at different rates. These masses are often circumscribed and may be lobulated, which is an appearance that is not adequately specific to confirm the diagnosis. Calcification is an additional radiologic finding that may be present in as many as 20% of hamartomas. In contrast to typical granulomatous calcifications, hamartomatous calcifications consist of rings and dots that may be scattered throughout the bulk of the tumor. This calcification resembles the calcified cartilaginous matrix seen in cartilaginous bone tumors and is, in fact, ossification of the cartilage contained within the tumor. CT reliably detects fat in the mass, which frequently confirms the diagnosis of hamartoma.[135]

Arteriovenous Malformation

An arteriovenous malformation (AVM)[135] is a lesion that may assume a characteristic shape (Fig 20.9, *A-C*). The presence of large vessels entering a nodule should strongly suggest the diagnosis. The definitive diagnostic procedure is a contrast-enhanced CT scan. It is imperative to rule out the possibility of AVM prior to transbronchial or percutaneous biopsy. Of the benign neoplasms, pulmonary AVMs may have strongly suggestive or diagnostic clinical associations. Patients with pulmonary AVMs may have dyspnea, hemoptysis, cyanosis, clubbing of the fingers, and polycythemia, which may be followed by congestive heart failure. Physical findings may include extracardiac humming sounds or bruits over the chest, particularly when the fistulas are large. Arteriovenous fistulas usually occur spontaneously but have also been reported to occur as sequelae to trauma. In addition, there are hereditary associations. The clinical syndrome of Rendu-Osler-Weber disease is characterized by multiple AVMs that may involve the skin, lips, gastrointestinal tract, urinary bladder, nose, central nervous system, and lungs. Hemorrhage is the most severe and life-threatening complication of a pulmonary AVM—hemoptysis is a common presentation. Associated gastrointestinal bleeding or signs of intracranial bleeding should suggest Rendu-Osler-Weber syndrome.[271]

INFLAMMATORY DISEASES

Granulomas are the most common cause of a solitary pulmonary nodule, but absolute certainty in the clinical diagnosis of a noncalcified inflammatory nodule is rarely possible, and they must be distinguished from malignant nodules. Certain clinical settings do occasionally permit an accurate diagnosis. The common granulomatous infections, mainly tuberculosis, histoplasmosis, and coccidioidomycosis, are occasionally diagnosed as the cause of a nodule on the basis of clinical and laboratory data. When a patient is seen during the acute exudative phase of the disease, and serial chest radiographs reveal that the exudate has organized with the formation of a nodule, the causal agent may be confirmed by growing the organism in culture from the acute exudate or by a definite rise in the patient's serologic titers. Cryptococcal infection is frequently an opportunistic infection that may mimic primary bronchogenic carcinoma.[380] It may require transbronchial, percutaneous, or open lung biopsy for diagnosis, but it may be associated with central nervous system symptoms, leading to a cerebrospinal fluid examination and identification of the infecting organism. *Nocardia* is another opportunistic organism that should be strongly considered when patients are known to be immunosuppressed because of neoplastic disease or organ transplantation and develop pulmonary nodules. The consideration of talc granuloma is largely reserved for drug abusers. In this clinical setting, the development of solitary or multiple pulmonary nodules is suggestive of septic emboli, which may frequently contain talc.

Calcifications detected on chest radiographs or CT scans that are central, laminated, or complete confirm the diagnosis of granuloma[135] (Fig 20.10, *A* and *B*). (Answer to question 5 is *c*.) Although concentric swirls of calcification in the center of the mass are virtually diagnostic of a granuloma, eccentric calcification in the periphery of a lesion should not be regarded as an indication of a benign process. Tumors occasionally arise around preexistent calcified scars, at times engulfing a healed granuloma. In such cases, the calcification is most likely to be eccentric. Another explanation for eccentric calcification is reactivation of an old granulomatous process. In either case, the presence of a mass with eccentric calcification warrants further diagnostic evaluation. In the case of multiple pulmonary nodules, it must be emphasized that patients may have calcified granulomas and also develop carcinomas. The presence of calcium in one nodule is meaningless with regard to the evaluation of a second soft tissue nodule. The detection of minimal calcification in a mass must also be cautiously evaluated. Microscopic calcifications in primary lung tumors and metastatic tumors, particularly from mucin-producing adenocarcinomas (Fig 20.11, *A* and *B*) and certainly from primary bone tumors, are not rare.[359] Calcification from metastases of osteosarcoma may be readily detected by conventional radiographic examinations, but the microscopic calcifications seen in primary lung tumors are very rarely detectable by conventional radiography. Detection of minimal calcification by thin-section CT or CT with a

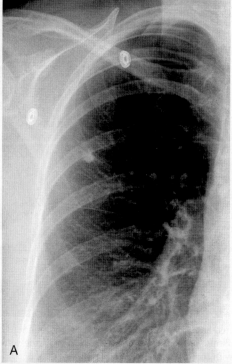

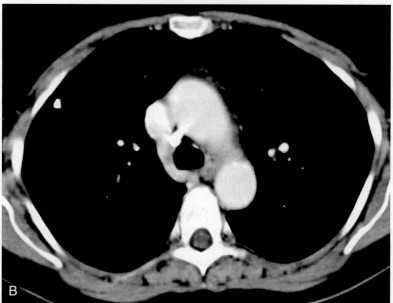

Fig. 20.10   A, This right upper lobe nodule is well visualized, but the chest radiograph is not adequate to confirm benign calcification. **B,** Thin-section computed tomography is ideal for confirmation of central, laminated, or complete calcification of granulomas.

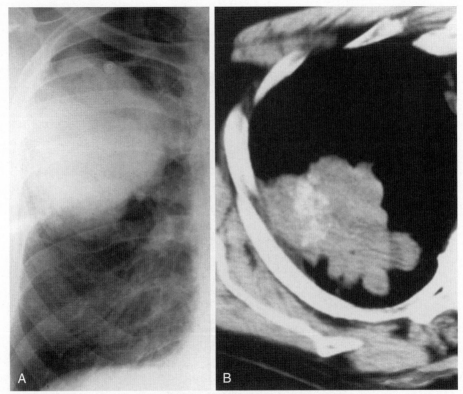

Fig. 20.11 A, This large lobulated adenocarcinoma appears to be homogenous on the chest radiograph. **B,** Computed tomography shows amorphous speckled areas of calcification in a large soft-tissue opacity mass. These calcifications should not be confused with the calcifications of a benign granuloma.

reference phantom may lead to an incorrect diagnosis of a benign process. The following criteria are recommended for avoiding the potential pitfalls of thin-section CT:

1. Benign calcifications should extend over 10% of the cross-sectional area of the nodule.

2. The calcification must have a symmetric pattern of deposition (e.g., diffuse, laminated, or central nidus).

3. Benign nodules have smooth margins.

4. Benign nodules should not be larger than 3 cm in diameter.

5. Nodules meeting the preceding criteria should show no change in 24 months of follow-up.

Aspergillus fungus balls (Fig 20.12) may present as solitary or multiple pulmonary nodules. They are a noninvasive saprophytic manifestation of aspergillosis. In contrast with healed granulomas, fungus balls colonize preexisting cysts, cavities, or bullae. They typically occur in chronic tuberculous cavities but do not indicate the cause of the cavitary lesion, and have even been reported in cavitary neoplasms. Although they are noninvasive, they could erode the walls of the cavities and may cause severe hemoptysis.

A pulmonary abscess is not clinically or radiologically suggested without evidence of a previous necrotizing pneumonia. An abscess usually causes cavitary opacities, but may be filled with fluid and appear as a nodule or mass on plain film. CT should confirm the liquefaction but is still limited for distinguishing an infectious versus a neoplastic cavitary opacity.

Atypical measles pneumonia is a cause of a solitary pulmonary nodule during childhood (Chart 20.3). These nodules occur in patients with an atypical form of measles

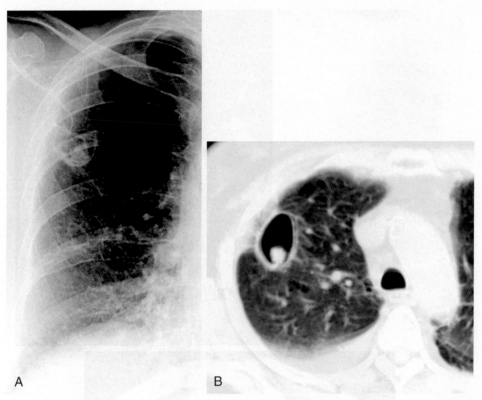

Fig. 20.12   A, *Aspergillus* fungus balls form in preexisting cavities and may resemble a solitary pulmonary nodule. The presence of a nodule or mass within a thin-walled lucent area may be a diagnostic appearance. **B,** Computed tomography is not always required to make this diagnosis but may be confirmatory.

characterized by a febrile illness with cough, headache, myalgias, abdominal pain, and peripheral maculopapular rash. However, the rash has been an inconsistent finding, making the diagnosis more difficult. A pneumonia developed in all the patients in the study by Young et al.,[661] frequently associated with hilar adenopathy and pleural effusion. Resolution of the pneumonia was atypical in that a solitary pulmonary nodule was left as a residual of the illness. The diagnosis of atypical measles is based on a rise in the hemagglutination inhibition and complement fixation titers of late convalescent sera. Young et al.[661] emphasized that immunization for measles with inactivated virus vaccine precedes the atypical measles infection by a period of 3 to 4½ years.

VASCULAR DISEASES

An organizing infarct may be suspected in patients who have a preceding history of pulmonary embolism weeks or months prior to the development of a nodule. This may be even more evident when the radiographs obtained during the period of the acute embolic episode show areas of increased radiologic opacity in the same area as the demonstrated pulmonary nodule. These nodules may safely be assumed to represent organized infarcts, and a more rigorous evaluation should not be necessary.

Pulmonary vein varix[38] is another vascular abnormality that may present as a solitary opacity. These lesions occur in the medial portion of the lung, just before the veins enter the left atrium. Fluoroscopy is a valuable procedure for their identification because the Valsalva maneuver will demonstrate a change in size, indicating a vascular mass. Pulmonary arteriography distinguishes pulmonary vein varix from AVM.

Bronchopulmonary sequestrations (Fig 20.13, *A-C*) most often occur in the lower lobes and often present as an incidental finding on a chest radiograph. They frequently

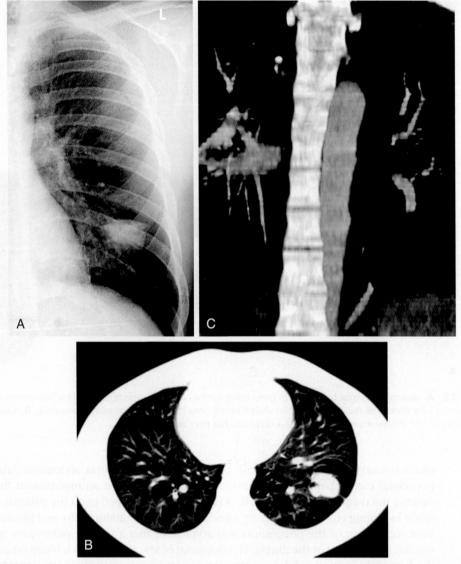

Fig. 20.13 A, This solitary nodular-appearing opacity in the left lower lobe has surrounding lucency, but this is not an appearance that permits a specific diagnosis. **B,** Axial computed tomography (CT) reveals a lobulated opacity with surrounding cystic lesions. **C,** Coronal CT reveals a vessel extending from the descending aorta toward the left lower lobe. This is an intralobar pulmonary sequestration.

appear as a solitary pulmonary nodule or mass. They are complex multicystic foregut anomalies and have a feeding vessel from the aorta rather than the pulmonary artery. These cysts may be filled with fluid, but after they develop communications with the bronchi they will appear as lucent multicystic lesions.

Top 5 Diagnoses: Solitary Pulmonary Nodule

1. Primary lung cancer
2. Solitary metastasis
3. Tuberculous granuloma
4. Fungal granuloma (e.g., histoplasmosis, coccidioidomycosis)
5. Hamartoma

Summary

Perception of the abnormality is the most important task of the radiologist in the management of a patient with a solitary nodule.

The optimal chest radiograph is performed using high-kilovoltage techniques (120–150 kVp).

The only disadvantage of the high-kilovoltage technique is the decreased visualization of calcium. Calcium is best visualized at 68 kVp. This may increase the number of patients requiring CT evaluation of nodules.

The differential diagnosis of a solitary nodule is lengthy, but consideration of lung cancer is a critical responsibility of the interpreting radiologist.

Care must be taken to recognize artifacts, skin lesions (e.g., moles), rib lesions (e.g., fractures), and calcified benign bone islands.

Fluoroscopy is an expeditious way of localizing rib lesions and artifacts.

Monitoring serial examinations is particularly useful for distinguishing pneumonias or infarcts from tumors. Infarcts and infections regress in size; tumors grow.

Clinical correlation may confirm infectious processes, infarcts, and metastases.

Pulmonary AVM and varix are suggested on the basis of their shape and location. CT should confirm the diagnosis.

CT is more sensitive than chest radiography for detection of small pulmonary nodules, but CT is not adequately specific to differentiate a benign from malignant noncalcified nodule.

Central laminated or total calcification is the most reliable feature for radiologic diagnosis of a benign granuloma.

Noncalcified nodules may be evaluated with contrast-enhanced CT scan or FDG-PET.

Because both neoplasms and active granulomas may take up iodinated contrast or FDG, a positive scan may be an indication for biopsy.

The ultimate diagnosis often requires biopsy.

ANSWER GUIDE

Legends for introductory figures

Fig. 20.1 A, This sharply circumscribed solitary pulmonary nodule requires consideration of both malignant and benign disease. **B, C**omputed tomography (CT) reveals this nodule to be solid and mildly lobulated. Biopsy confirmed invasive adenocarcinoma.
Fig. 20.2 A, This perihilar opacity has irregular spiculated borders. **B,** Examination 5 months later revealed the opacity to be larger and more irregular. This is a classic growth pattern for primary lung cancer.

ANSWERS

1. d   2. d   3. e   4. c   5. c

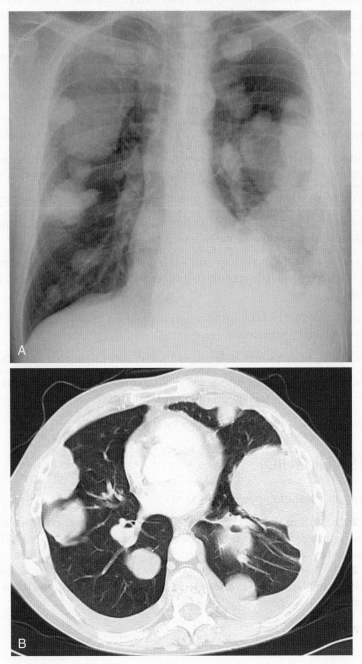

Fig. 21.1

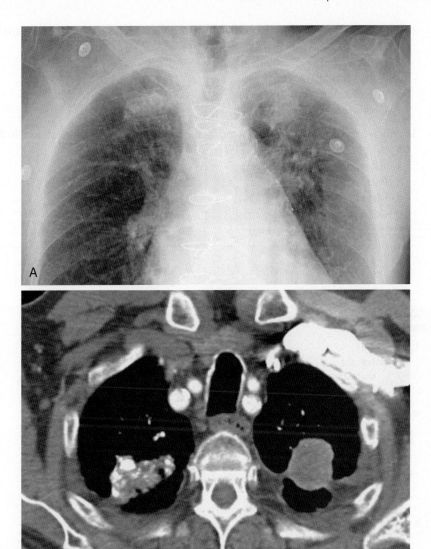

Fig. 21.2

QUESTIONS

1. A 50-year-old man admitted with a history of weight loss had the examinations shown
   in Fig. 21.1, *A* and *B*. Which one of the following procedures would most likely determine the site of a primary tumor?
   a. Physical examination of the testis.
   b. Total spine radiograph.
   c. Radionuclide bone scan.
   d. Computed tomography (CT) scan of the brain.
   e. Magnetic resonance imaging (MRI) of the knee.

2. Which one of the following primary tumors is least likely to metastasize to the lung?
   a. Melanoma.
   b. Osteosarcoma.
   c. Astrocytoma.
   d. Adenocarcinoma of the colon.
   e. Choriocarcinoma.

3. Which one of the following diagnoses is most likely in the patient shown in Fig. 21.2, *A* and *B*?
   a. Tuberculosis.
   b. Primary lung cancer.
   c. Metastases.
   d. Coal worker's pneumoconiosis.
   e. Histoplasmosis.

Chart 21.1	**MULTIPLE NODULES AND MASSES**

I. Neoplastic
   A. Malignant
      1. Metastases (kidney, gastrointestinal tract, uterus, ovary, testes; melanoma, sarcoma)
      2. Lymphoma[21,126,543]
      3. Posttransplantation lymphoproliferative disorder[119,224,474]
      4. Kaposi sarcoma (acquired immunodeficiency syndrome [AIDS] related)[126]
   B. Benign
      1. Hamartoma[510]
      2. Arteriovenous malformation[135] or hemangioma
      3. Amyloidosis[246,604]
      4. Benign metastasizing leiomyoma[7]
II. Inflammatory
   A. Fungal[371]
      1. Histoplasmosis[283]
      2. Coccidioidomycosis[283]
      3. Cryptococcosis[200]
      4. Invasive aspergillosis[224]
   B. Nocardiosis[29,208]
   C. Tuberculosis[388] (typical and atypical)
   D. Parasites
      1. Hydatid cysts[30,435]
      2. Paragonimiasis[260,262]
   E. Atypical measles[661]
   F. Inflammatory pseudotumors[10] (e.g., fibrous histiocytoma, plasma cell granuloma,[283] hyalinizing pulmonary nodules)
   G. Q fever[385]
   H. Sarcoidosis
III. Vascular
      1. Rheumatoid nodules and Caplan syndrome[59,283]
      2. Granulomatosis with polyangitis[4]
      3. Organizing infarcts[25,218]
      4. Septic emboli
IV. Posttraumatic (organizing hematoma)[499]
V. Chronic renal failure (calcified nodules)[77]

Discussion

One of the first decisions in the evaluation of the chest radiograph showing multiple pulmonary opacities is to distinguish multiple nodules and masses from areas of pulmonary consolidation. Nodules and masses are more circumscribed and homogenous, whereas consolidating lesions have less circumscribed borders and are less solid, often containing aerated alveoli and air bronchograms. Loss of definition of the border implies that the process is spreading into the lung parenchyma, either following interstitial planes or actually spilling into the alveolar spaces. Loss of definition is therefore more consistent with a consolidating process. High-resolution CT has been used to better characterize the borders of a variety of metastatic nodules and has shown that metastases may be locally invasive,[247] which would account for the phenomenon of nodules growing and becoming less circumscribed.

A second major problem confronting the radiologist in the evaluation of the patient with multiple pulmonary nodules is the perception of the nodules. Small, peripheral pulmonary nodules are often not detectable on the chest radiograph. These nodules are obscured by surrounding vascular opacities or may be incompletely surrounded by aerated lung. They are also obscured by overlying ribs. CT reliably detects peripheral subpleural nodules and nodules obscured by the heart, mediastinum, and vessels.[399,624] Spiral CT with a single breath-hold technique reduces artifacts and has reduced the risk of missing small nodules that change position with respiratory motion. CT is the most sensitive procedure available for detecting pulmonary nodules. By increasing the sensitivity of the procedure, it has become the optimal technique for staging a variety of cancers; however, as the sensitivity increases, the specificity decreases. Although CT detects more metastatic nodules than chest radiography, it also detects more benign nodules caused by granulomas and unrelated scars. The decision to perform a CT scan should be based on the primary diagnosis and the plan of therapy. When the radiographs show multiple, bilateral pulmonary nodules, the value of detecting an additional number of nodules depends on the mode of therapy planned for the patient. If the therapy will not be influenced by the detection of additional nodules, it is doubtful whether the more expensive and complicated procedure is justified. When resection of a metastatic nodule is contemplated, the detection of additional nodules will change the treatment plan, and the preoperative CT scan is essential.

NEOPLASMS

From the preceding discussion, it should be apparent that metastatic disease is the most important cause of multiple pulmonary nodules in today's practice. The list of primary tumors that metastasize to the lung is long (Chart 21.1).[197,361] In most cases, multiple pulmonary metastases are detected after the primary lesion, thus making the presumptive diagnosis of metastases from the known primary lesion a very secure diagnosis (Fig. 21.3). Although this is a reliable assumption for larger masses that are detected by chest radiograph, very small occult opacities detected by CT may often represent benign nodules. These very small opacities must be cautiously evaluated when their detection may influence the choice of therapy, sometimes even justifying biopsy. Multiple pulmonary metastases constitute a relatively unusual presenting complaint that is sometimes followed by an extensive search for an occult primary tumor. One primary tumor that is well known for this presentation is testicular carcinoma. When a male patient's chest radiograph shows multiple pulmonary nodules and masses of varying size, testicular carcinoma should be one of the first considerations. Physical examination may confirm the diagnosis (answer to question1 is *a*), but detection of very small occult tumors often requires testicular ultrasound. Other primary tumors that may be occult but metastasize to the lungs include melanoma, ovarian carcinoma, breast cancer, renal cell carcinoma, colon cancer, and gastrointestinal tumors. Most other tumors that have a high rate of

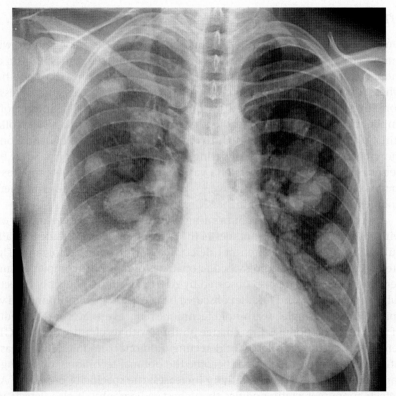

Fig. 21.3   Multiple, well-circumscribed pulmonary masses in this patient with a small right breast and a history of treated right breast cancer virtually ensures the diagnosis of metastatic breast cancer.

pulmonary metastases have local findings and are less likely to present as an occult primary. Spontaneous pneumothorax and multiple pulmonary nodules together are an unusual combination that is nearly diagnostic of osteosarcoma (Fig. 21.4), although it has been encountered with other tumors (e.g., Wilms tumor). This combination should suggest the diagnosis of osteosarcoma, but primary bone tumors are rarely occult. They usually cause pain and are diagnosed via radiography and combinations of CT, MRI, and radionuclide bone scans. Patients with primary bone tumors are more likely to have occult pulmonary metastases at the time of diagnosis. The unsuspected metastases may be diagnosed by radiography or may require CT.

Some tumors that frequently metastasize to the chest often produce patterns other than nodules. Patients with a late stage of pancreatic carcinoma frequently have malignant pleural effusions and pulmonary interstitial spread with a reticular or fine nodular pattern, but they infrequently have multiple larger nodules and masses. Central nervous system tumors are distinctive for their rarity as a cause of metastases to the lung. Furthermore, the rare pulmonary metastases from these tumors apparently occur only after the blood-brain barrier has been violated. (Answer to question 2 is *c*.) Of all the malignant conditions considered in Chart 21.1, lymphoma may be the least likely to present with multiple, well-circumscribed masses. This is because lymphoma tends to be invasive and spreads along the alveolar walls and interlobular septa; therefore lymphoma usually has the more ill-defined appearance of multifocal consolidations.[21]

Benign neoplasms presenting as multiple masses are rare. The two neoplasms best known for this presentation are multiple pulmonary hamartomas and multiple arteriovenous malformations (AVMs).[135] As mentioned in the discussion of solitary nodules, hamartomas occasionally have a characteristic cartilage calcification, but they more commonly appear as a homogeneous nodule on the chest radiograph (though CT detection of fat or characteristic calcifications usually confirms the diagnosis).

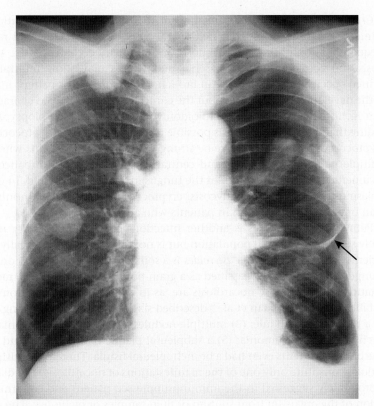

Fig. 21.4 A combination of multiple pulmonary nodules and spontaneous pneumothorax is nearly diagnostic of metastatic osteosarcoma. Pneumothorax is detected by identification of a pleural line *(arrow)*. The air-fluid level above the diaphragm indicates associated hydropneumothorax.

Multiple AVMs may be even more characteristic than the solitary AVM because there are more opportunities for the radiologist to identify the feeding and draining vessels. As with solitary lesions, the diagnosis is usually confirmed by CT with identification of the vessels. The diagnosis of multiple AVMs may be further suggested by the family history. Hereditary telangiectasia (Rendu-Osler-Weber syndrome) is a rare autosomal dominant condition with multiple AVMs. Patients with this condition may have cyanosis, hemoptysis, and cerebrovascular accidents.

INFLAMMATORY DISEASES

Histoplasmosis[283] may be one of the most easily confirmed causes of multiple inflammatory nodules. After inhalation of a large quantity of organisms, patients often present with a chest radiograph showing multiple ill-defined opacities during the acute stage of the disease, which is followed by healing of the nodules to well-circumscribed nodules. This appearance may be even more specific when the nodules are subsequently noted to calcify. The diagnosis of histoplasmosis may be confirmed by the conversion of skin tests and by positive serologic studies for histoplasmosis. Coccidioidomycosis is another fungal disease that can occasionally be diagnosed during its acute phase, at which time the patient has a febrile illness associated with a flu-like syndrome, and the chest radiograph demonstrates multiple patchy opacities similar to those of bronchopneumonia. These opacities may resolve over a period of weeks or may undergo organization, leading to the pattern of multiple nodules. Some of the nodules may undergo central necrosis and subsequent cavitation. If the patient is in an endemic area and serologic tests demonstrate rising titers, the diagnosis is easily documented. The nodules of histoplasmosis and coccidioidomycosis tend to be small and would not be an expected cause of the apical masses seen in Fig. 21.2.

Cryptococcus[200] is another fungal agent that may cause the formation of multiple pulmonary nodules. However, neither the clinical course nor serial radiographs are adequate for confirming the diagnosis of pulmonary cryptococcosis. As in histoplasmosis and coccidioidomycosis, serial radiographs may show multiple areas of ill-defined opacity, similar to those in bronchopneumonia. This pattern may be followed by the development of nodules, but the clinical setting is rarely as characteristic as that seen in histoplasmosis and coccidioidomycosis. Short of lung biopsy, one associated finding that makes the diagnosis possible is the association of cryptococcal meningitis. Cryptococcosis should therefore be strongly considered in patients who are seen with multiple pulmonary opacities and central nervous system disturbances. This is best documented by demonstration of the fungus in cerebrospinal fluid. In contrast to histoplasmosis and coccidioidomycosis, cryptococcosis is most commonly encountered as an opportunistic infection in patients who are immunosuppressed.

Pulmonary nocardiosis is another infectious cause of pulmonary nodules that is rarely seen in the general population but is not rare in immunologically compromised patients. The agent *Nocardia asteroides* is a soil contaminant that was once classified as a fungus but is currently classified as a gram-positive bacterium. The radiologic manifestations of pulmonary nocardiosis are, as in the other granulomatous diseases, predictably variable. Balikian et al.[29] described six cases with the following presentations: (1) a tiny solitary nodule; (2) multiple nodules; (3) cavitary pneumonias; (4) bilateral patchy bronchopneumonia; (5) a subpleural plaque-like infiltrate; and (6) empyema. One of these patients even had a bronchopleural fistula. Therefore multiple pulmonary nodules constitute only one of the manifestations of nocardiosis. The diagnosis is most appropriately suggested in the immunosuppressed patient and confirmed by identification of the organism from sputum or fluid samples or by biopsy. The use of percutaneous needle biopsy and transbronchial biopsy has greatly increased the confirmation of this diagnosis. Because specific antibiotic therapy is essential for cure, an aggressive approach and early diagnosis are essential.

Tuberculosis is an uncommon cause of multiple pulmonary nodules. As in histoplasmosis, central calcification is one of the most diagnostic features of an old, healed tuberculous nodule. Calcification does not indicate a precise bacteriologic diagnosis, but it does indicate that the histology is one of a granuloma that has undergone central necrosis and calcification, thus limiting the differential to histoplasmoma versus tuberculoma. A major problem in evaluating patients with known previous tuberculosis and multiple pulmonary nodules is identifying coexistent tumors. Because tuberculomas may vary in size and shape, and calcium may not be detectable in all of the nodules, the evaluation of old radiographs is essential. A change in one of the nodules or the development of a new nodule indicates reactivation of the tuberculosis or a new process, such as carcinoma. Because of the frequency of carcinoma arising around old tuberculous scars, even calcified nodules must be carefully evaluated. Eccentric calcification in a nodule is not adequate for confirming that the nodule is a completely benign process, and neither can the coexistence of calcified and noncalcified nodules be accepted as evidence that all of the nodules are benign (Fig. 21.5).

Sarcoidosis is frequently described as having a nodular presentation, but the descriptive terminology must be carefully chosen. The fine miliary nodules (see Chapter 17) are not generally considered to represent the nodular form of sarcoidosis, and the larger opacities seen in sarcoidosis commonly have ill-defined borders that make them rather distinct from the pattern seen in patients with multiple metastases. This pattern is more like that discussed in Chapter 16, but occasionally, patients do have discrete opacities that are the result of sarcoidosis (Fig. 21.6, *A* and *B*). The histologic character of these nodules is somewhat variable. Sarcoidosis may have massive accumulations of interstitial granulomas that may account for the large opacities. These large accumulations of granulomas may understandably present in a more circumscribed manner than the obstructive

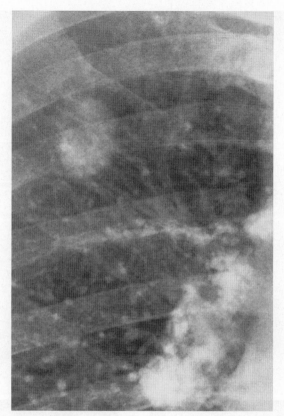

Fig. 21.5 Multiple, small, scattered nodules with calcified hilar nodes are consistent with prior granulomatous infection. The presence of granulomas does not ensure that the larger soft tissue mass in the right upper lobe is benign. This patient has multiple granulomas and a primary lung cancer.

pneumonia that was described in Chapter 16 as a cause of the ill-defined opacities more typical of sarcoidosis. The most diagnostic radiologic information is sometimes obtained by comparison with old radiographs, which may reconstruct the course of a process that initially entailed bilateral and symmetric hilar adenopathy, followed by the development of multiple pulmonary nodules or masses. There may also be a marked disparity between the radiologic and clinical severity of the disease, with the patient appearing to be relatively asymptomatic at a time when there may be many large opacities in the lung. This is very helpful in excluding metastatic and lymphomatous processes.

Parasites as a cause of multiple pulmonary opacities are relatively uncommon in the United States, but are of great importance in the worldwide population. The classic parasite to produce single or multiple, well-circumscribed pulmonary opacities is *Echinococcus granulosus* (dog tapeworm), which causes hydatid disease. Because hydatid disease results in the formation of fluid-filled cysts, the presentation may be that of multiple opacities; more commonly, some of the cysts will have drained their watery fluid, leading to the radiologic appearance of thin-walled, circumscribed lucent spaces[175] (see Chapter 23).

Paragonimiasis[260,262] is another parasitic disease that is reported to be the cause of multiple pulmonary opacities. Paragonimiasis is rare in the West but is encountered in patients who have traveled extensively. Elsewhere, it is a widespread endemic disease with a low mortality, occurring in Korea, Japan, China, the Philippine Islands, Indonesia, Papua New Guinea, and Thailand. An African variety of paragonimiasis is found in eastern Nigeria and the Democratic Republic of the Congo. Paragonimiasis is also encountered in Peru, Ecuador, Brazil, and Venezuela. The most likely patient population in the United States to contract paragonimiasis is the military population, in particular those who have been in Southeast Asia. The life cycle of the adult fluke includes

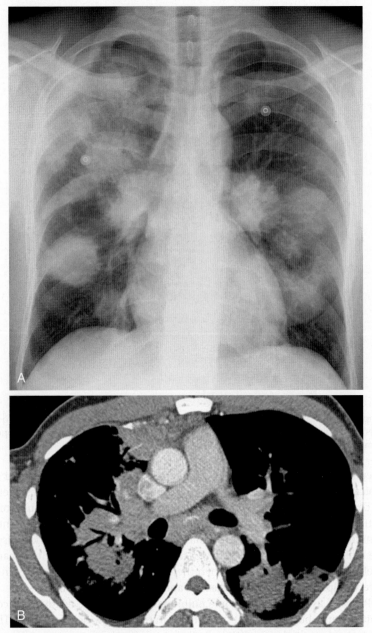

Fig. 21.6   A, Multiple bilateral masses could suggest metastases. **B,** Computed tomography scan with lung windows reveals the masses to have poorly defined borders and air bronchograms with the appearance of consolidations rather than solid masses. Lymphoma cannot be easily excluded by this radiologic presentation. Clinical correlation revealing the patient to have minimal symptoms would strongly support the diagnosis of sarcoidosis, but biopsy confirmation is essential.

humans, snails, and certain crayfish and crabs. Crabs are the usual source of human infection. The fluke normally burrows into the lungs of humans and animals to form small granulomatous cysts. Eggs are shed from the cysts into the air passages on coughing or swallowing and are excreted in the feces. When these eggs contaminate fresh water, snails become infected, developing a sporocyst and radial stage, followed by the liberation of cercariae. The latter are actively motile parasites that penetrate the soft periarticular tissues of crayfish and crabs. These parasites are consumed by humans when the crabs are eaten. An adult cercaria is liberated in the bowel and penetrates the wall of the jejunum, crossing the peritoneal cavity to the tendinous portion of the diaphragm, through which it burrows into the pleural space. It crosses the pleural space, penetrates the visceral pleura, and burrows into the lung. It then reaches maturity and begins to produce eggs, thus beginning the life cycle of the parasite once again. Patients with paragonimiasis clinically have chronic hemoptysis, slight dyspnea, mild fever, severe anorexia, and weight loss. They gradually become accustomed to their symptoms and may have hemoptysis for years. The radiologic consequence of the disease is the emergence of multiple pulmonary opacities, which, as in hydatid disease, may appear as masses or as cystic or cavitary lesions.

Septic emboli are another important cause of inflammatory nodules. Like many of the inflammatory conditions described herein, septic emboli frequently present with multiple ill-defined opacities that frequently cavitate but, as they heal, they may become solid and more circumscribed. The healed nodules actually represent organized infarcts. Clinical correlation is essential in suggesting and confirming this diagnosis. Most patients have an identifiable source of infection such as sepsis, osteomyelitis, cellulitis, or extrapulmonary abscess. Another source of septic emboli is bacterial endocarditis involving the right side of the heart. This is particularly common in intravenous drug abusers.

VASCULAR AND COLLAGEN VASCULAR DISEASES

The vascular diseases that result in multiple pulmonary opacities include venous thromboembolism and the collagen vascular diseases. As has been noted above, the nodules that appear following thromboembolism are organizing infarcts. This diagnosis is usually verified by a history of documented emboli weeks to months prior to the development of the nodules. Chest radiographs obtained at the time of the acute embolic event sometimes reveal areas of ill-defined opacity. Because the infarcts heal by organization of the nodules, the nodules should be smaller than the preceding ill-defined opacities, which were caused primarily by hemorrhagic edema

Granulomatosis with polyangiitis[4,146] results in a diffuse vasculitis involving most of the vessels of the lung. As these vessels become occluded, infarcts develop in the areas of vascular occlusion, with the radiologic result of multiple areas of increased opacity. These opacities are ill defined in the early phases of the process and become circumscribed as the infarcts organize. Clinical correlation is extremely helpful when a history of coexistent renal or sinus disease is uncovered. The classic triad of granulomatosis with polyangiitis consists of lung, kidney, and sinus disease. A limited form of the disease is usually confined to the lung and requires biopsy for confirmation.

Rheumatoid nodules[146] are the least common of the various thoracic manifestations of rheumatoid disease, but are a cause of multiple pulmonary nodules. These nodules tend to occur in the periphery of the lung, are frequently pleural-based, and occasionally cavitate. Histologically, they are necrobiotic nodules, similar to the subcutaneous nodules of rheumatoid arthritis.

PNEUMOCONIOSIS

Silicosis and coal workers' pneumoconiosis both cause nodular scarring of the lungs with an upper lobe predominance. As the fibrosis advances, the nodules are drawn together forming apical masses (see Fig. 21.2, A and B). (Answer to question 3 is d.) These masses vary in size and are usually bilateral but may be asymmetric. They are described as progressive massive fibrosis. This patient population is also at risk for tuberculosis, and many are at risk for lung cancer. The masses may calcify, resembling granulomas, and they may rarely cavitate, which requires laboratory evaluation to exclude superimposed tuberculosis.

ACQUIRED IMMUNODEFICIENCY SYNDROME

Multiple nodules in patients with AIDS may be infectious or neoplastic. Size, number, and distribution are features that influence the most likely diagnoses. Numerous

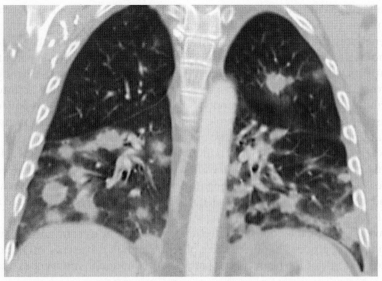

Fig. 21.7 Coronal computed tomography scan of this patient with AIDS reveals multiple nodules, which were confirmed to be B cell lymphoma.

nodules smaller than 1 cm are most likely the result of infections, which include bacterial bronchopneumonia, tuberculosis, or fungi. Multiple nodules larger than 1 cm are usually neoplastic, with Kaposi sarcoma or lymphoma being most likely (Fig. 21.7).[126]

Top 5 Diagnoses: Multiple Nodules and Masses

1. Metastases
2. Tuberculosis
3. Fungal infections
4. Septic emboli
5. Sarcoidosis

Summary

Multiple pulmonary nodules are distinguished from multifocal infiltrative diseases by their homogeneous appearance and sharply defined borders.

Multiple pulmonary nodules and masses are usually the result of metastatic disease.

The list of primary tumors that metastasize to the lung is long. Least commonly, central nervous system tumors lead to pulmonary metastases.

The presence of calcification may be virtually diagnostic of a benign granuloma, but this must be carefully considered. The presence of one calcified granuloma does not prove that other noncalcified nodules are benign granulomas.

Evaluation of old examinations is imperative. The pattern of large, multifocal, ill-defined opacities that evolve to smaller, sharply defined nodules over a period of weeks to months indicates healing granulomas or organizing infarcts as the cause of the nodules. The evolution excludes the diagnosis of metastases.

Clinical correlation is essential when suggesting parasitic disease as a cause of pulmonary nodules.

ANSWER GUIDE

Legends for introductory figures

Fig. 21.1   A, These masses are distinguished from the multifocal opacities seen in Chapter 16 by their sharp borders, but they are more confluent in the right upper lobe and left lower lobe. Metastatic disease is the most common cause of this pattern, but is most often seen late in the course of a known malignant tumor. In this patient, the chest radiograph revealed an unexpected finding of multiple masses, and the physical examination detected a testicular mass that was the primary tumor. **B,** Computed tomography confirms that the more confluent areas are the result of superimposition of multiple, large masses.

Fig. 21.2   A, Bilateral apical masses would be unusual for all the diagnoses offered in question 3, except for coal workers' pneumoconiosis. **B,** Computed tomography shows bilateral apical masses that are mildly irregular and extend to the pleura. The right-sided mass has internal calcifications, and the patient had a long history of working in a coal mine. This is the appearance of progressive massive fibrosis. Sarcoidosis is another cause of masses that resemble progressive massive fibrosis.

ANSWERS

1. a   2. c   3. d

PART 3

Hyperlucent Abnormalities

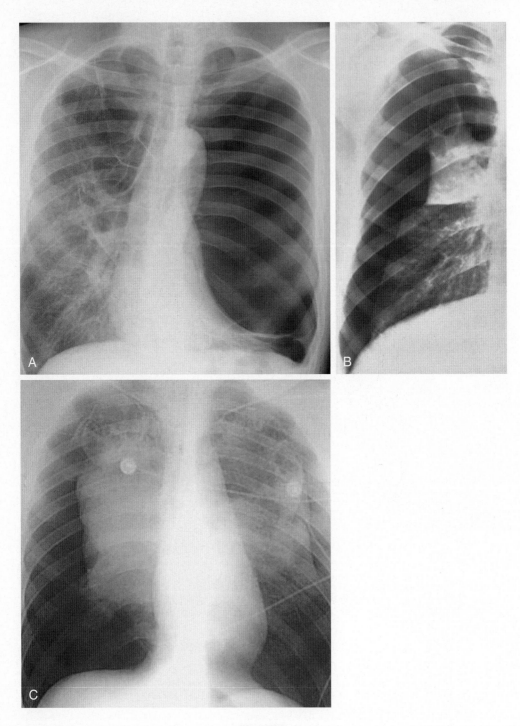

Fig. 22.1

QUESTIONS

1. Match the abnormal thoracic lucencies seen in Fig. 22.1, *A* to *C*, with the following diagnoses.
   ____ Bilateral pneumothorax.
   ____ Bullous emphysema.
   ____ Ruptured subpleural bullae with pneumothorax.

2. Asymmetric air trapping may be confirmed by which of the following radiographic techniques?
   a. Lateral decubitus view.
   b. Forced inspiratory view.
   c. Forced expiratory view.
   d. Overpenetrated view.
   e. Oblique view.

3. Mosaic attenuation on high-resolution computed tomography (HRCT) is a common finding in patients with which one of the following diagnoses?
   a. Constrictive bronchiolitis.
   b. Pulmonary embolism.
   c. Panacinar emphysema.
   d. Centrilobular emphysema.
   e. Asthma.

Chart 22.1	**HYPERLUCENT LUNGS**

I. Bilateral
   A. Faulty radiologic technique (overpenetrated examination)
   B. Thin body habitus
   C. Bilateral mastectomy
   D. Right-to-left cardiac shunts (e.g., tetralogy of Fallot, pseudotruncus arteriosus, truncus type IV)
   E. Pulmonary embolism[396]
   F. Emphysema[169,174,593,594]
   G. Acute asthmatic attack[175]
   H. Acute bronchiolitis (usually in pediatric patients)
   I. Interstitial emphysema[649]
II. Unilateral
   A. Mastectomy
   B. Absent pectoralis muscles
   C. Faulty radiologic technique, including rotation of patient
   D. Extrapulmonary air collections (e.g., pneumothorax, mediastinal emphysema, subcutaneous emphysema)
   E. Pulmonary embolism (acute or chronic)[660]
   F. Emphysema (particularly bullous emphysema)[235]
   G. Atrophy of trapezius muscle (after radical neck dissection)[568]
   H. Bronchial obstruction
      1. Neoplastic
         a. Bronchogenic carcinoma (rare)
         b. Metastatic (rare, but most common primary tumors are breast, thyroid, pancreas, colon, melanoma)[36]
      2. Granulomatous masses, including broncholith

Continued

Chart 22.1	HYPERLUCENT LUNGS—cont'd

3. Bronchial stenosis with mucocele[574]
4. Foreign body (common in children)
J. Hilar mass (e.g., adenopathy, bronchogenic cyst)
K. Constrictive bronchiolitis (Swyer-James, or MacLeod, syndrome)
L. Compensatory overaeration
M. Congenital lobar overdistension
N. Cardiomegaly (left lower lobe)

Discussion

The first step in the evaluation of the apparently hyperlucent lung (Chart 22.1) is to check on radiologic technique. A high-contrast, low-kilovoltage (low-kVp) technique may result in a high-contrast chest film and thus obscure the normal vascular markings of the lung, leading to the false impression of hyperlucent lungs. Such highly contrasted radiographs are readily identified by the marked contrast between the soft tissue opacities and the lucency of the lung. This is a particularly common problem with the portable examination, for which high-kVp techniques are more difficult to obtain. The radiologic technique may also result in the appearance of a unilateral hyperlucent lung when the patient is rotated. Rotation produces the unilateral hyperlucent appearance by projecting soft tissues over one side of the chest while rotating the soft tissues off the opposite side of the chest. This latter problem is particularly noticeable in female patients with large pendulous breasts, which add considerably to the opacity over the lower lung fields. Improper centering of the radiographic beam may also cause asymmetric exposure.

Anatomic variations also result in the appearance of hyperlucent lungs. The best-known example is the patient with a very thin body habitus, which results in an over-penetrated chest radiograph. Asymmetric absence of soft tissues can likewise result in unilateral hyperlucent lungs. Radical mastectomy is the most common source of this problem. Rarely, congenital asymmetry of the chest wall results in a similar appearance. This is noted in patients who have hypoplastic or absent pectoralis muscles.

Extrapulmonary air collections, including subcutaneous emphysema, mediastinal emphysema, and pneumothoraces (see Fig. 22.1, B and C), produce lucent abnormalities that are usually recognized on the basis of their location and are not usually confused with hyperlucent lungs. Most of these conditions result in differences in the opacity of the lung because of overlying soft tissues or their absence. It is important to remember that the radiologic opacity of the normal lung is produced by the pulmonary vascularity. The pulmonary vessels are radiologically identifiable because they contain blood, which is of soft tissue opacity, and are surrounded by air. Therefore, any loss of opacity of the lung reflects a change in the pulmonary vascularity. This should be detected by noting diminution in the size and number of radiologically identifiable vessels (Fig. 22.2). The size and number of radiologically visible vessels are directly related to pulmonary blood flow, supporting the observation that a truly hyperlucent lung is a reflection of decreased blood flow through the lung. This may be the result of cardiac or primary pulmonary disease.

EMPHYSEMA

Emphysema is a very important cause of loss of pulmonary vascularity (see Fig. 22.1, A).[169,174] Severe cases of emphysema will produce marked attenuation and stretching of pulmonary vessels. This process may be diffuse to such an extent that there may even be nearly complete absence of vessels. The diagnosis of emphysema by evaluation of the pulmonary vascularity requires a subjective evaluation of the vascular

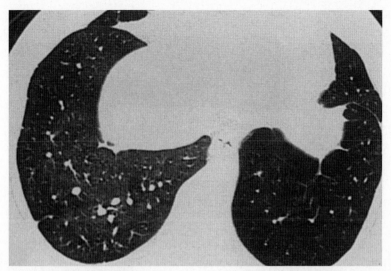

Fig. 22.2 High-resolution computed tomography of a patient with a unilateral, hyperlucent, left lower lobe. Note the asymmetry of the pulmonary vessels with decreased size and number of vessels in the hyperlucent area.

patterns. Thurlbeck and Simon[594] evaluated 700 patients in an effort to correlate paper-mounted, whole-lung sections with posteroanterior and lateral view roentgenograms to determine the accuracy of the radiologic diagnosis of emphysema. They measured lung length and width, size of the retrosternal clear space, heart size, and position of the diaphragm. They observed that lung length and the size of the retrosternal clear space increased, the level of the diaphragm was lowered, the heart size decreased, and the lung width was unchanged as the emphysema became more severe. They believed that lung length and diaphragm level were the most discriminating measurements for diagnostic accuracy, followed by size of the retrosternal clear space. However, they identified no combination of these radiologic variables that identified emphysema better than the subjective diagnosis of the disease based on arterial deficiency. They also emphasized that radiologic lung dimensions are related to stature and must therefore be interpreted cautiously. For example, kyphosis of the thoracic spine causes an increase in the anteroposterior diameter of the chest. They further divided vascular patterns into three main categories of abnormality: (1) the vessels are present but narrowed in most of the lung; (2) there is a normal axial pathway but fewer side branches; and (3) there may be complete absence of vessels. While these vascular alterations may be subtle on chest radiograph, HRCT is very sensitive for the detection of variations in regional perfusion and detection of emphysema (Fig. 22.3, *A* and *B*).

There is hardly any aspect of chest disease that generates more controversy than the role of the radiologist in the diagnosis of emphysema, but most agree that the alterations in pulmonary vascularity are the most reliable radiologic criteria for this diagnosis. When the foregoing criteria are applied, the chest radiograph (Fig. 22.4) is highly specific for the diagnosis of emphysema in patients with advanced disease, but it is not sensitive. HRCT has been shown to be much more sensitive for the diagnosis of early emphysema by demonstrating vascular attenuation, areas of hyperlucency, and small bullae that may be subtle or not detectable by chest radiography.[187,593]

It is important to emphasize that emphysema is an anatomic diagnosis. The morphologic definition of emphysema requires the presence of destruction of alveolar walls and obstruction of small airways. This destruction results in increased size of the distal air spaces. Emphysema is further subdivided into two main types, panlobular (panacinar) and centrilobular (centriacinar). An emphysematous process that destroys all of the lung that is distal to the terminal bronchiole is termed *panlobular emphysema*, whereas incomplete destruction of lung distal to the terminal bronchiole

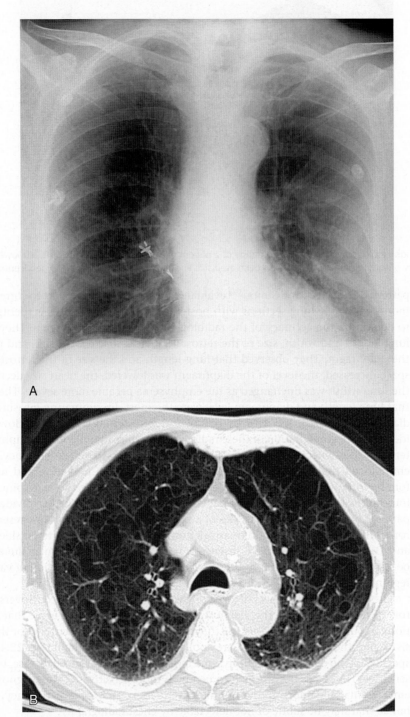

Fig. 22.3 **A,** Centrilobular emphysema destroys normal lung parenchyma and decreases the pulmonary vasculature. The loss of vasculature accounts for the increased lucency of the lungs on plain film. Plain film is not a sensitive test for the diagnosis of emphysema. **B,** High-resolution computed tomography (HRCT) of the same patient with centrilobular emphysema shows multiple lucent spaces and minimal vascularity in the anterior lungs, although there are moderately large vessels in the posterior lungs. Also, compare the hyperlucent areas with the opacity of the more normally perfused areas. This makes HRCT a sensitive test for emphysema.

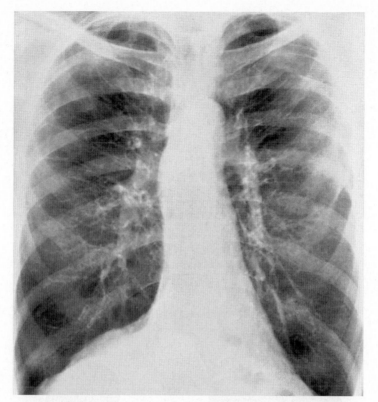

Fig. 22.4 Depression of the diaphragm, a vertically positioned small heart, and hyperlucent lungs caused by the loss of normal vasculature constitute a highly specific appearance for emphysema. These findings indicate advanced disease and are not sensitive for the diagnosis of early emphysema by plain film radiography.

is termed *centrilobular emphysema*. The destruction in centrilobular emphysema may occur in the center of the lobule, but may also be eccentrically located. Of the two types, centrilobular is the more common. Other terms frequently confused in the discussion of emphysema are *bulla* and *bleb*. A bleb is a collection of air within the layers of visceral pleura, and a bulla is an emphysematous space in the lung parenchyma with a diameter of more than 1 cm; however, these terms are frequently used interchangeably. A bulla represents a distended secondary pulmonary lobule or group of lobules involved by paraseptal or panacinar emphysema.[235] Bullous lesions have a rounded or oval configuration, indicating that there is a significant element of air trapping in the bulla (Fig. 22.5, *A* and *B*). Bullae must be carefully evaluated because they may be misdiagnosed as pneumothorax (see Fig. 22.1, *A*). They may also rupture, causing pneumothorax and a bronchopleural communication, which may be difficult to manage (see Fig. 22.1, *B*).

Radiologic distinction of the types of emphysema is frequently impossible, but there are differences in the distribution. Centrilobular emphysema (see Fig. 22.3, *A* and *B*) tends to involve the upper lobes, whereas panacinar emphysema tends to be more severe in the bases (Fig. 22.6). Bullous emphysema may accompany paraseptal or panacinar emphysema (see Fig. 22.1, *A* and *B*).

The term *chronic obstructive pulmonary disease* (COPD) should not be used interchangeably with the term *emphysema*.[169,174] The diagnosis of COPD is a clinical diagnosis encompassing the entire group of obstructive pulmonary diseases, including chronic bronchitis, asthma, bronchiolitis obliterans, bronchiectasis, and emphysema. Of these entities, only emphysema results in chronic bilateral loss of pulmonary vascularity and thus results in hyperlucent lungs.

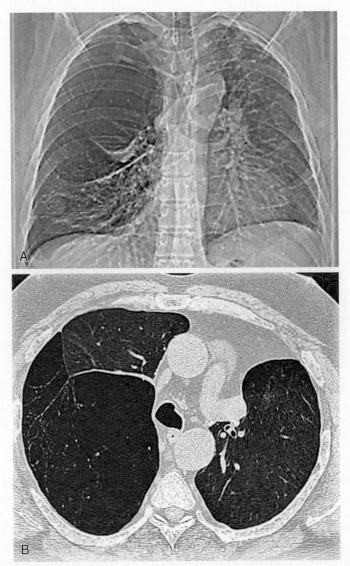

Fig. 22.5 **A,** Bullous emphysema is a common cause of unilateral or localized hyperlucency. Note attenuation of the right upper vasculature and compression of the right lower lobe. **B,** Computed tomography confirms the large lucent space replacing the right upper lobe and compressing the middle and lower lobes.

In contrast to the foregoing situation, a severe acute asthmatic attack may cause bilateral air trapping with depression of the diaphragm and hyperlucent lungs, but these changes are reversible.

AIR TRAPPING

Air trapping is an important cause of hyperlucent lung. Air trapping has the effect of stretching the alveoli, compressing the capillaries and arterioles, and thus decreasing the pulmonary blood flow. However, this is undoubtedly an oversimplification of the pathologic mechanisms whereby air trapping leads to a decrease in the size of pulmonary vessels.

The acute asthmatic attack is one of the most striking examples of transient air trapping. It is well known that bronchial asthma usually produces little radiologic abnormality except during acute attacks, at which time there may be significant air trapping with hyperlucency, attenuation of the vascular markings, and depression of the diaphragm. Acute bronchiolitis is another important cause of diffuse air trapping,

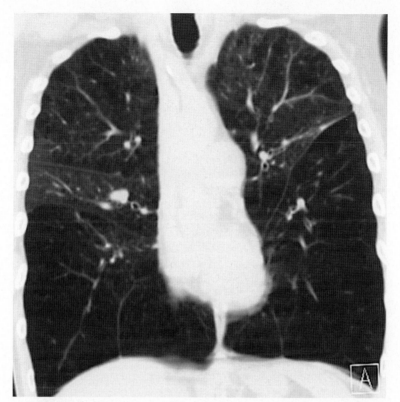

Fig. 22.6   Coronal computed tomography of a patient with panacinar emphysema, which was caused by alpha-1 antitrypsin deficiency, shows the characteristic basilar distribution of the severe emphysema.

but is primarily a disease of the pediatric age group. In both of these situations, the air trapping is transient. Confirmation of air trapping is established with examinations carried out during the expiratory phase of respiration.

UNILATERAL HYPERLUCENT LUNG

The preceding discussion of hyperlucent lung focused primarily on diseases that result in bilaterally hyperlucent lungs, but it must be emphasized that bilateral diseases may lead to the radiologic appearance of unilaterally hyperlucent lungs (Figs. 22.7 and 22.8). In such cases, chest radiography is unfortunately not sensitive enough to detect all areas of involvement, but it can be assumed that areas of hyperlucency reflect areas of the most severe involvement.

The nonpulmonary causes of hyperlucent lung, including faulty radiologic technique, mastectomy, absent pectoralis muscles, and extrapulmonary air collections, are more likely to be unilateral than bilateral. Besides excluding the nonpulmonary causes of hyperlucent lung, the radiologic evaluation of a unilateral hyperlucent lung requires the additional determination of whether the lucent lung or opaque lung is abnormal. This is particularly true in the case of large airway obstruction, which may result in air trapping. Because the overdistention of the lung in these cases results in decreased perfusion of the vascular bed, the additional flow is directed to the normal lung, resulting in a truly increased opacity of the normal lung. In addition, the bronchial obstruction results in overinflation of the lung with a shift of the mediastinum toward the normal side in a manner resembling compensatory overaeration, as is seen in cases of atelectasis. Flattening of the diaphragm on the side of the hyperlucency should be a clue that the bronchial obstruction is producing air trapping rather than atelectasis with compensatory overaeration of the opposite side. The presence of air trapping can be readily confirmed by a number of procedures, including: (1) an expiratory examination,

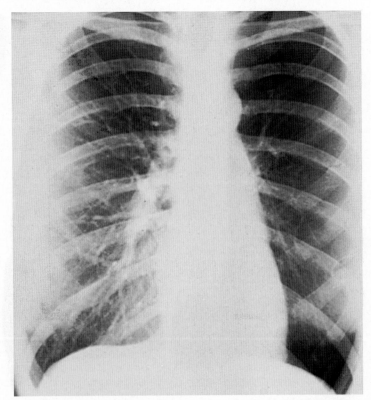

Fig. 22.7 Swyer-James syndrome was originally described as unilateral hyperlucent lung. In this case, the hyperlucent left lung is the result of constrictive bronchiolitis, which is a late complication of viral infection of the bronchi and bronchioles.

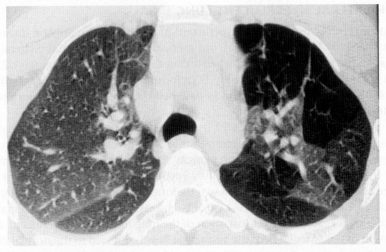

Fig. 22.8 High-resolution computed tomography shows extensive hyperlucency with marked loss of peripheral vasculature of the left lung. This is the pattern of mosaic attenuation, and in this case it is the result of severe constrictive bronchiolitis that resulted from a previous viral infection.

which reveals the volume of the hyperlucent lung to be unchanged; (2) fluoroscopy, which likewise reveals the volume of the overinflated lung to be unchanged; and (3) a lateral decubitus view with the overinflated side down. (Answers to question 2 are *a* and *c*.)

The lateral decubitus view is particularly helpful in infants, small children, and uncooperative patients because it has the effect of splinting the side that is down and is therefore the equivalent of an expiratory view for that side. A suspected endobronchial mass may result in bronchial obstruction with atelectasis or bronchial obstruction with air trapping. It is generally agreed that collateral air drift contributes to air trapping beyond bronchial obstructions. This collateral air drift is irreversible and therefore permits air to enter the area of lung distal to the obstruction, where the air is then trapped, resulting in hyperexpansion. Atelectasis probably occurs distal to bronchial obstructions in those patients who have underlying diseases that prevent normal collateral air drift. Felson[150] emphasized that bronchial obstruction in an adult is more likely to result in atelectasis, whereas bronchial obstruction in a child most frequently leads to air trapping. The primary diagnostic considerations are quite different in these two cases. An endobronchial mass is the most frequent cause of bronchial obstruction in an adult, whereas a foreign body is the most common cause of bronchial obstruction in a child.

Swyer-James syndrome (Macleod syndrome)[536,564] deserves special mention because it was originally described as a radiologic syndrome consisting of a unilateral hyperlucent lung (see Fig. 22.7). There is considerable evidence that cases of the syndrome are the late sequelae of a viral or mycoplasma pneumonia, particularly an adenoviral bronchiolitis. Histologic examination of patients with this diagnosis has demonstrated a constrictive bronchiolitis. (Answer to question 3 is *a*.) HRCT shows that the hyperlucent areas of mosaic attenuation are bilateral but often asymmetric (see Fig. 22.8).[185] HRCT scans taken in the expiratory phase of respiration confirm that the areas of hyperattenuation are the result of air trapping. Bronchiectasis is not a common associated finding, but some viral infections cause central bronchiectasis with peripheral constrictive bronchiolitis, which may be asymmetric with the appearance of unilateral hyperlucent lung on the radiograph and mosaic attenuation on an HRCT scan. The most exaggerated cases of air trapping may demonstrate additional radiograph findings that include flattening of the diaphragm, herniation of lung through the mediastinum, and even compression of the normal lung.

The observation of a mass with associated air trapping is rare. Because of the frequency of bronchial obstruction by carcinoma of the lung, hyperlucent lung might be an anticipated abnormality; however, as stated previously, atelectasis is much more commonly observed. Because of the possibility of detecting air trapping from an early bronchogenic carcinoma, studies using inspiratory and expiratory films have been performed as a possible means for the early detection of bronchogenic tumor, but this approach has not been of value.

Other lesions, including adenopathy, fibrosing mediastinitis, benign masses, and bronchial stenosis with a mucocele, may rarely cause bronchial obstruction and result in a unilateral hyperlucent lung (Fig. 22.9).[574]

PULMONARY EMBOLISM

Massive pulmonary emboli may obstruct blood flow through the main pulmonary artery, producing bilaterally hyperlucent lungs, but fortunately this is a rare occurrence. More localized areas of hyperlucency (Westermark sign)[660] may result from lobar or segmental pulmonary emboli (Fig. 22.10, *A* and *B*). These areas of hyperlucency are likely segmental or lobar, but the hyperlucency may involve an entire lung.

The diagnosis is usually suggested by the clinical setting. These patients frequently present with acute pleuritic chest pain, dyspnea, and extreme apprehension. A ventilation and

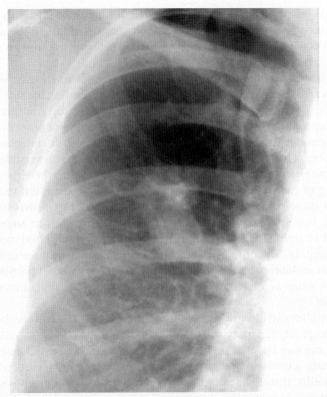

Fig. 22.9   Bronchial stenosis has caused a bronchocele with collateral air drift expanding the right upper lobe distal to the bronchial obstruction.

perfusion scan may confirm the diagnosis by demonstrating that the hyperlucent areas on the chest radiograph are poorly perfused but normally ventilated. The combination of perfusion and ventilation scanning is extremely important in distinguishing pulmonary emboli from emphysema, another important cause of hyperlucent lung and poor pulmonary vascular perfusion. In the case of emphysema, the ventilation scan will demonstrate significant trapping of the radionuclide imaging agent with delayed activity. Computed tomography (CT) angiography is currently the most definitive procedure for the diagnosis of pulmonary embolism. There is often good correlation of the hyperlucent areas on the chest radiograph, with the arterial obstructions demonstrated by CT angiography.

CARDIAC DISEASE

The cardiac diseases that result in decreased pulmonary blood flow are the right-to-left cardiac shunts. These shunts usually occur in combination with obstruction of pulmonary blood flow from the right side of the heart at the pulmonary valve, right ventricle, or tricuspid valve. The most common of these conditions is the tetralogy of Fallot. The combination of infundibular pulmonary stenosis with a ventricular septal defect forms a bypass for the blood to enter directly into the high-pressure left ventricular system, thereby bypassing the pulmonary circulation. With this arrangement, both the peripheral and proximal pulmonary vessels will be abnormally small. Although the vascularity is decreased, this appearance is not often perceived as hyperlucent lungs. Tetralogy of Fallot is a congenital heart disease that results clinically in cyanosis and is usually identified in early childhood. Other right-to-left shunts, such as pseudotruncus arteriosus, type 4 truncus arteriosus, Ebstein malformation of the tricuspid valve, and tricuspid atresia, may produce decreased pulmonary vasculature by a similar mechanism. Cardiac catheterization or magnetic resonance imaging (MRI) is essential for accurate diagnosis of these congenital heart lesions.

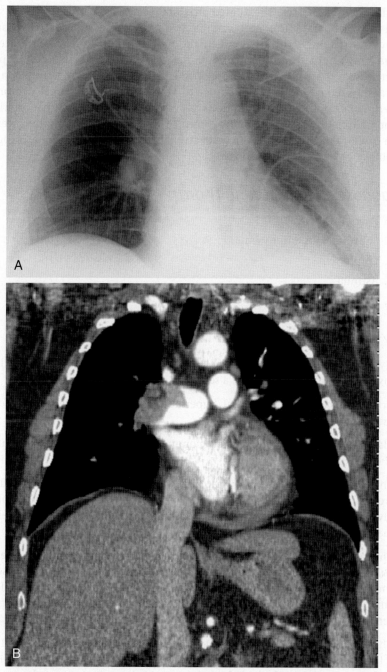

Fig. 22.10 **A,** Development of a hyperlucent, right lower lobe with any of the clinical signs of pulmonary embolic disease should strongly suggest the correct diagnosis. This is the classic Westermark sign of pulmonary embolism. Compare the vascular markings of the normal left lung with the hypovascular right lower lobe. **B,** Computed tomography angiogram reveals a large thrombus occluding the right pulmonary artery.

In addition to the right-to-left shunts, long-standing left-to-right shunts may result in the Eisenmenger complex, which is an endarteritis obliterans of the small pulmonary arteries that decreases peripheral vasculature and thus may cause hyperlucent lungs. Eisenmenger complex can be radiologically distinguished from right-to-left shunts by observing progressive enlargement of the proximal pulmonary arteries. Frequently, the Eisenmenger response to a left-to-right shunt results in pulmonary arteries that are massively dilated proximally and may even suggest bilateral hilar masses. The dilated proximal vessels are caused by increased resistance in the peripheral pulmonary vascular bed. Serial chest radiographs should therefore reveal a striking contrast between the primary right-to-left shunts (tetralogy) and the left-to-right shunts (atrial septal defect, ventricular septal defect, patent ductus arteriosus) that precipitate the Eisenmenger response. For example, a chest radiograph obtained early in the course of ventricular septal defect demonstrates large peripheral and proximal pulmonary vessels. As the obliterative arteritis develops, the peripheral vessels gradually diminish in size, and the proximal vessels enlarge. In this late stage, the shunt may reverse. The latter complication is recognized by the clinical observation of cyanosis.

Top 5 Diagnoses: Hyperlucent Thorax

1. Pneumothorax
2. Subcutaneous emphysema
3. Emphysema
4. Asthma
5. Mastectomy

Summary

Hyperlucency of the lung may be a bilateral or unilateral process. If unilateral, it may involve an entire lung, a lobe, a segment, or even a lobule.

Artifactual causes of unilateral hyperlucent lung, including faulty radiologic technique, must always be excluded.

Mastectomy is probably the most common cause of unilateral hyperlucency of the chest.

The true pulmonary diseases that result in hyperlucent lung are a reflection of decreased pulmonary blood flow. The causes for decreased pulmonary blood flow are diverse and include cardiac shunts, pulmonary emboli, emphysema, endobronchial masses, and bronchiolitis obliterans.

The radiologic diagnosis of emphysema is controversial, but most agree that the vascular changes correlate well with the pathologic diagnosis of emphysema. Most of these controversies concern the sensitivity of the chest radiograph for detecting early emphysema. HRCT is very specific and very sensitive for the diagnosis of early emphysema.

The term *chronic obstructive pulmonary disease* should be used as a clinical term because it includes emphysema, chronic bronchitis, bronchial asthma, bronchiolitis obliterans, and bronchiectasis. The radiologic features of these diseases are diverse. The areas of hyperlucency are the result of destruction of lung parenchyma. The radiologic result is the appearance of decreased pulmonary vasculature. Loss of pulmonary vascularity is a reliable radiologic sign of emphysema.

Although pulmonary emboli are frequently multiple and bilateral, they may result in localized areas of hyperlucency (Westermark sign).

In the case of large airway obstruction, the first decision is to determine whether the hyperlucent or the opaque side is abnormal. This is easily accomplished by confirming air trapping with expiratory films, fluoroscopy, or lateral decubitus films.

ANSWER GUIDE

Legends for introductory figures

Fig. 22.1   A, Bullous emphysema causes loss of pulmonary vasculature and hyperlucent lungs. The bullae have very thin walls that appear as linear opacities. Very large bullae, as seen on the *left,* may sometimes be difficult to distinguish from a pneumothorax. **B,** Subpleural bullae are a frequent cause of spontaneous pneumothorax. This patient has cystic fibrosis with early development of apical bullae. **C,** Large pneumothoraces increase the lucency of the chest with complete loss of pulmonary vascular opacity, and are most reliably identified by recognition of the visceral pleural lines. This patient has bilateral pneumothoraces.

ANSWERS

1. c, a, b   2. a, c   3. a

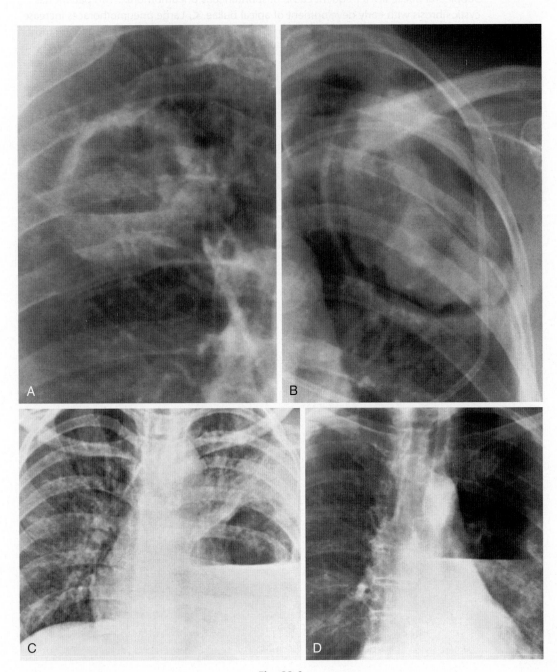

Fig. 23.1

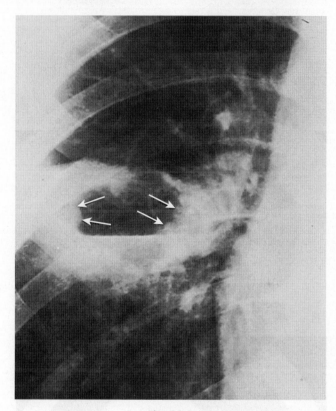

Fig. 23.2

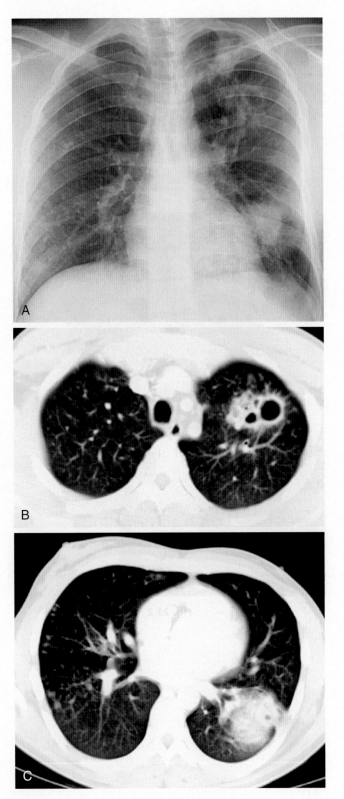

Fig. 23.3

QUESTIONS

1. Match the cases shown in Fig. 23.1, *A-D*, with the following diagnoses:
   _____ Bronchogenic carcinoma.
   _____ Pneumonia with abscess.
   _____ Bronchopleural fistula with hydropneumothorax.
   _____ Pulmonary gangrene.

2. Which one of the following pulmonary infections is least likely cause of necrotizing pneumonia?
   a. *Streptococcus pneumoniae.*
   b. *Pseudomonas.*
   c. *Klebsiella.*
   d. *Staphylococcus aureus.*
   e. Mixed gram-negative pneumonia.

3. Refer to Fig. 23.2. Which one of the following diagnoses is least likely?
   a. Bronchogenic carcinoma.
   b. Metastatic nasopharyngeal carcinoma.
   c. Chronic anaerobic abscess.
   d. Bronchogenic cyst.
   e. Tuberculous cavity.

4. Which one of the following best explains the radiologic presentation in Fig. 23.3, *A-C*?
   a. Metastatic melanoma.
   b. Tuberculosis with bronchogenic spread.
   c. Bronchogenic carcinoma.
   d. Coccidioidomycosis.
   e. Metastatic nasopharyngeal carcinoma.

Chart 23.1	**SOLITARY LUCENT DEFECT**

I. Cavity
  A. Inflammation
    1. Abscess, acute or chronic
       a. Pyogenic infection[207] (staphylococcal and gram-negative pneumonia)
       b. Aspiration pneumonia (common source of anaerobes)
       c. Mycoplasma pneumonia[338,540] (rare)
    2. Fungal infection[371]
       a. Histoplasmosis[97,110]
       b. Coccidioidomycosis[373]
       c. Blastomycosis[216,450]
       d. Cryptococcosis[200,229]
       e. Mucormycosis[33,662]
       f. Aspergillosis[172]
    3. Mycobacterial infection
       a. Tuberculosis (typical and atypical)[54,82,366,388,612]
       b. Nocardiosis[29,208]
  B. Neoplasms
    1. Primary lung tumor[587]
    2. Metastases (usually multiple)[118]
       a. Squamous cell (e.g., nasopharynx, esophagus, cervix)

Continued

Chart 23.1	SOLITARY LUCENT DEFECT—cont'd

    b. Adenocarcinoma (e.g., lung, breast, gastrointestinal tract)
    c. Osteosarcoma (rare)
    d. Melanoma
  C. Vascular (commonly multiple)
    1. Rheumatoid[146,468]
    2. Granulomatosis with polyangiitis[4]
    3. Infarct (thromboemboli or septic emboli)
  D. Environmental
    1. Silicosis and coal workers' pneumoconiosis (most commonly owing to complicating tuberculosis)
II. Pneumatocele
  A. Postinfectious[212,226]
  B. Posttraumatic[139,204]
III. Congenital cyst[463,464]
  A. Bronchogenic cyst
  B. Intrapulmonary sequestration[149,233]
IV. Parasitic cysts (hydatid cyst)[30,435]
V. Bronchiectatic cyst[464]
VI. Bullous emphysema[169]

Discussion

The radiologic presentation of a localized, avascular, lucent lung defect surrounded by a band of opacity might best be described as a hole in the lung, although this is a non-medical term. Chart 23.1 lists a number of causes for a solitary hole in the lung that differ considerably in their pathogenesis. For this reason, such terms as *cavity, cyst,* and *pneumatocele* constitute the differential diagnosis for a hole in the lung.[317] This chapter examines differences in the pathogenesis of these lesions as a basis for understanding the similarities and differences in their radiologic presentations.

CAVITY

The radiologic appearance of a pulmonary cavity is the result of necrosis of lung parenchyma with evacuation of the necrotic tissue via the tracheobronchial tree. A communication with the tracheobronchial tree permits air to enter the area of necrosis, with the radiologic result of a lucent defect. The necrosis causes near-complete destruction of the alveolar walls, interlobular septa, and bronchovascular bundles in the area of the cavity, resulting in loss of normal vascular markings throughout the area of lucency. The surrounding normal lung parenchyma reacts to the necrosis by forming a band of inflammation around the necrotic material, with local edema and hemorrhage. When the cavity expands under tension, as frequently happens in patients who are on positive-pressure ventilator therapy, there may even be compression of normal surrounding lung. The surrounding inflammatory cellular infiltrate, edema, hemorrhage, and compressed normal lung all contribute to the cavity wall. Central necrosis of a preexisting nodule or mass with drainage of its liquefied contents is a second mechanism for the development of a cavity. Central necrosis with liquefaction of a pulmonary lesion cannot be detected on a chest radiograph prior to drainage of a portion of the liquid. However, computed tomography (CT) is sensitive to the difference in opacity caused by liquefaction and may be useful for detecting early necrosis of a pulmonary infection or neoplasm (Fig. 23.4, *A* and *B*).

The radiologic characteristics of the wall of a cavity are determined by the reaction of the lung parenchyma to the pathologic process. A surrounding air space consolidation indicates acute edema, hemorrhage, or exudate, whereas irregular reticular strands

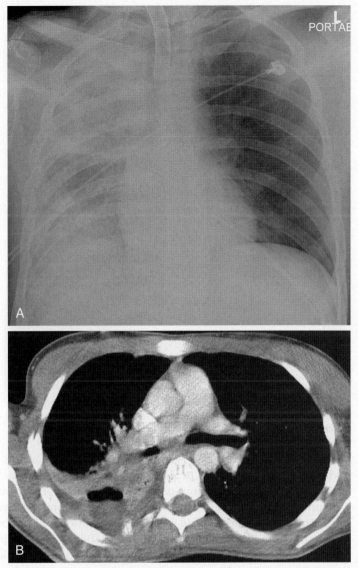

Fig. 23.4   A, Posteroanterior chest radiograph demonstrates diffuse opacification of the right lung but no evidence of cavitation. **B,** Computed tomography (CT) scan reveals a well-localized area of liquefaction of tissue, with an air-fluid level. CT is more sensitive for the detection of early cavitation of pneumonias and often permits the early diagnosis of necrotizing pneumonias.

are suggestive of chronic fibrotic scars. Therefore, wall characteristics may be helpful in establishing the age of the cavity. In addition, necrosis of an inflammatory or neoplastic mass may leave thick nodular walls (Fig. 23.5, *A* and *B*; see Fig. 23.1, *A*).

Pyogenic Infection

The term *abscess* is usually reserved for cavities that are caused by pyogenic infections. This complication indicates a virulent process that results in vasculitis with thrombosis of small vessels, which leads to necrosis of lung tissue. The abscess, which is made up of necrotic material, will appear to be of tissue opacity until communications with airways are established. These communications permit drainage of the necrotic debris. This liquefied necrotic material is coughed up, with the radiologic result of a lucent defect or cavity. The presence of cavitation in the acute phase of a pulmonary infection is a significant radiologic finding that narrows the differential considerations; viral and mycoplasma pneumonia are virtually eliminated, and pneumococcal pneumonia (infection

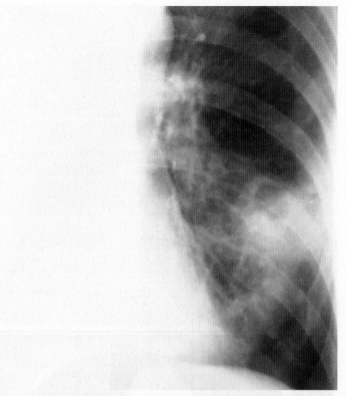

Fig. 23.5 Tuberculous cavities are most typically in the apical segments of the upper lobes, but cavities in other locations are not rare. *Mycobacterium tuberculosis* was cultured from this cavity in the left lower lobe.

with *Streptococcus pneumoniae*) would be a rarity. The organisms most likely to lead to cavitation are *Staphylococcus*, beta-hemolytic streptococci, *Klebsiella, Pseudomonas, Escherichia coli,* mixed gram-negative organisms, and anaerobes. (Answer to question 2 is *a.*)

Aspiration is frequently the source of the mixed gram-negative and anaerobic infections. This may be the result of subclinical aspiration and has been described as gravitational pneumonia. Aspiration pneumonia should be particularly suspected when the cavity occurs in a dependent portion of the lung. The clinical setting of a condition such as poor oral hygiene, alcoholism, or a tumor in the nasopharynx, larynx, or mouth supports the diagnosis. The patient typically experiences a febrile response with productive cough, similar to that of other patients with necrotizing pneumonia.

On occasion, the cavities resulting from a necrotizing pneumonia rupture into the pleura, forming a bronchopleural fistula. This leads to the radiologic appearance of a hydropneumothorax, which is usually recognized by an air-fluid level in the pleural space. Pleural air-fluid collections are often elliptic, may lack an identifiable wall, and have air-fluid levels that differ in length depending on the radiographic projection. Abscesses tend to have spherical thick walls and air-fluid levels that are equal in length, regardless of the radiographic projection[458,519,557] (Fig. 23.6, *A* and *B*; see Fig. 23.1, *C* and *D*). CT may be required to distinguish an abscess from a loculated hydropneumothorax secondary to bronchopleural fistula.[318,625] The clinical presentation of pyogenic pneumonia is usually dramatic with the patient being profoundly ill, running a toxic febrile course, and having an elevated white blood cell (WBC) count. Because of the necrosis of lung tissue, hemoptysis is not a rare complication of these more virulent infections. Culture of the organism is required for definitive diagnosis.

Pulmonary gangrene[662] results from the very acute ischemic necrosis of lung tissue. It differs from lung abscess in that a region of lung undergoes necrosis, detaches from

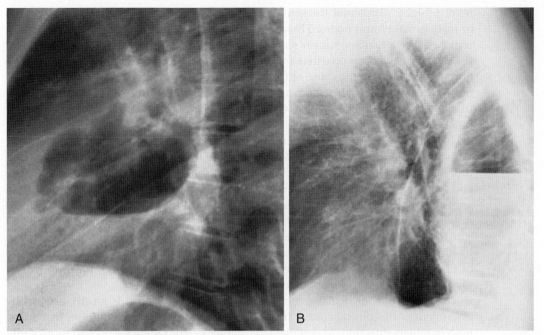

Fig. 23.6 A, Lateral view of the patient shown in Fig. 23.1, *C,* demonstrates a spherical cavity with an air-fluid level in the lingular segment of the left upper lobe. This confirms the diagnosis of pneumonia with lung abscess. **B,** Lateral view of the patient seen in Fig. 23.1, *D,* demonstrates a posterior, vertically oriented, elliptic structure with an air-fluid level. This confirms a pleural air-fluid collection consistent with hydropneumothorax. This resulted from pneumonia with a bronchopleural fistula.

viable lung, and forms a mass of devitalized tissue lying within a cavity. Organisms to be considered when gangrene is identified include *Staphylococcus aureus, Streptococcus* spp., *Klebsiella pneumoniae, Haemophilus influenzae, Mucor* fungi, and *Aspergillus.* The characteristic radiographic appearance is that of a mass surrounded by eccentric lucency (see Fig. 23.1, *B*). Radiographically, pulmonary gangrene may resemble a fungus ball in a cavity, but the latter is due to a solid mass of fungus that has colonized a preexisting cavity or cystic space. CT may be helpful in demonstrating that the intracavitary mass consists of lung. Early diagnosis of gangrene is important because it may require surgical resection.

Granulomatous Disease

Tuberculosis is the prototypical cause of an infectious pulmonary cavity. The cavitary phase of tuberculosis rarely occurs at the time of the initial infection but is a secondary phenomenon resulting from a hyperimmune response.[82,641] The necrosis of lung tissue liberates organisms previously isolated by a surrounding fibrotic reaction. The cavities of tuberculosis are usually quite distinctive because of their proclivity to the apical or the posterior segments of the upper lobes. Approximately 10% of tuberculous cavities are found in atypical locations. A cavity in an anterior segment of an upper lobe as the sole manifestation of pulmonary tuberculosis is very rare. Isolated lower lobe cavities are rarely caused by tuberculosis, but lower lobe tuberculosis in association with upper lobe disease is not rare. Although these latter locations should be considered more suggestive of some of the other causes of cavitary disease, such as acute necrotizing pneumonias or fungal infections, an unusual location should not be cause for rejecting the diagnosis of tuberculosis (see Fig. 23.5).[54,82,215,388,641]

Other radiologic features that aid in the identification of a tuberculous cavity include the following: (1) associated reticular pulmonary scars; (2) volume loss in the involved lobe; (3) pleural thickening; (4) pleural calcification; and (5) calcified hilar or mediastinal lymph nodes. These are all the result of a long-standing inflammatory response. The reticular or linear scars cause a very irregular margin of the outer wall of the cavity. These linear opacities are the result of granulomas and fibrotic scarring. The fibrotic scars are also the cause of the volume loss, which is radiologically detected by noting an elevation of the hilum and shift of the mediastinum (see discussion of cicatrizing atelectasis in Chapter 13). Calcified nodular opacities in the area of the cavity indicate a previous granulomatous infection. Associated homogeneous nodules are less diagnostic but may occur in clusters and indicate transbronchial spread of infection.

Reactivation of tuberculosis indicates a failure in host defenses. Older patients and those with chronic illnesses, including acquired immunodeficiency syndrome (AIDS) and a variety of neoplasms[342]—in particular, lung cancer, leukemia, and lymphoma—are at increased risk for developing active tuberculosis. The failure of an immune response results in liberation of organisms that may have been isolated for years. Exposure to a person with cavitary tuberculosis accounts for most new cases of tuberculosis. In addition to the possibility of spreading the infection to others, patients in this phase of tuberculosis are at considerable risk of developing disseminated infection, which may be bronchogenic or hematogenous.

The distinction of hematogenous and bronchogenic spread is greatly assisted by assessment of the clinical course. Involvement of multiple organs indicates hematogenous or miliary infection. As described in Chapter 17, the radiologic presentation of miliary tuberculosis is that of a diffuse fine nodular pattern, with the nodules being sharply defined. The association of cavitary tuberculosis with disseminated larger opacities in the range of 2 to 5 mm and that have ill-defined borders is more suggestive of bronchogenic spread, with the opacities representing peribronchial inflammatory infiltrates and exudation into the terminal air spaces. The latter has been termed *acinar tuberculosis*.[175] The combination of a large, irregular, upper lobe cavity and ill-defined opacities in the lower lobe strongly suggests the diagnosis. A primary or secondary tumor is unlikely to produce such a pattern; the irregular nodules with ill-defined borders are certainly not typical metastatic nodules. Bronchogenic carcinoma might produce a similar cavity but is an unlikely cause for the disseminated opacities. Coccidioidomycosis is a granulomatous infection that can mimic tuberculosis and cannot be entirely eliminated by radiologic criteria alone, but the case shown in Fig. 23.3, *A-C*, would not represent a classic appearance for cavitary coccidioidomycosis and is a case of cavitary tuberculosis with transbronchial spread of the infection. (Answer to question 4 is *b*.)

Atypical mycobacterial infections (Fig. 23.7, *A* and *B*) produce a variety of patterns including cavities that are indistinguishable from tuberculosis, nodules, masses, and bronchiectasis, as well as the small diffuse nodules of hypersensitivity pneumonitis. *Mycobacterium avium* complex (MAC) is the most common of the nontuberculous mycobacteria. When conventional laboratory examinations fail to isolate the cause of an apical cavity, atypical mycobacteria must be considered. Although the radiologic features of the cavity are often identical to those in typical tuberculosis, some differences in the radiologic presentation of the two infections have been described. The atypical organisms are more likely to produce multiple, thin-walled, apical cavities with only minimal surrounding parenchymal disease and with minimal or no pleural reaction. Nodules surrounding a cavity are uncommon. Nodules or masses without a cavity may mimic the appearance of lung cancer or metastases. Patients with chronic lung diseases, including chronic obstructive pulmonary disease, interstitial lung disease, cystic fibrosis, and bronchiectasis, are at increased risk for atypical mycobacterial infection. MAC is also a common cause of opportunistic infection, especially in patients with AIDS. It occurs in the setting of a CD4 count of less than 100 cells/mm^3 and causes cavities, nodules, endobronchial nodules, pericardial effusion, and extensive hilar or mediastinal adenopathy.[366]

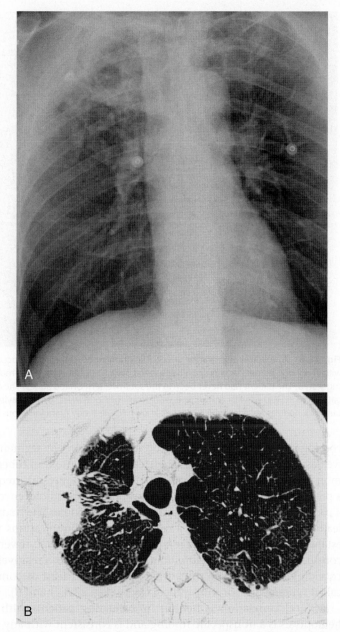

Fig. 23.7   A, This right apical opacity has a lucency suggesting an apical cavity. Cultures for *Mycobacterium tuberculosis* were negative. **B,** Computed tomography scan confirms a peripheral opacity with a small lucent center, but the lucency seen on the chest radiograph is probably accounted for by the associated bullae. This patient also has linear scarring of the right upper lobe. Chronic lung disease is a risk factor for atypical mycobacterial infection, and cultures confirmed *Mycobacterium avium* complex.

Histoplasmosis[97,110,371] is another consideration in the differential diagnosis of an apical cavity that may completely mimic the appearance of tuberculosis. In fact, histoplasmosis was originally discovered because of its similarities to tuberculosis.[108] There may even be extensive, associated parenchymal scarring, volume loss, and calcifications involving the lung parenchyma and hilar lymph nodes. This diagnosis should be considered most likely in patients who have negative reactions to skin or serologic tests for tuberculosis and who have positive reactions to skin or serologic tests for histoplasmosis.

Cavitary coccidioidomycosis[373] is much more variable in terms of location of the cavities than is tuberculosis or histoplasmosis. In contrast to tuberculosis,

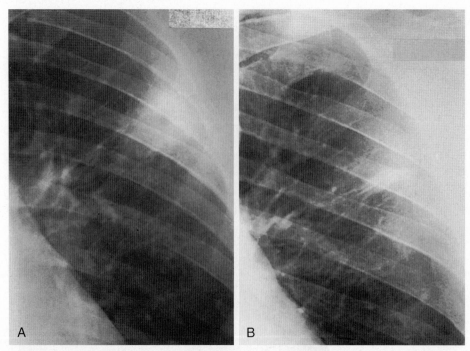

Fig. 23.8   **A,** Atypical appearance of coccidioidomycosis. A small cavity occurred in a large focal opacity with ill-defined borders. It was not a thin-walled cavity, but this is probably more common than sometimes suggested. The patient had never been in the southwestern United States. The organism was brought to the patient, who worked with cotton and wool from the Southwest. **B,** The cavity did not completely resolve but left a nodular residual, which is a well-known result of any granulomatous infection.

coccidioidomycotic cavities may occur in the anterior segment of the upper lobes as well as in the lower lobes, but these cavities, like those of tuberculosis, are more common in the upper lobes. The cavities of coccidioidomycosis frequently form in areas of a preexisting nodule. The classic evolution of a coccidioidomycotic cavity begins with a parenchymal infiltrate that organizes into a nodule. The nodule undergoes necrosis, leading to the formation of a cavity when communications with small airways are established to permit drainage of the necrotic material. A very thin-walled cavity is considered classic for coccidioidomycosis, but this is a relatively late stage of cavitary coccidioidomycosis. The thick-walled cavity is at least as common as the classic so-called "grape skin," or thin-walled, cavity (Fig. 23.8, *A* and *B*).

Clinical correlation is helpful in evaluating patients with cavities. As expected, hemoptysis is a nonspecific finding and is consistent with any cavitary process. A history of having been in an area where coccidioidomycosis is endemic supports the diagnosis. Patients who have not been in an endemic area are usually not suspected of having this infection, but on occasion the organism can be transported to the patient. This has been documented in patients working with cotton, wool, and other farm products from the desert Southwest. The results of skin and serologic tests add valuable data to the diagnosis of coccidioidomycosis.

Other fungal agents, including *Blastomyces dermatitidis* (North American blastomycosis), *Cryptococcus neoformans* (cryptococcosis), and actinomycosis, are less common causes of pulmonary cavities that produce patterns similar to those of tuberculosis and histoplasmosis. These diagnoses require laboratory confirmation.

Nocardia spp. are gram-positive organisms that were previously classified as fungi. Nocardiosis frequently results in consolidation or in pulmonary nodules, which may cavitate. It is rarely encountered in normal patients but is not rare in patients who are immunologically suppressed. Nocardiosis is a well-known cause of pulmonary infection

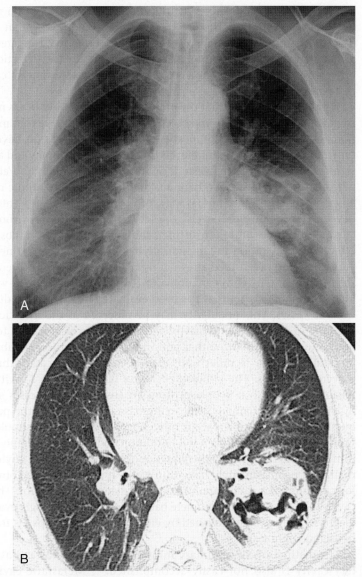

Fig. 23.9   A, This large, left lower lobe opacity has internal lucencies, which suggest that this is a thick-walled cavity. This appearance might be seen with a lung abscess, but is more suggestive of a cavitary mass. **B,** Computed tomography (CT) scan confirms a thick-walled cavitary mass in the left lower lobe. Even with this CT appearance, an abscess might be considered, but this is a squamous cell carcinoma.

in renal transplant patients and in patients with alveolar proteinosis. It should not lead to chronic cavities with the surrounding scars typical of tuberculosis and histoplasmosis.

NEOPLASM

Cavitation of pulmonary neoplasms is not rare. Approximately 16%[587] of all peripheral primary carcinomas show radiologic evidence of cavitation. This is most frequent in epidermoid carcinomas, with approximately 30% of the peripheral epidermoid carcinomas showing cavitation. Well-differentiated adenocarcinoma is the second most common cell type of tumor to cavitate, whereas invasive mucinous adenocarcinoma has been reported to undergo a variety of cystic changes that resemble cavities and are often described as *pseudocavities*.[621,623]

The radiologist's first responsibility in the assessment of a possible cavitating neoplasm is to verify the presence of cavitation (Fig. 23.9, *A* and *B*). This is frequently accomplished by the simple identification of a large hole in a mass. When there is doubt about cavitation, the presence of an air-fluid level on an upright view should be confirmatory. When such views cannot be obtained, the lateral decubitus view is an alternative examination. CT is very sensitive for the detection of cavitation and often reveals liquefaction of a mass before the lesion appears cavitary on the chest radiograph.

It has been suggested that the presence and size of fluid levels may be helpful in distinguishing carcinomas from abscesses. Although it is true that many cavitating carcinomas do not contain a significant amount of fluid and thus have no air-fluid level or only modest fluid levels, fluid levels do occur in carcinomas and are not a trustworthy sign for distinguishing between a cavitating neoplasm and an abscess. Bleeding into a neoplasm may result in a high air-fluid level and may mimic the appearance of an abscess. Cavitating carcinomas may also become secondarily infected, leading to the development of air-fluid levels. The location of the cavity within the mass has been cited as another feature for distinguishing carcinomas from abscesses. The presence of eccentric cavitation might indicate malignancy, but an Armed Forces Institute of Pathology study identified an equal number of eccentric and central cavities in more than 1200 patients with carcinoma.[587] A lobulated or nodular wall is another radiologic feature of cavities that has been evaluated in an effort to distinguish neoplasms from abscesses. This nodularity may be observed at the interface of the cavity with the lung or with the inner cavity wall. The walls of abscesses tend to be smoother, but it must be emphasized that both tuberculous cavities and abscesses may produce a nodular margin. Nodular walls may be seen in any cavity that has resulted from a necrotic process. The radiologic features of the wall of a cavity cannot be used to reliably distinguish a neoplasm from an abscess.[652] The cases shown in Figs. 23.1, A, and 23.3 are squamous cell carcinomas of the lung. All the possibilities offered in question 3 are plausible except bronchogenic cyst, which should have smooth thin walls. (Answer to question 3 is d.) Additionally, it must be emphasized that a smooth thin wall does not exclude the presence of tumor. Dodd and Boyle[118] emphasized that cavitating neoplasms may have thin walls. It should now be obvious that the radiologic features of a cavity are infrequently diagnostic of tumor. The identification of a cavity therefore requires complete bacteriologic and cytologic evaluation. If a positive diagnosis cannot be established by either technique, biopsy is frequently mandatory to exclude tumor.

The distinction of a primary lung tumor from metastasis as the cause of a solitary cavity is also not easily accomplished.[118] Metastatic cavities are more commonly multiple or at least associated with multiple pulmonary nodules. A solitary metastasis may present a particularly difficult diagnostic problem because metastases that cavitate are frequently of squamous cell origin and may therefore mimic the histologic features of a primary lung tumor. Cavitary lung metastases are most likely to be from the head and neck in men and from the gynecologic tract in women.

VASCULAR LESIONS

Granulomatosis with polyangiitis (Fig. 23.10, A and B)[4,177] and rheumatoid arthritis[468] are the two most likely collagen vascular diseases to result in a perivascular inflammatory reaction and thus cause necrosis of lung tissue with subsequent cavitation. Both entities are likely to result in multiple pulmonary opacities or multiple cavities. These lesions are considered in greater detail in the chapters elsewhere in this text that discuss multifocal opacities and multiple cavities (see Chapters 16 and 24).

Thromboemboli and septic emboli[664] also produce vascular occlusion that may lead to ischemic necrosis with cavitation. They are also more likely to produce multiple areas of opacity with multiple cavities.

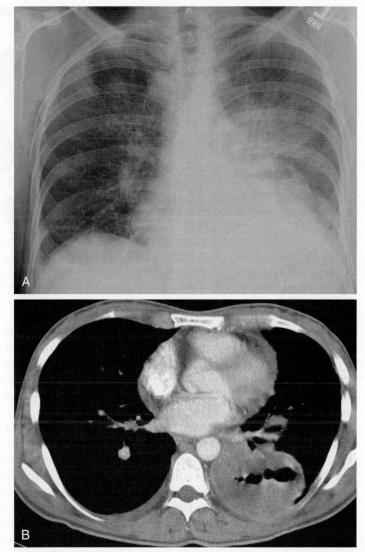

Fig. 23.10   A, Bilateral air space opacities are more severe on the left. A more circumscribed opacity behind the heart has an air-fluid level that indicates cavitation. This could be an abscess in an area of pneumonia, but the patient had no symptoms of infection; rather, the patient had severe hemoptysis. **B,** Computed tomography scan confirms a large thick-walled cavity in the left lower lobe. This resulted from vasculitis with ischemic necrosis caused by granulomatosis with polyangiitis.

ENVIRONMENTAL DISEASES

Both silicosis and coal workers' pneumoconiosis have been reported to result in cavitation, most often in one of the conglomerate masses seen in these diseases. These cavities have been postulated to result from ischemic necrosis of the center of the mass; this is a rare complication of silicosis. The most likely cause of a cavity occurring in a patient with silicosis or coal workers' pneumoconiosis is complicating tuberculosis.[641] Tuberculosis must be ruled out in all patients with either condition who develop subsequent cavitation. The associated reticular changes in these patients may also result from the primary disease or the associated tuberculosis. Serial examinations documenting a change require complete clinical evaluation to exclude active tuberculosis.

PNEUMATOCELES

Pneumatoceles could have been appropriately discussed with the pyogenic infections that result in holes in the lung, but it is important to distinguish pneumatoceles

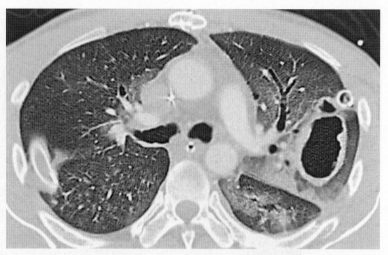

Fig. 23.11 Axial computed tomography scan of a patient following a motor vehicle accident reveals an area of consolidation with a ground-glass opacity and an oval lucent area with a thick wall in the periphery of the left upper lobe. This is a posttraumatic pneumatocele, which was the result of a pulmonary laceration.

from necrotic cavities. The appearance of a lucency in the midst of extensive air space consolidation does not always indicate a necrotic cavity. The development of pneumatoceles, particularly in staphylococcal and hydrocarbon aspiration pneumonias,[226] represents a well-known example of a lucency that mimics the radiologic appearance of cavitation. In the early stages of infection, these cystic spaces are virtually indistinguishable from cavities. Clinical and laboratory correlation are frequently the only ways to establish the correct cause of the holes. Pneumatoceles characteristically occur in the healing phase of the disease, and they appear radiologically to enlarge and increase in number while the patient appears to be clinically improving. They are more frequently multiple than solitary. The pathologic mechanism for the development of pneumatoceles has not been clearly defined. One postulate is that they are secondary to small airway obstructive disease with a sleeve valve mechanism that results in localized air trapping. Other researchers believe that pneumatoceles result from an alteration of the normal pulmonary elasticity. Their importance is that they do not indicate destruction of lung parenchyma and are usually transient, although their resolution may take weeks to months.

The term *traumatic pneumatocele*[139] is applied to lesions that follow blunt injury to the chest (Fig. 23.11). These injuries initially result in an area of pulmonary contusion. The development of a cystic structure following in an area of pulmonary contusion is generally thought to result from laceration of the lung. The situation is therefore somewhat different from the pneumatocele that results from an infectious process and is clearly different from a true cavity in its pathogenesis. A history of trauma and serial chest radiographs usually confirm the origin of the cyst. CT is often useful for early detection and for confirming the diagnosis of posttraumatic pneumatoceles.[204,609]

CONGENITAL CYST

The congenital lesions that may result in the radiologic appearance of a solitary hole in the lung include the bronchogenic[464] cyst and bronchopulmonary sequestration. Although these structures are considered to be congenital or developmental, they are frequently seen in young adults.

The bronchopulmonary sequestration may assume a very characteristic radiologic appearance[150] (Fig. 23.12, *A*). It is a complex foregut anomaly found medially in either

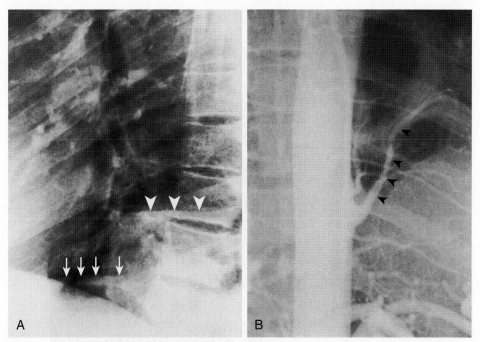

Fig. 23.12   A, Lateral chest radiograph reveals an air-fluid level in the left lower lobe (large arrowheads). Note that the posterior portion of the left hemidiaphragm is obscured, confirming the location. The anterior left hemidiaphragm is outlined by *small white arrows*. This raises the differential diagnosis of a hiatal hernia, abscess, cystic bronchiectasis, or intralobar sequestration. **B,** Aortogram from the same case reveals a large artery arising from the abdominal aorta *(arrowheads)* that feed to the left lower lobe cyst. This confirms the diagnosis of pulmonary sequestration.

lower lobe, almost always in the posterior basal segment.[233,516,640] It is somewhat more frequent on the left and may present as a cystic lesion posterior to the heart.[175] This appearance may casually resemble that of a hiatal hernia, except that a hiatal hernia is usually more of a midline structure. The distinction is easily made after a barium swallow. There are two types of bronchopulmonary sequestration, intralobar and extralobar. The extralobar variety is totally isolated from the lung by its own pleura and is therefore unlikely to present as a cystic lesion. The development of a lucent defect requires the development of communications with airways that permit the drainage of fluid from the cystic structure. This is a common presentation for the intralobar sequestration that may occur spontaneously or as a result of superimposed infection. Prior to development of the communication, the sequestration is more likely to have the radiologic appearance of a mass or ill-defined opacity. The clinical presentation is often that of recurrent infection in the area of sequestration. This may suggest the differential diagnosis of chronic, recurrent, lower lobe infection, including cystic bronchiectasis, chronic abscess, and intrapulmonary sequestration. Radiologic confirmation of the diagnosis requires aortography or CT angiography for demonstration of the anomalous artery from the aorta to the sequestered lung (Fig. 23.12, *B*). Histologically, the sequestration consists of a multicystic structure. The linings of the cysts frequently contain multiple elements that resemble alveolar walls, bronchioles, and even bronchi. The bronchus-like structures do not have normal communications with the tracheobronchial tree. Occasionally, some of the cyst may continue to be fluid filled and may even give rise to the appearance of a mass within a cystic structure. Because of the multicystic nature of the lesion, the radiologic appearance of the hole in the lung may be that of a large cystic structure with multiple loculations and even multiple air-fluid levels.

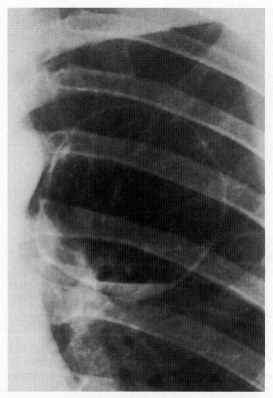

Fig. 23.13   A very thin-walled, circumscribed lucent lesion is a typical appearance for a congenital bronchogenic cyst that has drained its fluid content. (From Reed JC, Sobonya RE. Congenital respiratory cyst. RPC from the AFIP. *Radiology.* 1975;117:315-319. Used by permission.)

A bronchogenic cyst,[464] in contrast to a pulmonary sequestration, is a simple cyst (Fig. 23.13). The majority of bronchogenic cysts occur as mediastinal opacities. Of the small number that occur in the lung (approximately 14%), the radiologic presentation is usually that of a well-circumscribed, homogeneous, soft-tissue opacity. Approximately 36% of bronchogenic cysts occurring in the lung will be contain air and therefore present a lucent defect. The differentiation of these cysts from acquired inflammatory cysts usually presents a diagnostic dilemma, with the latter being chronic lung abscesses or a dominant cyst of cystic bronchiectasis. Bronchogenic cysts are not expected in the apices and are therefore unlikely to be confused with a tuberculous cavity. Because the inflammatory causes of a hole in the lung are much more common, a bronchogenic cyst frequently becomes a diagnosis of exclusion. It is often easier for the radiologist to reject the diagnosis of a bronchogenic cyst than to actually make the diagnosis. Ill-defined borders with surrounding irregular opacities, reticular strands radiating away from the lucent space, loculations (coarse bands of opacity) within the hole, and associated pleural reactions all strongly suggest an infectious causal agent rather than a congenital cyst. Only those cases with very thin, sharply defined walls should be considered as possible bronchogenic cysts. This appearance might be mimicked by coccidioidomycosis and may also be confused with a pneumatocele or bullous lesion. It must be emphasized that bullous lesions are frequently multiple and are associated with stretching and attenuation of the pulmonary vasculature. Pneumatocele is best excluded on the basis of history because it typically follows staphylococcal pneumonia, hydrocarbon pneumonia, or trauma. A bronchogenic cyst is therefore suggested by exclusion of the more likely causes of a localized lucent space.

BRONCHIECTATIC CYSTS

Cystic bronchiectasis is not a rare cause of multiple holes in the lung and is considered in detail in Chapter 24. Occasionally, a very large, dominant cyst may result from cystic bronchiectasis and mimic an abscess or congenital cyst.[464]

PARASITIC CYSTS

Hydatid cysts are the result of infection with *Echinococcus granulosus* or *Echinococcus multilocularis*. Dogs or other carnivores are the primary host of these parasites, and sheep may be intermediate hosts. Humans are infected by the ingestion of contaminated food, and the parasite embryo passes through the duodenal mucosa into the portal vein to the liver.

The wall of a hydatid cyst has three layers. The inner layer is a very thin, unicellular layer from which arise the scolices; the middle layer is a laminated, chitinous layer, which is the parasite (endocyst); and the third layer is a fibrous reaction of the host to the parasite. When they are intact, cysts may be filled with fluid and appear as a nodule or mass on the chest radiograph and a low attenuation cyst on CT. After a cyst develops a communication with a bronchus, the radiologic appearance changes. Introduction of air into the cyst causes separation of the fibrous and laminated layers of the cyst. A small amount of air between the two layers leads to a lucent crescent, or the air meniscus sign. This appearance might be mimicked by the development of a fungus ball in a preexisting cavity, but examination of previous studies should resolve this differential because the previous existence of a homogeneous circumscribed opacity would be evidence against the diagnosis of a fungus ball.

When the endocyst ruptures, the fluid drains into the tracheobronchial tree, leading to the radiologic appearance of an air-fluid level in a sharply defined lucent space. After the fluid has partially drained, the laminated, chitinous middle layer of the cyst separates from the fibrous layer. This permits the endocyst layer to separate from the outer wall and float on the remaining fluid. It has a very characteristic chest radiographic and CT appearance that permits a specific diagnosis (Fig. 23.14, *A-C*). This radiologic presentation has been described as the "water lily" sign and is distinctive for hydatid disease. It is very common for the scolices to disseminate through the bronchi with the development of multiple cysts.[435] A history of having lived in an area of the world where hydatid disease is endemic is essential if the diagnosis is to be suspected. The incidence of the disease is particularly high in Russia, Eastern Europe, Italy, Greece, Iran, the Middle East, Spain, North Africa, Argentina, Uruguay, Australia, New Zealand, and Ireland. In North America, the disease is seen mainly in Canada, Alaska, and the southwestern United States, particularly in New Mexico, Arizona, and Nevada.

BULLOUS EMPHYSEMA

Bullous emphysema[235] is another process that rarely presents with a solitary cystic structure or hole in the lung. However, these defects may vary considerably in size and result in the appearance of a large hole in the lung. Other associated bullae may produce only minimal changes on the chest radiograph. These holes tend to have very thin walls and are frequently surrounded by attenuated, elongated pulmonary vessels. The cyst itself should appear to be avascular. Cysts of bullous emphysema may be distinguished from thin-walled bronchogenic cysts by their peripheral location, as opposed to a more central location for the bronchogenic cyst. They are commonly encountered in the apices or the bases of the lungs and are often the cause of recurrent pneumothorax.

DIAPHRAGMATIC HERNIAS

Diaphragmatic hernias through the foramen of Morgagni (Fig. 23.15, *A* and *B*) or Bochdalek may mimic the appearance of elevation of one side of the diaphragm on

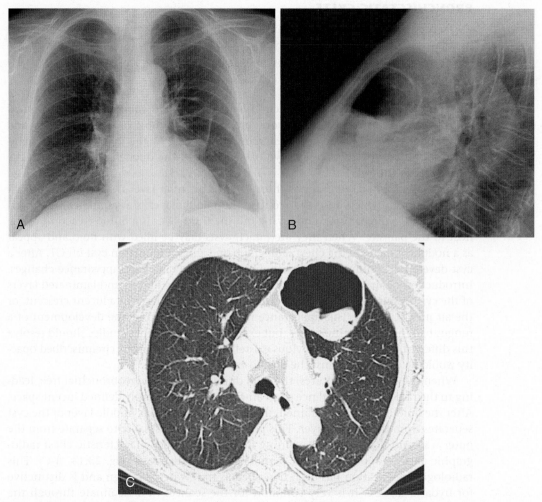

Fig. 23.14   A, This large, thin-walled lucent space in the medial left lung has an inferior opacity that might suggest the presence of fluid in a cyst or cavity. **B,** Lateral view confirms the presence of a thin-walled lucent space with fluid or tissue in its base. **C,** Computed tomography scan confirms that the opacity in the base is solid tissue that has layered in the dependent portion of the cyst. This is the typical appearance for a hydatid cyst.

a single view. However, the lateral view reveals the characteristic anterior location of a Morgagni hernia or the posterior location of a Bochdalek hernia. Hiatal hernias are near the midline and are more likely to be confused with cavities or masses than with elevation of the diaphragm. Paraesophageal hernias (Fig. 23.16, *A* and *B*) often contain most of the stomach and produce a large lucent structure in the left lower chest. The diagnosis can be confirmed with an upper gastrointestinal series or CT scan. Large paraesophageal hernias do have an increased risk of gastric volvulus.

Top 5 Diagnoses: Solitary Lucent Defect

1. Abscess
2. Cavitary lung cancer
3. Tuberculosis
4. Metastasis
5. Loculated hydropneumothorax

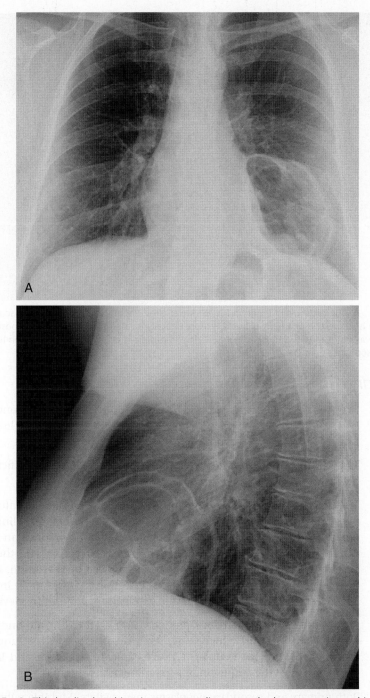

Fig. 23.15 A, This localized multicystic structure adjacent to the heart contains multiple loops of bowel that have herniated into the chest. **B,** The lateral view reveals that the hernia is anterior and is therefore a Morgagni hernia.

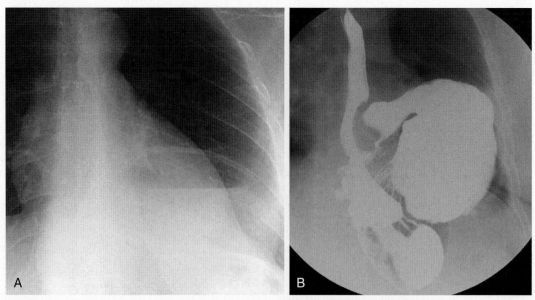

Fig. 23.16 **A,** The large lucent lesion in the left lower chest has an air-fluid level and obscures the diaphragm. The appearance is suggestive of a hernia, but it is more laterally located than the expected position for a hiatal hernia, and there was no history of trauma to suggest diaphragmatic rupture. **B,** Upper gastrointestinal series confirms a large paraesophageal hernia.

Summary

Holes in the lung may be caused by cavities, pneumatoceles, bronchiectatic cysts, bullous emphysema, and even congenital cysts, including bronchogenic cysts and intrapulmonary sequestration.

True cavities are the result of infection, tumor, or vascular insufficiency with ischemic necrosis.

The processes that lead to infectious cavities may be divided into two categories: (1) pyogenic infection; and (2) granulomatous inflammation. The clinical course is usually quite distinct for each category. Pyogenic infections produce an acute febrile illness with elevation and a shift to the left of the WBC count, and the radiologic appearance of extensive air space consolidation followed by cavitation. In contrast, cavitary diseases resulting from granulomatous infection follow a more indolent course, with a low-grade temperature, less sputum production, and mildly elevated WBC counts.

The granulomatous infections produce associated radiologic findings of chronic disease, including pleural thickening, reticular opacities in the lung, cicatrizing atelectasis, and pulmonary nodules. Careful clinical correlation and laboratory diagnosis usually confirm the suspicion of a granulomatous process.

Both primary and secondary neoplasms may cavitate. Multiple pulmonary nodules with cavitation strongly suggest metastatic disease. A solitary cavity with thick nodular walls must be considered to be tumor until proven otherwise. Approximately two-thirds of cavitating tumors are of squamous cell origin and either primary or secondary in the lung.

Of the vascular diseases that result in ischemic necrosis and thus a solitary cavity, thromboembolism is the most common. These diseases frequently produce multiple radiologic opacities, although they may occasionally produce only one cavity. Clinical correlation is particularly important. For example, granulomatosis with polyangiitis may be associated with renal disease or sinus disease that virtually confirms the diagnosis. Although the clinical setting of thromboemboli can be nonspecific, an association of thrombophlebitis, pleuritic chest pain, and pleural effusion followed by the development of a cavity is virtually diagnostic.

Cavitation of a conglomerate mass of silicosis or coal workers' pneumoconiosis may result from ischemic necrosis, but this complication must be considered to be superimposed tuberculosis until proven otherwise.

Infectious pneumatoceles must be distinguished from abscesses. Both result from a necrotizing pneumonia. Clinical correlation is essential because pneumatoceles tend to occur in the healing phases of pneumonia when the patient appears to have passed the crisis. Differentiating between an abscess and a pneumatocele is definitely important because pneumatoceles resolve spontaneously after a period of weeks to months without any notable residual effect. Abscesses may persist as a source of recurrent infection or leave parenchymal scars.

Traumatic pneumatocele is the result of pulmonary laceration with the development of a cystic space.

Intrapulmonary sequestration is a complex foregut anomaly that may result in a cystic lesion in the base of the lung. It frequently appears as a localized multilocular cyst and may be associated with recurrent basilar pulmonary infections. It may therefore be confused with cystic bronchiectasis. Aortography or CT angiography is the confirmatory diagnostic procedure. Bilateral pulmonary sequestrations are very rare.[640]

Cystic bronchiectasis is more commonly the cause of multiple holes in the lung; however, one cystic structure may be dominant and therefore mimic the appearance of a solitary cyst. Of the entities considered in this differential diagnosis, sequestration most closely mimics cystic bronchiectasis because both occur in the bases of the lung.

Bullous emphysema may also result in a dominant cyst with very thin walls. There is usually an associated attenuation of pulmonary vasculature. The cysts tend to be in the periphery of the lung and are frequently pleural based. Because of their characteristic location and associated findings, they should not be easily confused with the other entities considered in this chapter.

ANSWER GUIDE

Legends for introductory figures

Fig. 23.1 A, Squamous cell carcinoma of the lung caused this cavity with thick nodular walls and a low air-fluid level. Compare its appearance with the tuberculosis case seen in Fig. 23.6, *A* and *B*. **B,** Another cavity with thick, irregular walls contains a large soft-tissue mass. This is the expected appearance for pulmonary gangrene. It results from a virulent infection that has invaded the pulmonary vessels. This is a case of mucormycosis. **C,** A large, lucent lesion with a long air-fluid level is surrounded by a large area of air space consolidation. An earlier lateral view (see Fig. 23.7, *A*) confirmed the location of the lesion to be in the lingula. This is a necrotizing pneumonia with pulmonary abscess. **D,** Compare this lucent lesion with the one shown in **C**. It also contains a high fluid level but lacks a well-defined wall or surrounding pulmonary consolidation. These are clues to a loculated hydropneumothorax. The lateral view (see Fig. 23.7, *B*) confirmed the extrapulmonary location of the lesion. This is an empyema with a bronchopleural fistula. (**B** from Zagoria RJ, Choplin RH, Karstaedt N. Pulmonary gangrene as a complication of mucormycosis. *Am J Roentgenol* 1985;114:1195-1196. Used by permission.)

Fig. 23.2 Nodularity of the inner wall *(arrows)* of a cavity should suggest a necrotic tumor. This is a primary carcinoma of the lung. (From Theros EG. Varying manifestations of peripheral pulmonary neoplasms: a radiologic-pathologic correlative study. *Am J Roent-genol* 1977;128:893-914. Used by permission.)

Fig. 23.3 A, Upper lobe cavities should always be considered suspicious for tuberculosis. **B,** Computed tomography scan confirms a multiloculated, left upper lobe cavity. **C,** The focal consolidation in the left lower lobe is evidence of transbronchial spread of the infection. This is a highly infectious stage of tuberculosis.

ANSWERS
1. a, c, d, b   2. a   3. d   4. b

24 | MULTIPLE LUCENT LESIONS

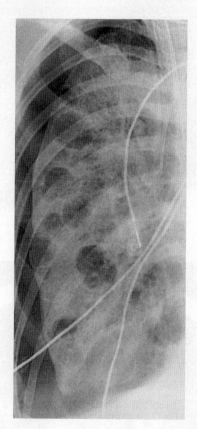

Fig. 24.1

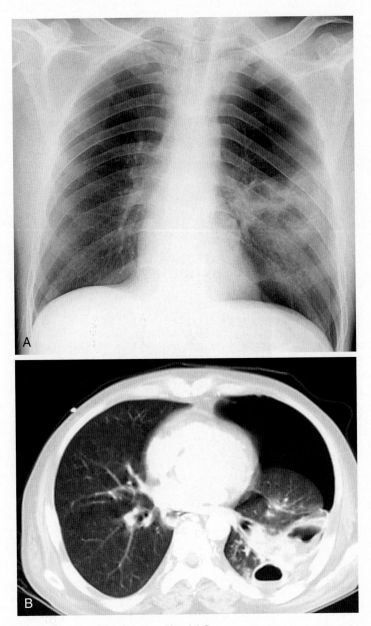

Fig. 24.2

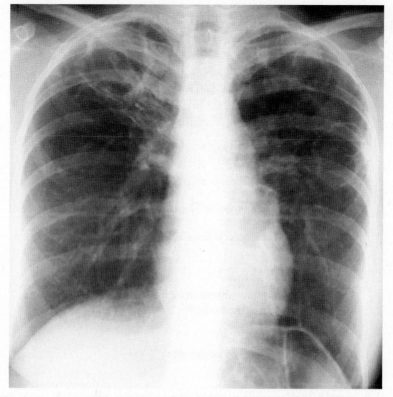

Fig. 24.3

QUESTIONS

1. Refer to Fig. 24.1. Which of the following is the best diagnosis?
   a. Adult respiratory distress syndrome.
   b. Pneumatoceles.
   c. Multiple abscesses.
   d. Bronchopleural fistula.
   e. Necrotizing pneumonia, abscesses, and bronchopleural fistula.

2. Which is the most likely diagnosis in the case illustrated in Fig. 24.2, *A* and *B*?
   a. Metastatic squamous cell carcinoma.
   b. Histoplasmosis.
   c. Tuberculosis.
   d. Necrotizing pneumonia.
   e. *Mycoplasma pneumoniae.*

3. The multiple cavities with surrounding reticular opacities shown in Fig. 24.3 are consistent with which of the following diagnoses?
   a. *Klebsiella pneumoniae.*
   b. Metastases.
   c. Coccidioidomycosis.
   d. *Mycoplasma pneumoniae.*
   e. Pseudomonas *aeruginosa.*

| Chart 24.1 | **MULTIPLE LUCENT LESIONS** |

I. Cavities
  A. Infection
    1. Bacterial pneumonias[207] (Staphylococcus, Klebsiella, mixed gram-negative organisms, anaerobes, and Nocardia)
    2. Fungal infections
      a. Histoplasmosis[97,110]
      b. Blastomycosis[450]
      c. Coccidioidomycosis[373]
      d. Cryptococcosis[200,229,293]
      e. Mucormycosis[33]
      f. Sporotrichosis[89]
      g. Aspergillosis (invasive)[591]
    3. Tuberculosis[54,641]
    4. Parasites (echinococcal disease)[435]
  B. Neoplasms
    1. Metastases[118]
    2. Lymphoma (rare)[356]
    3. Invasive mucinous adenocarcinoma (pseudocavities)[621,623]
    4. Pulmonary papillomatosis[190]
  C. Vascular
    1. Rheumatoid disease[468]
    2. Granulomatosis with polyangiitis
    3. Infarcts
    4. Septic emboli[664]
II. Cystic bronchiectasis (e.g., recurrent pneumonias, tuberculosis, cystic fibrosis, agammaglobulinemia, allergic aspergillosis)
III. Tracheobronchomegaly (Mounier-Kuhn syndrome)[381]
IV. Pneumatoceles[139,226]
V. Bullous emphysema (see Chapter 22)
VI. Honeycomb lung (see Chapter 19)
VII. Cystic pulmonary airway malformation (CPAM)[357,626]
VIII. Herniation of small bowel (congenital or traumatic)
IX. Idiopathic lung diseases with cysts
  1. Langerhans cell histiocytosis[20]
  2. Lymphangioleiomyomatosis[424]
  3. Lymphocytic interstitial pneumonia[398]
  4. Amyloidosis[175]

| Chart 24.2 | **ILL-DEFINED OPACITIES WITH HOLES** |

I. Infections
  A. Necrotizing pneumonias[207]
    1. *Staphylococcus aureus*
    2. Beta-hemolytic streptococci
    3. *Klebsiella pneumoniae*
    4. *Escherichia coli*
    5. *Proteus, Aerobacter*
    6. *Pseudomonas*
    7. Anaerobes
  B. Aspiration pneumonia (usually mixed gram-negative organisms)
  C. Septic emboli[664]
  D. Fungus

Chart 24.2   ILL-DEFINED OPACITIES WITH HOLES—cont'd

    1. Histoplasmosis
    2. Blastomycosis
    3. Coccidioidomycosis
    4. Cryptococcosis[252,293]
  E. Tuberculosis[641]
II. Neoplasms
  A. Primary carcinomas
  B. Invasive mucinous adenocarcinoma[597,621,623]
  C. Lymphoma
III. Vascular and collagen vascular diseases
  A. Emboli with infarction
  B. Granulomatosis with polyangiitis
IV. Trauma
  A. Contusion with pneumatoceles[139]

Chart 24.3   CAVITATING NODULES

I. Neoplasms
  A. Primary lung
    1. Squamous cell carcinoma
    2. Adenocarcinoma
    3. Invasive mucinous adenocarcinoma (pseudocavitation)[597,621,623]
  B. Metastasis
    1. Squamous cell (e.g., head and neck, cervix, esophagus)
    2. Adenocarcinoma
    3. Melanoma
    4. Sarcoma (e.g., osteosarcoma)
  C. Lymphoma[356]
II. Infections
  A. Septic emboli[664] (*Staphylococcus aureus*, including MRSA)
  B. Nocardiosis
  C. Cryptococcosis[255,293]
  D. Coccidioidomycosis
  E. Aspergillosis
III. Vascular and collagen vascular diseases
  A. Pulmonary embolism with infarction
  B. Vasculitis (e.g., granulomatosis with polyangiitis)
  C. Rheumatoid nodules and Caplan syndrome[146,468]
  D. Lupus erythematosus[615]

Chart 24.4   PULMONARY LUCENT LESIONS RELATED TO ACQUIRED IMMUNODEFICIENCY SYNDROME (AIDS)

  I. *Pneumocystis jiroveci* pneumonia–related lung cysts[81]
 II. Premature bullous emphysema[212,316] (periphery of upper lobe)
III. Pneumatoceles
IV. Necrotizing pneumonias (e.g., pyogenic bacteria, *Pneumocystis*)[156,304,348]
 V. Tuberculosis[198]
VI. Atypical mycobacterial infection
VII. Fungal infections[93] (fewer than 5% of patients with AIDS[406])
  A. Cryptococcosis
  B. Coccidioidomycosis
  C. Histoplasmosis
VIII. Nocardiosis
 IX. Mixed infections (common)

Discussion

Many of the entities considered in Chapters 19, 22, and 23 also result in multiple lucent lesions. In fact, some entities more typically produce multiple lesions. The latter include necrotizing pneumonias, septic emboli, cystic bronchiectasis, pneumatoceles, bullous emphysema, honeycomb lung, and metastatic tumor. Although the precise location of the solitary lucent defect is important, the distribution of multiple lucencies assumes an even greater importance in their radiologic analysis (Chart 24.1).

CAVITIES

Infection

As in solitary cavities, infection is the most common cause of multiple pulmonary cavities (see Fig. 24.1). Acute pyogenic infections are radiologically characterized by areas of air space consolidation, a clinical course of elevated temperature, and often diagnostic laboratory findings, including elevation of the white blood cell (WBC) count with an associated shift to the left and positive sputum cultures. The development of multiple lucencies in the midst of an acute pneumonia (see Fig. 24.2, *A* and *B*) is the expected appearance of necrotizing pneumonias. Peripheral cavities from necrotizing pneumonias and septic emboli are at high risk for rupture into the pleural space with bronchopleural fistulas causing pneumothorax. (Answer to question 1 is *e*.) Other causes of lucent spaces in the consolidations caused by pneumonia include the following: (1) resolution of the process with intervening normal lung; and (2) pneumatoceles. The pathogenesis of these processes was considered in Chapter 23. Clinical correlation is extremely valuable in making this distinction. When the patient appears to be recovering from illness, the holes likely represent normal aerated lung or pneumatoceles. The radiologic observation of a round, sharply defined lucency with a discrete smooth wall suggests that the lucencies represent pneumatoceles. Ill-defined lucencies without a distinct margin are more typical of reaerated lung. The development of air-fluid levels in the midst of an area of consolidation indicates the development of spaces in the lung parenchyma that are most probably the result of tissue necrosis and abscess formation.

Air-fluid levels are not encountered in normally aerated lung or pneumatoceles; they are likely to appear when the patient is profoundly ill. In such cases, they are diagnostic of a virulent necrotizing pneumonia. The most common organisms to result in such a process include *Staphylococcus, Klebsiella, Pseudomonas*, anaerobes, and mixed gram-negative organisms (Chart 24.2). (Answer to question 2 is *d*.) As emphasized earlier, it is exceptional for pneumococcal pneumonia, *Mycoplasma* pneumonia, or viral pneumonias to cavitate, but cavitary *Mycoplasma* has been reported.[338,540]

Septic emboli (Fig. 24.4, *A* and *B*) are another cause of necrotizing pulmonary infection that may result from infection with some of the same organisms that cause necrotizing pneumonia, especially staphylococcus and, more recently, methicillin-resistant *Staphylococcus aureus* (MRSA).[411] Septic emboli may result from any cause of systemic sepsis. Bacterial endocarditis of the right heart is a complication of intravenous (IV) drug abuse that places the patient at high risk for MRSA septic emboli.[312] Other sources of septic emboli include long-term indwelling vascular lines, pacemaker wires, septic thrombophlebitis, and organ transplants.[491]

Tuberculous cavities may be distinctive with apical cavities and associated reticular or nodular scarring. The clinical findings and radiologic patterns of chronic tuberculosis are substantially different from that of the acute necrotizing pneumonias, but reactivation of tuberculosis may be more difficult to distinguish from a bacterial pneumonia and the air space consolidations may obscure the cavities on the chest radiograph (Fig. 24.5, *A-C*). Reactivation of tuberculosis may cause cavities, air space consolidations, and clusters of small nodules from transbronchial spread of the infection.

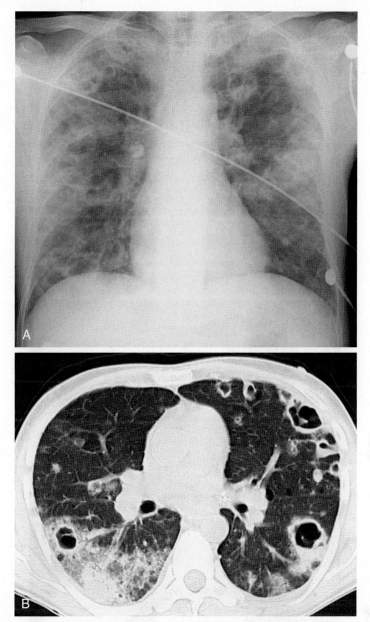

Fig. 24.4   A, Numerous bilateral cavities are scattered though out the lungs. **B,** Computed tomography scan reveals the cavities to have a peripheral distribution and vary in size. There is some surrounding air space consolidation and ground-glass opacity in the superior segment of the right lower lobe. This is the result of methicillin-resistant *Staphylococcus aureus* (MRSA) septic emboli from an infected dialysis catheter.

Histoplasmosis, blastomycosis, coccidioidomycosis, and tuberculosis are frequently radiologically indistinguishable. The chronic cavities from these granulomatous infections may be associated with considerable parenchymal reaction, but the parenchymal reaction is often a reticular or reticulonodular reaction and is usually distinctive when compared with the consolidations of acute necrotizing pneumonias (see Fig. 24.2, *A* and *B*). The marked tendency to apical distribution is likewise characteristic but is not absolutely diagnostic of these infections. In tuberculosis and histoplasmosis, cavities may develop months to years after the primary infection. There is, however, a rare form of tuberculosis—primary progressive tuberculosis—in which there is progression

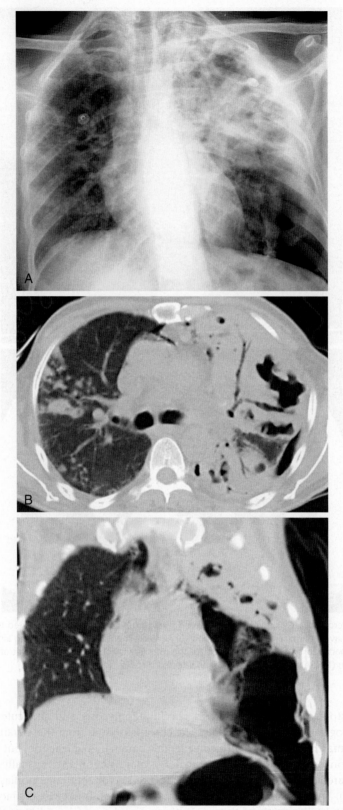

Fig. 24.5 **A,** Left upper lobe consolidation with multiple lucent cavities. **B,** Axial computed tomography (CT) scan confirms consolidation with air bronchograms and large cavities with multiple nodules in the right lung with peripheral tree-in-bud nodules. **C,** Coronal CT scan reveals a large inferior pneumothorax in this patient with cavitary tuberculosis, with transbronchial spread to the right lung and left bronchopleural fistula.

from primary air space consolidation to cavitary tuberculosis over a short period without an asymptomatic interval between the two phases of the disease.

Blastomycosis and coccidioidomycosis, in contrast to histoplasmosis and tuberculosis, are more difficult to define in terms of primary and secondary disease.[450] The cavities of blastomycosis may be apical and mimic the appearance of postprimary tuberculosis, but the cavitation may occur during the acute alveolar exudative phase of the disease with an appearance more like that of a necrotizing pneumonia. The radiologic course of such cases of blastomycosis is more protracted than that of necrotizing pneumonia, and the clearing of the exudate sometimes requires 2 to 3 months. The clinical course is also more indolent than that of the necrotizing pneumonias, with characteristic low-grade temperatures.

Coccidioidomycosis (see Fig. 24.3) is known for producing very thin-walled cavities that may lack the surrounding parenchymal reaction that is expected in the other granulomatous infections. The radiologic presentation of thin-walled cavities occurs as a late sequela of the infection. (Answer to question 3 is *c*.) In the early stages of the process, cavities may occur in areas of air space consolidation. This early acute cavitation results from central necrosis and liquefaction of parenchyma. As the infection is contained, there is organization with circumscription of the opacity. The radiologic sequence may thus be that of a process that begins with an air space consolidation followed by cavitation, leading to the appearance of a thick-walled cavity. When air is trapped in the cavity, it expands under tension. As the surrounding inflammatory response resolves, the characteristic thin-walled cavity appears. The cavities of coccidioidomycosis are also much less likely to follow the characteristic apical distribution of tuberculosis or histoplasmosis. The combination of a typical radiologic presentation of multiple thin-walled cavities and a definite history of exposure to *Coccidioides*, with positive serologic studies, frequently makes possible a precise diagnosis.

Neoplasms

Multiple cavities are not rare in patients with pulmonary metastases. This radiologic appearance makes the diagnosis of primary lung cancer less likely, but lucent cystic lesions have been described as so-called "pseudocavitation" and reported as a possible presentation of invasive mucinous adenocarcinoma of the lung.[621,623] The diagnosis of metastasis is frequently aided by knowledge of a distant primary tumor. The typical radiologic appearance is that of sharply circumscribed multiple opacities with some having central lucencies (Chart 24.3). These cavities frequently have thick nodular walls, although occasionally the wall may be very thin and smooth. Wall characteristics are not reliable for distinguishing metastases from other causes of multiple cavities. Approximately two-thirds of cavitating metastases are of the epidermoid variety. Squamous cell tumors of the head and neck, esophagus, and uterine cervix are best known for producing cavitary metastases, but as many as one-third of cavitary metastases may be from adenocarcinoma. Even malignant melanoma and osteosarcoma have been reported to cavitate. Lymphoma is an infrequent cause of cavitary pulmonary nodules. The exact pathologic mechanism for the cavitation of metastases is not always easily determined, but most cavitating metastases seem to represent tumors that have undergone central necrosis.

Vascular Diseases

Cavitation is generally considered to be a secondary result of infectious and neoplastic diseases, but primary diseases of the pulmonary blood vessels also result in cavitation. These include thromboembolism, septic emboli, and the collagen vascular diseases that cause vasculitis and thus result in small vessel occlusions. The radiologic diagnosis of thromboembolism with infarction is not easily achieved. Most patients with venous thromboemboli may have a normal chest radiograph. Those patients who do exhibit radiologic abnormalities have extremely variable patterns that include: (1) localized areas of hyperlucency that

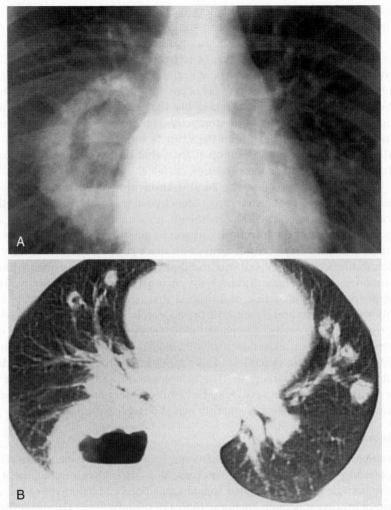

Fig. 24.6 **A,** Granulomatosis with polyangiitis is the cause of this large, thick-walled cavity with an air-fluid level. Additional nodules are minimally visible on the chest radiograph. **B,** Computed tomography scan of the same patient shows additional nodules, some of which are cavitary. This appearance of multiple cavitary nodules with a large dominant cavity is more typical of granulomatosis with polyangiitis than a solitary cavity would be.

result from decreased perfusion of an area of lung (Westermark sign); (2) nonspecific areas of atelectasis; (3) air space consolidation by hemorrhage and edema; (4) pleural effusion; and (5) rarely, cavitation. Of these radiologic presentations, only cavitation can be considered diagnostic of a true infarction of lung tissue. Patients with significant amounts of hemorrhage and edema may have had infarction of lung tissue. Infarction cannot be detected during the acute phase of the illness, but the development of cavitation indicates necrosis of lung tissue. It has been stated that cavitating infarcts are usually secondarily infected, but sterile infarcts have been observed to cavitate. Septic emboli, in contrast to embolic venous thrombi, commonly cause multiple bilateral cavities.

Granulomatosis with polyangiitis (formerly Wegener granulomatosis; Fig. 24.6, *A* and *B*) and rheumatoid arthritis are the two collagen vascular diseases that are most likely to result in multiple cavitary lesions. The pulmonary radiologic patterns of classic granulomatosis with polyangiitis and the variants (limited form and lymphomatoid granulomatosis) are identical. These entities were all mentioned as causes of solitary cavities, but they are more likely to result in multiple parenchymal opacities with one or more of the opacities progressing to cavitation. Granulomatosis with polyangiitis frequently results in pulmonary hemorrhage with multifocal areas of ground-glass opacity and ill-defined consolidations that may undergo cavitation. However, in some cases the cavitating lesions may be observed as discrete, well-defined cavities, some of which have thick walls and resemble cavitating nodules or masses. These cavities all result from the diffuse vasculitis and localized areas of ischemic necrosis. Rheumatoid nodules are a well-documented cause of cavitary nodules, but this is an infrequent manifestation of rheumatoid lung. Lupus erythematosus is a collagen vascular disease that usually causes pleural effusion, but has been observed to involve the lung with pulmonary hemorrhage, so-called "lupus pneumonitis," and has been reported as a very rare cause of multiple cavitary nodules.[615]

CYSTS

Cystic Bronchiectasis

Cystic bronchiectasis (Fig. 24.7, *A* and *B*) is a complication of either recurrent or chronic infection that may completely mimic the appearance of multiple cavities. This is not true cavitation, but rather dilation of multiple bronchi with the appearance of cystic spaces. Cystic fibrosis is one of the most common underlying causes for severe cystic bronchiectasis. Patients with cystic fibrosis have a defect in mucus production, with an unusually thick mucus that predisposes to recurrent pulmonary infections. The recurrent pulmonary infections lead to extensive inflammatory reaction in the bronchial walls (chronic bronchitis), which is followed by cystic bronchiectasis. Ring shadows around the hila are an important radiologic clue to a bronchial origin for the cystic spaces. These rings represent abnormally dilated and thickened bronchi rather than true cavitation. They are frequently more obvious in the upper lobes and may be associated with signs of air trapping in the lower lobes, including loss of peripheral vascularity and flattening of the diaphragm. Another process that may produce a similar effect is agammaglobulinemia. Patients with agammaglobulinemia are also predisposed to recurrent bacterial infections and may have secondary obstructive airway disease and bronchiectasis.

Recurrent bacterial pneumonias, even with no apparent underlying predisposing condition, are prone to the development of bronchiectasis. In the early phases, this bronchiectasis may be cylindric and even reversible, but after many episodes of pneumonia, the bronchial damage may progress to the form of bronchiectasis described as varicose or cystic bronchiectasis. This is most characteristically encountered in the lower lobes. During the early phases of this process, chest radiographs obtained during the intervals between infection may be normal. This is followed by the gradual accumulation of linear opacities in the bases. At this stage, high-resolution computed tomography (HRCT) may reveal cylindric bronchiectasis. As the bronchiectasis progresses, there may be saccular dilation of the bronchi, with lucent areas appearing in the bases as ring shadows, again representing abnormally dilated and thickened bronchi. Multiple thin-walled lucencies with low air-fluid levels are very suggestive of cystic bronchiectasis. HRCT is a reliable method for confirming the cause of these lucent areas and showing the extent of the disease.

Tuberculosis is another cause of cystic bronchiectasis.[641] When multiple cavities are encountered in the apices or throughout a lung after long-standing infection with tuberculosis, the possibility that these lucencies represent bronchiectasis in addition to necrotic cavities must be considered. This distinction can occasionally be made by chest radiographs demonstrating tubular lucencies that appear to connect with the hila. Such an appearance may be verified by HRCT. When the cystic spaces are very large, the distinction of true cavities from dilated bronchi may not be possible by chest radiography or CT. Severe destruction of the lung by tuberculosis may include both necrotic cavities and cystic bronchiectasis. Cultures are required to determine activity.

Allergic bronchopulmonary aspergillosis occurs primarily in asthmatic patients and is often associated with bronchiectasis. The perihilar cystic spaces that may develop in these patients are often the result of a unique form of cystic bronchiectasis that involves the proximal bronchi but appears to spare the smaller distal bronchi. Mucus

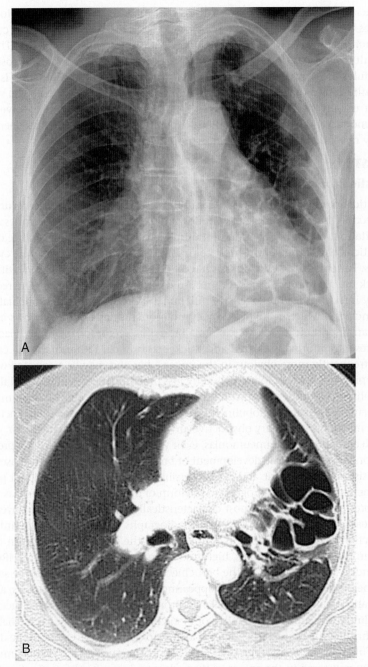

Fig. 24.7   A, The numerous thin-walled lucent lesions in the left lower lung appear cystic and contain a small amount of fluid. **B,** Computed tomography scan shows the extent of these cystic lesions that extend from the hilum to the periphery of the lung. This is cystic bronchiectasis that has developed as a result of a prior pneumonia.

plugs in these dilated bronchi produce areas of increased opacity that often have a typical branching pattern. When the plugs are coughed up, the cystic spaces may become visible on the chest radiograph. A history of chronic asthma and laboratory identification of elevated precipitin levels to *Aspergillus fumigatus* should confirm the diagnosis.

Tracheobronchomegaly (Mounier Kuhn syndrome)[381] is a rare developmental condition that results in dilation of the trachea with cystic dilation of the bronchi resembling that of cystic bronchiectasis (Fig. 24.8). Like bronchiectasis from other causes, this is a source of recurrent infections.

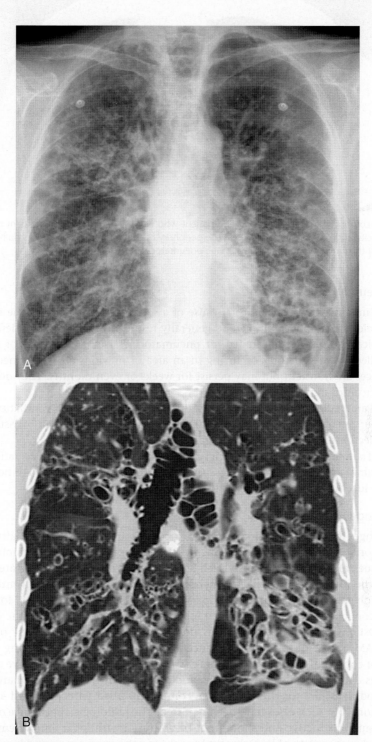

Fig. 24.8   A, Posteroanterior chest radiograph shows multiple diffuse bilateral lucent spaces and dilation of the trachea. **B,** Coronal computed tomography scan confirms that the lucent spaces in the lung are dilated bronchi resembling cystic bronchiectasis with associated dilation of the main stem bronchi and trachea. This is tracheobronchomegaly, also known as Mounier Kuhn syndrome.

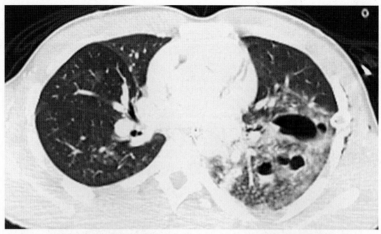

Fig. 24.9 Axial computed tomography scan of a patient who was in a motor vehicle accident reveals an area of ground-glass opacity and multiple lucent areas in the periphery of the left lower lobe. This is pulmonary contusion with lacerations of the lung resulting in posttraumatic pneumatoceles.

Pneumatoceles

Pneumatoceles are an unusual cause of a solitary lucent space in the lung. Pneumatoceles are usually multiple and generally result in multiple lucent defects. The most typical radiologic appearance for pneumatoceles is therefore that of multiple thin-walled cystic structures occurring in an area of previous air space pneumonia. These spaces are transient but may persist for weeks or even months. They do not represent necrosis of lung tissue.

Paramediastinal pneumatoceles that follow mechanical ventilation differ from other pneumatoceles in location and cause. They were previously assumed to be air collections in the inferior pulmonary ligament.[610]

Traumatic pneumatoceles (Fig. 24.9) result from pulmonary lacerations that often occur in areas of contusion. The spaces may initially fill with blood or hematoma, with the lucent lesions appearing as the blood is replaced with air.[204,609]

Congenital Lesions

Congenital causes of circumscribed lucencies in the lung are relatively rare, and reports of multiple bronchogenic cysts are exceedingly rare. Intralobar pulmonary sequestrations are frequently seen as multicystic structures in one area, particularly in the lower lobe but, like bronchogenic cysts, they rarely entail multiple areas of involvement. Congenital pulmonary airway malformation (CPAM, formerly known as congenital cystic adenomatoid malformation)[357,626] is possibly the only true multicystic congenital disease of the lung. The most typical radiologic presentation of CPAM is that of multiple large lucencies that have walls of varying thickness and that commonly fill one hemithorax. These cystic structures may have air-fluid levels. This entity is seen in the newborn and is infrequently encountered after early childhood. It is rare for the cysts to be completely filled with fluid and appear as solid lesions, but such cases have been reported. The radiologic appearance of these lesions is quite distinctive and should not be confused with lobar emphysema, which may produce a unilateral hyperlucent lung during the newborn period but lacks the thick reticular bands separating the multicystic spaces of CPAM. Radiologically, CPAM is most likely to be confused with herniation of the small bowel through a congenital hernia of the diaphragm, but the abdominal findings in herniation of the small bowel are usually distinctive because of the absence of gas-containing bowel loops in the abdomen. Staphylococcal pneumonia with multiple cystic spaces might also

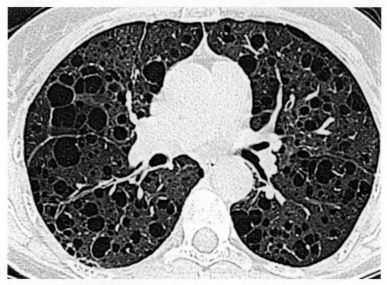

Fig. 24.10 Computed tomography scan of a woman with multiple circumscribed cysts and a history of chylous pleural effusions, confirming the diagnosis of lymphangioleiomyomatosis.

mimic the appearance of CPAM, but pleural effusion, which commonly accompanies staphylococcal pneumonia, has not been reported with CPAM. The clinical history of high fever and sepsis in staphylococcal pneumonia should make distinction of these entities relatively simple.

Birt-Hogg-Dubé syndrome is a rare congenital syndrome with skin lesions on the face and neck with multiple, bilateral, thin-walled lung cysts and increased risk for kidney cancer.[552]

Idiopathic Lung Diseases with Cysts

Cysts are often differentiated from cavities and bullae by wall thickness, with cavities having walls larger than 2 to 3 mm and bullae having no measurable walls, whereas cysts have very thin walls of 1 to 2 mm. Pneumatoceles and cysts both have very thin walls and may be indistinguishable, except that pneumatoceles are likely to be transient, whereas cysts are expected to persist. The distinction of cavities from cysts is limited on chest radiographs and often requires HRCT. Multiple cysts may result from the following idiopathic lung diseases: Langerhans cell histiocytosis (LCH),[1] lymphangioleiomyomatosis (LAM),[401,424] lymphocytic interstitial pneumonia (LIP),[398] and amyloidosis.[175]

LCH is a smoking-related disease that causes multiple cysts, nodules with an upper lobe distribution, and may be complicated by pneumothorax. When the cysts are extensive, the pattern may resemble honeycombing fibrosis.

LAM (Fig. 24.10) and tuberous sclerosis are also causes of multiple thin-walled cysts that may be complicated by chylous pleural effusions and pneumothorax.

LIP is a rare lymphocytic infiltrate of the interstitium that may be a prelymphomatous condition. There is a strong association with Sjögren syndrome, and it may also be a complication of human immunodeficiency virus (HIV) infection. The radiologic patterns include fine reticular opacities with a mixture of multiple cysts.

Amyloidosis may be primary or secondary. The secondary form is more common and complicates hematologic diseases, in particular multiple myeloma. It may cause diffuse, fine, reticular opacities or a combination of soft tissue nodules, calcified nodules, and multiple cysts.

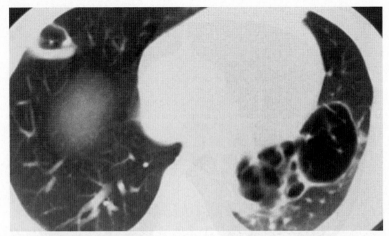

Fig. 24.11 AIDS-related lucent lesions include abscesses, pneumatoceles, and premature bullous emphysema. This computed tomography scan shows a peripheral lucent lesion in the right lung, with an air-fluid level and multiple, thin-walled lucent lesions in the left lower lobe. This patient had a necrotizing pneumonia with abscesses and pneumatoceles.

AIDS-RELATED LUCENT LESIONS

A variety of lucent lesions have been observed in patients with AIDS (Chart 24.4) and have been described as bullae, pneumatoceles, cysts, and cavities.[a]

Pyogenic pneumonias are most common in the early stages of HIV infection and in patients receiving antiretroviral therapy. The patterns of pyogenic pneumonia in patients with HIV are essentially the same as those seen in patients with normal immunity. Virulent organisms, such as staphylococci, are not frequent but are likely to cause necrosis. Lung abscesses (Fig. 24.11) occur in the acute stages of necrotizing pneumonias, whereas pneumatoceles occur during the healing phase.

Postprimary tuberculosis is another cause of necrotic cavities. This manifestation of tuberculosis is identical to that of postprimary tuberculosis in patients with normal immunity and, like the pyogenic pneumonias, occurs during the early stages of HIV infection. This is usually before the onset of AIDS. Other granulomatous infections, including nocardiosis, coccidioidomycosis, cryptococcosis, and *Mycobacterium avium* complex, are less frequent but must be considered as possible causes of cavities (Fig. 24.12, *A* and *B*).

Pneumocystis jiroveci pneumonia is a reported cause of localized opacities that may undergo necrosis and cavitate, but this is uncommon. *Pneumocystis* more typically causes diffuse interstitial or air space opacities that may develop cystic-appearing lucent spaces. Like necrotizing cavities, these spaces are often randomly scattered throughout the lungs. They rarely contain fluid and in many cases probably represent pneumatoceles. These lucent spaces may be obscured by the diffuse opacities and are therefore not well visualized on the chest radiograph, but they are often confirmed with computed tomography (CT) (Fig. 24.13). When *Pneumocystis* fails to clear, it may leave a coarse reticular pattern with intervening cystic spaces and a radiologic appearance resembling the pattern of honeycombing fibrosis. Bullous lesions have also been reported as a late complication of *Pneumocystis*. These lesions are usually distinguished from postinflammatory cysts and pneumatoceles by their locations. Cysts and pneumatoceles are randomly scattered throughout the lungs, whereas bullae are subpleural and most frequently found in the apices (Fig. 24.14). This complication appears to be particularly common in patients with recurrent *Pneumocystis* infections. The pathologic mechanism for this so-called premature bullous emphysema has not been well

[a]References 81, 156, 212, 304, 348, 508.

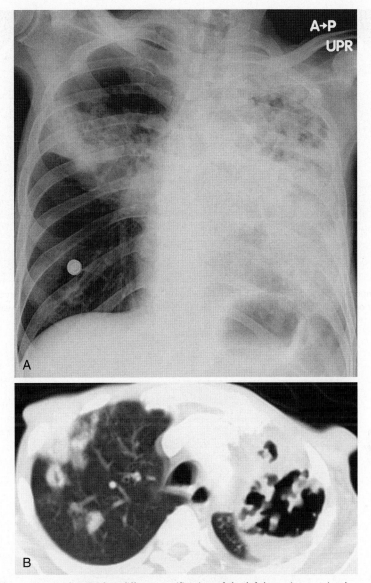

Fig. 24.12   A, This patient with AIDS has diffuse opacification of the left lung, intervening lucencies in the left upper lobe, and air space opacification in a portion of the right upper lobe. **B,** Computed tomography scan through the apex reveals a large irregular cavity with a smaller anterior cavity in the left upper lobe and multiple small nodules with a cavitary nodule in the right upper lobe. This appearance resembles tuberculosis but was caused by nocardiosis.

defined, but the complication has also been observed in IV drug abusers. There is a high incidence of pneumothorax, which is often complicated by a persistent air leak caused by rupture of bullae into the pleural space.

Top 5 Diagnoses: Multiple Lucent Lesions

1. Abscesses
2. Septic emboli
3. Tuberculosis
4. Cystic bronchiectasis
5. Metastases

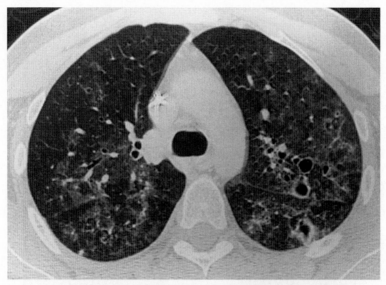

Fig. 24.13   Computed tomography scan of a patient with AIDS and *Pneumocystis* shows scattered areas of ground-glass and reticular opacities. There are also multiple lucent cystic spaces with some variation in wall thickness.

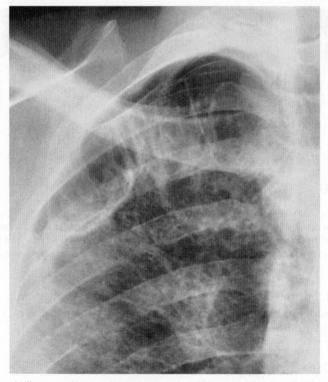

Fig. 24.14   Premature bullous emphysema in patients with AIDS causes subpleural and apical lucent lesions; in addition, it is often complicated by recurrent pneumothoraces.

Summary

Multiple cavities most commonly result from pulmonary infections that lead to necrosis of lung tissue. Acute necrotizing pneumonias usually result in multiple cavities in one area of the lung, with associated air space consolidation and an acute toxic febrile course.

The granulomatous infections, including tuberculosis, histoplasmosis, blastomycosis, and coccidioidomycosis, follow a more indolent course with low-grade temperatures. Cavities in these diseases are usually seen in the secondary hyperimmune phases of the disease and may develop from months to years after the primary infection.

Metastases are the most common neoplasms to result in multiple cavities. These cavities may vary in size and shape. Wall thickness is not a good criterion for distinguishing benign from malignant cavitary lesions, although thick nodular walls do favor a neoplastic process rather than an inflammatory reaction.

True cavities also result from vascular occlusions. This differential diagnosis includes thromboembolism with infarction, septic embolism with infarction, and vasculitis with infarction. The most common cause of vasculitis that may lead to necrotic cavities is granulomatosis with polyangiitis. This is less frequently encountered in rheumatoid arthritis.

Cystic bronchiectasis is a severe form of end-stage bronchiectasis that may result in multiple holes in the lung. It is frequently associated with a history of recurrent infection. Predisposing factors may include agammaglobulinemia and cystic fibrosis.

Tuberculosis and histoplasmosis may also result in cystic bronchiectasis. These diagnoses should be particularly considered when the lucent spaces are primarily in the upper lobes and when there are other radiologic findings of previous granulomatous infection.

Pneumatoceles typically present with multiple thin-walled cystic spaces in the lung. They occur during the healing phases of acute necrotizing pneumonias, particularly staphylococcal pneumonia.

AIDS-related lucent lesions include abscesses, pneumatoceles, and bullae. Pneumothorax is a frequent complication.

ANSWER GUIDE

Legends for introductory figures

Fig. 24.1 Diffuse coalescent opacities with multiple, interspersed, circumscribed lucent lesions, and a spontaneous pneumothorax are the result of necrotizing staphylococcal pneumonia with abscesses and bronchopleural fistula.

Fig. 24.2 **A,** Localized area of air space consolidation with multiple, eccentric lucent spaces and left pneumothorax in this patient with an elevated white blood cell count; productive sputum is most suggestive of a necrotizing pneumonia. **B,** Computed tomography scan confirms consolidation with multiple cavities and a large pneumothorax. This is a gram-negative pneumonia, which is complicated by cavitation with bronchopleural fistula.

Fig. 24.3 Multiple, bilateral, upper lobe thin-walled cavities with surrounding reticular opacities are nearly diagnostic of a granulomatous process. Infections that lead to this response include tuberculosis, histoplasmosis, and coccidioidomycosis. This patient had coccidioidomycosis.

ANSWERS

1. e   2. d   3. c

BIBLIOGRAPHY

1. Abbott GF, Rosado-de-Christenson ML, Franks TJ, et al.: From the archives of the AFIP: pulmonary langerhans cell histiocytosis, *Radiographics* 24:821–841, 2004.
2. Abdallah PS, Mark JBD, Merigan TC: Diagnosis of cytomegalovirus pneumonia in com promised hosts, *Am J Med* 61:326–332, 1976.
3. Aberle DR, Adams AM, Berg CD, et al.: (National Lung Screening Trial Research Team). Reduced lung-cancer mortality with low-dose computed tomographic screening, *N Engl J Med* 365(5):395–409, 2011.
4. Aberle DR, Gamsu G, Lynch D: Thoracic manifestations of Wegener granulomatosis: diagnosis and course, *Radiology* 174:703–709, 1990.
5. Aberle DR, Gamsu G, Ray CS, et al.: Asbestos-related pleural and parenchymal fibrosis: detection with high-resolution CT, *Radiology* 166:729–734, 1988.
6. Aberle DR, Wiener-Kronish JP, Webb WR, et al.: Hydrostatic versus increased permeability pulmonary edema: diagnosis based on radiographic criteria in critically ill patients, *Radiology* 168:73–79, 1988.
7. Abramson S, Gilkeson RC, Goldstein JD, et al.: Benign metastasizing leiomyoma: clinical, imaging, and pathologic correlation, *AJR Am J Roentgenol* 176:1409–1413, 2001.
8. Ackerman LV, Taylor FH: Neurogenous tumors within the thorax, *Cancer* 4:669–691, 1951.
9. Adler B, Padley S, Miller RR, et al.: High-resolution CT of bronchioloalveolar carcinoma, *AJR Am J Roentgenol* 159:275–277, 1992.
10. Agrons GA, Rosado-de-Christenson ML, Kirejczyk WM, et al.: Pulmonary inflammatory pseudotumor: radiologic features, *Radiology* 206:511–518, 1998.
11. Ahn JM, Im JG, Ryoo JW, et al.: Thoracic manifestations of Behcet syndrome: radiographic and CT findings in nine patients, *Radiology* 194:199–203, 1995.
12. Akira M: Computed tomography and pathologic findings in fulminant forms of idiopathic interstitial pneumonia, *J Thorac Imaging* 14:76–84, 1999.
13. Alexander E, Clark RA, Colley DP, et al.: CT of malignant pleural mesothelioma, *AJR Am J Roentgenol* 137:287–291, 1981.
14. Altman AR: Thoracic wall invasion secondary to pulmonary aspergillosis: a complication of chronic granulomatous disease of childhood, *Am J Roentgenol* 129:140–142, 1977.
15. Amendola MA, Shirazi KK, Brooks J, et al.: Transdiaphragmatic bronchopulmonary foregut anomaly: "dumbbell" bronchogenic cyst, *AJR Am J Roentgenol* 138:1165–1167, 1982.
16. Aoki T, Nakata H, Watanabe H, et al.: Evolution of peripheral lung adenocarcinomas: CT findings correlated with histology and tumor doubling time, *AJR Am J Roentgenol* 174:763–768, 2000.
17. Arcasoy SM, Jett JR: Superior pulmonary sulcus tumors and Pancoast's syndrome, *New E J Med* 37(19):1370–1376, 1997.
18. Aronchick JM, Gefter WB: Drug-induced pulmonary disease: an update, *J Thorac Imaging* 6(1):19–29, 1991.
19. Arroliga AC, Podell DN, Matthay RA: Pulmonary manifestations of scleroderma, *J Thorac Imaging* 7(2):30–45, 1992.
20. Attili AK, Kazerooni EA, Gross BH, et al.: Smoking-related interstitial lung disease: radiologic-clinical-pathologic correlation, *Radiographics* 28:1383–1396, 2008.

21. Au V, Leung AN: Radiologic manifestations of lymphoma in the thorax, *AJR Am J Roentgenol* 168:93–98, 1997.

22. Austin JHM, Müller NL, Friedman PJ, et al.: Glossary of terms for CT of the lungs: recommendations of the nomenclature committee of the Fleischner Society, *Radiology* 200:327–331, 1996.

23. Austin JHM, Romney BM, Goldsmith LS: Missed bronchogenic carcinoma: radiographic findings in 27 patients with a potentially resectable lesion evident in retrospect, *Radiology* 182:115–122, 1992.

24. Avila NA, Dwyer AJ, Rabel A, et al.: Sporadic lymphangioleiomyomatosis and tuberous sclerosis complex with lymphangioleiomyomatosis: comparison of CT features, *Radiology* 242(1):277–285, 2006.

25. Balakrishnan J, Meziane MA, Siegelman SS, et al.: Pulmonary infarction: CT appearance with pathologic correlation, *J Comput Assist Tomogr* 13:941–945, 1989.

26. Balikian JP, Cheng TH, Costello P, et al.: Pulmonary actinomycosis, *Radiology* 128:613–616, 1978.

27. Balikian JP, Herman PG: Non-Hodgkin lymphoma of the lungs, *Radiology* 132:569–572, 1979.

28. Balikian JP, Herman PG, Godleski JJ: Serratia pneumonia, *Radiology* 137:309–311, 1980.

29. Balikian JP, Herman PG, Kopit S: Pulmonary nocardiosis, *Radiology* 126:569–573, 1978.

30. Balikian JP, Mudarris FF: Hydatid disease of the lungs, *AJR Am J Roentgenol* 122:692–707, 1974.

31. Baron RL, Stark DD, McClennan BL, et al.: Intrathoracic extension of retroperitoneal urine collections, *AJR Am J Roentgenol* 137:37–41, 1981.

32. Barry Jr WF: Infrapulmonary pleural effusion, *Radiology* 66:740–743, 1956.

33. Bartrum Jr RJ, Watnick M, Herman PG: Roentgenographic findings in pulmonary mucormycosis, *AJR Am J Roentgenol* 117:810–815, 1973.

34. Bar-Ziv J, Nogrady MB: Mediastinal neuroblastoma and ganglioneuroma, *AJR Am J Roentgenol* 125:380–390, 1975.

35. Batra P, Brown K, Hayashi K, Mori M: Rounded atelectasis, *J Thorac Imaging* 11:187–197, 1996.

36. Baumgartner WA, Mark JBD: Metastatic malignancies from distant sites to the tracheobronchial tree, *J Thorac Cardiovas Surg* 79:499–503, 1980.

37. Becklake MR: Asbestos-related diseases of the lung and other organs: their epidemiology and implications for clinical practice, *Am Rev Respir Dis* 114:187–227, 1976.

38. Ben-Menachem Y, Kuroda K, Kyger III ER, et al.: The various forms of pulmonary varices, *AJR Am J Roentgenol* 125:881–889, 1975.

39. Benson REC, Rosado-de-Christenson ML, Martinez-Jimenez S, et al.: Spectrum of pulmonary neuroendocrine proliferations and neoplasms, *Radiographics* 33:1631–1649, 2013.

40. Berg HK, Petrelli NJ, Herrera L, et al.: Endobronchial metastasis from colorectal carcinoma, *Dis Colon Rectum* 27:745–748, 1984.

41. Berger HW, Samortin TG: Miliary tuberculosis: diagnostic methods with emphasis on the chest roentgenogram, *Chest* 58:586–589, 1970.

42. Bergin CJ, Coblentz CL, Chiles C, et al.: Chronic lung diseases: specific diagnosis by using CT, *AJR Am J Roentgenol* 152:1183–1188, 1989.

43. Berne AS, Heitzman ER: The roentgenologic signs of pedunculated pleural tumors, *Am J Roentgenol* 87:892–895, 1962.

44. Bitar R, Weiser WJ, Avendaño M, et al.: Chest radigraphic manifestations of severe acute respiratory syndrome in health care workers: the Toronto experience, *AJR Am J Roentgenol* 182:45–48, 2004.

45. Blankenbaker DG: The Luftsichel sign, *Radiology* 319–320, 2008.

46. Blum J, Reed JC, Pizzo SV, et al.: Miliary aspergillosis associated with alcoholism, *AJR Am J Roentgenol* 131:707–709, 1978.

47. Borow M, Conston A, Livornese L, et al.: Mesothelioma following exposure to asbestos: a review of 72 cases, *Chest* 64:641–646, 1973.

48. Boushea DK, Sundstrom WR: The pleuropulmonary manifestations of ankylosing spondylitis, *Semin Arthritis Rheum* 18:277–281, 1989.

49. Bragg DG, Chor PJ, Murray KA, et al.: Lymphoproliferative disorders of the lung: histopathology, clinical manifestations, and imaging features, *AJR Am J Roentgenol* 163:273–281, 1994.

50. Bragg DG, Janis B: The roentgenographic manifestations of pulmonary opportunistic infections, *AJR Am J Roentgenol* 117:798–809, 1973.

51. Brereton HD, Johnson RE: Calcification in mediastinal lymph nodes after radiation therapy of Hodgkin's disease, *Radiology* 112:705–707, 1974.

52. Brettner A, Heitzman R, Woodin WG: Pulmonary complications of drug therapy, *Radiology* 96:3138, 1970.

53. Bryk D: Infrapulmonary effusion: effect of expiration on the pseudodiaphragmatic contour, *Radiology* 120:30–36, 1976.

54. Buckner CB, Walker CW: Radiologic manifestations of adult tuberculosis, *J Thorac Imaging* 5:28–37, 1990.

55. Buckner CB, Walker CW, Purnell GL: Pulmonary embolism: chest radiographic abnormalities, *J Thorac Imaging* 4:23–27, 1989.

56. Buff SJ, McLelland R, Gallis HA, et al.: Candida albicans pneumonia: radiographic appearance, *AJR Am J Roentgenol* 138:645–648, 1982.

57. Burdon JGW, Sinclair RA, Henderson MM: Small cell carcinoma of the lung, *Chest* 76:302–304, 1979.

58. Buschman DL, Gamsu G, Waldron Jr JA, et al.: Chronic hypersensitivity pneumonitis: use of CT in diagnosis, *AJR Am J Roentgenol* 159:957–960, 1992.

59. Capobianco J, Grimberg A, Thompson BM, et al.: Thoracic manifestations of collagen vascular diseases, *Radiographics* 32:33–50, 2012.

60. Cardenose G, Deluca SA: Rounded atelectasis, *Am Fam Physician* 39:135–136, 1989.

61. Carey LS, Ellis Jr FH, Good CA, et al.: Neurogenic tumors of the mediastinum: a clinicopathologic study, *AJR Am J Roentgenol* 84:189–205, 1960.

62. Carilli AD, Ramanamurty MV, Chang Y, et al.: Noncardiogenic pulmonary edema following blood transfusion, *Chest* 74:310–312, 1978.

63. Carter BW, Benveniste MF, Betancourt SL, et al.: Imaging evaluation of malignant chest wall neoplasms, *Radiographics* 36:1285–1306, 2016.

64. Carvalho PM, Carr DH: Computed tomography of folded lung, *Clin Radiol* 41:86–91, 1990.

65. Castañer E, Gallardo X, Ballesteros E, et al.: CT diagnosis of chronic pulmonary thromboembolism, *Radiographics* 29:31–53, 2009.

66. Castañer E, Gallardo X, Rimola J, et al.: Congenital and acquired pulmonary artery anomalies in the adult: radiologic overview, *Radiographics* 26:349–371, 2006.

67. Castellino RA, Blank N: Adenopathy of the cardiophrenic angle (diaphragmatic) lymph nodes, *AJR Am J Roentgenol* 114:509–515, 1972.

68. Cayea PD, Rubin E, Teixidor HS: Atypical pulmonary malaria, *AJR Am J Roentgenol* 137:51–55, 1981.

69. Chaffey MH, Klein JS, Gamsu G, et al.: Radiographic distribution of pneumocystis carinii pneumonia in patients with AIDS treated with prophylactic inhaled pentamidine, *Radiology* 175:715–719, 1990.

70. Chan MSM, Chan IYF, Fung KH, et al.: High-resolution CT findings in patients with severe acute respiratory syndrome: a pattern-based approach, *AJR Am J Roentgenol* 182:49–56, 2004.

71. Chan T, Palevsky HI, Miller WT: Pulmonary hypertension complicating portal hypertension: findings on chest radiographs, *AJR Am J Roentgenol* 151:909–914, 1988.

72. Chang CH: The normal roentgenographic measurement of the right descending pulmonary artery in 1,085 cases, *AJR Am J Roentgenol* 87:929–935, 1962.

73. Chang CH, Zinn TW: Roentgen recognition of enlarged hilar lymph nodes: an anatomical review, *Radiology* 120:291–296, 1976.

74. Charan NB, Myers CG, Lakshminarayan S, et al.: Pulmonary injuries associated with acute sulfur dioxide inhalation, *Am Rev Respir Dis* 119:555–560, 1979.

75. Chen JTT: *Essentials of cardiac roentgenology*, Boston, 1987, Little, Brown and Company.
76. Chen JTT, Dahmash NS, Ravin CE, et al.: Metastatic melanoma to the thorax: report of 130 patients, *AJR Am J Roentgenol* 137:293–298, 1981.
77. Chinn DH, Gamsu G, Webb WR, et al.: Calcified pulmonary nodules in chronic renal failure, *AJR Am J Roentgenol* 137:402–405, 1981.
78. Choi YW, Munden RF, Erasmus JJ, et al.: Effects of radiation therapy on the lung: radiologic appearances and differential diagnosis, *Radiographics* 24:985–998, 2004.
79. Chong S, Lee KS, Chung MJ, et al.: Neuroendocrine tumors of the lung: clinical, pathologic, and imaging findings, *Radiographics* 26:41–58, 2006.
80. Chong S, Lee KS, Chung MJ, et al.: Pneumoconiosis: comparison of imaging and pathologic findings, *Radiographics* 26:59–77, 2006.
81. Chow C, Templeton PA, White CS: Lung cysts associated with pneumocystis carinii pneumonia: radiographic characteristics, natural history, and complications, *AJR Am J Roentgenol* 161:527–531, 1993.
82. Choyke PL, Sostman HD, Curtis AM, et al.: Adult-onset pulmonary tuberculosis, *Radiology* 148:357–362, 1983.
83. Christensen EE, Dietz GW, Murry RC, et al.: Effect of kilovoltage on detectability of pulmonary nodules in a chest phantom, *AJR Am J Roentgenol* 128:789–793, 1977.
84. Cimmino CV: Contacts of the left lung with the mediastinum, *AJR Am J Roentgenol* 124:412–416, 1975.
85. Citro LA, Gordon ME, Miller WT: Eosinophilic lung disease (or how to slice P.I.E.), *AJR Am J Roentgenol* 117:787–797, 1973.
86. Colby TV, Swensen SJ: Anatomic distribution and histopathologic patterns in diffuse lung disease: correlation with HRCT, *J Thorac Imaging* 11:1–26, 1996.
87. Collins J, Stern EJ: *Chest radiology: the essentials*, Philadelphia, 1999, Lippincott Williams and Wilkins.
88. Collins JD, Pagani JJ: Extrathoracic musculature mimicking pleural lesions, *Radiology* 129:21–22, 1978.
89. Comstock C, Wolson AH: Roentgenology of sporotrichosis, *AJR Am J Roentgenol* 125:651–655, 1975.
90. Conant EF, Fox KR, Miller WT: Pulmonary edema as a complication of interleukin-2 therapy, *AJR Am J Roentgenol* 152:749–752, 1989.
91. Conant EF, Wechsler RJ: Actinomycosis and nocardiosis of the lung, *J Thorac Imaging* 7(4):75–84, 1992.
92. Conces Jr DJ: Bacterial pneumonia in immunocompromised patients, *J Thorac Imaging* 13:261–270, 1998.
93. Conces Jr DJ: Endemic fungal pneumonia in immunocompromised patients, *J Thorac Imaging* 14:1–8, 1999.
94. Conces Jr DJ: Noninfectious lung disease in immunocompromised patients, *J Thorac Imaging* 14:9–24, 1999.
95. Conces Jr DJ: Pulmonary infections in immunocompromised patients who do not have acquired immunodeficiency syndrome: a systematic approach, *J Thorac Imaging* 13:234–246, 1998.
96. Conces Jr DJ, Kraft JL, Vix VA, et al.: Apical pneumocystis carinii pneumonia after inhaled pentamidine prophylaxis, *AJR Am J Roentgenol* 152:1193–1194, 1989.
97. Connell Jr JV, Muhm JR: Radiographic manifestations of pulmonary histoplasmosis: a 10–year review, *Radiology* 121:281–285, 1976.
98. Connolly Jr JE, McAdams HP, Erasmus JJ, Rosado-de-Christenson ML: Opportunistic fungal pneumonia, *J Thorac Imaging* 14:51–62, 1999.
99. Copley SJ, Lee YC, Hansell DM, et al.: Asbestos-induced and smoking-related disease: apportioning pulmonary function deficit by using thin-section CT, *Radiology* 242:258–266, 2007.
100. Copley SJ, Wells AU, Rubens MB, et al.: Asbestosis and idiopathic pulmonary fibrosis: comparison of thin-section CT features, *Radiology* 229:731–736, 2003.
101. Coppage L, Shaw C, Curtis AM: Metastatic disease to the chest in patients with extrathoracic malignancy, *J Thorac Imaging* 2:24–37, 1987.

102. Creasy JD, Chiles C, Routh WD, Dyer RB: Overview of traumatic injury of the thoracic aorta, *Radiographics* 17:27–45, 1997.

103. Criado E, Sanchez M, Ramirez J: Pulmonary sarcoidosis: typical and atypical manifestations at high-resolution CT with pathologic correlation (ATS/ERS/WASOG), *Radiographics* 30:1567–1586, 2010.

104. Crystal RG, Fulmer JD, Roberts WC, et al.: Idiopathic pulmonary fibrosis, *Ann Intern Med* 85:769–788, 1976.

105. Cushing H, Wolbach SB: The transformation of a malignant paravertebral sympathicoblastoma into a benign ganglioneuroma, *Am J Pathol* 3:203–216, 1927.

106. Daley CL: Pyogenic bacterial pneumonia in the acquired immunodeficiency syndrome, *J Thorac Imaging* 6(4):36–42, 1991.

107. Daly BD, Leung SF, Cheung H, et al.: Thoracic metastases from carcinoma of the nasopharynx: high frequency of hilar and mediastinal lymphadenopathy, *AJR Am J Roentgenol* 160:241–244, 1993.

108. Darling ST: A protozoan general infection producing pseudotubercles in the lungs and focal necroses in the liver, spleen and lymph nodes, *JAMA* 46:1283–1285, 1906.

109. Dashiell TG, Payne WS, Hepper NGG, et al.: Desmoid tumors of the chest wall, *Chest* 74:157–162, 1978.

110. Davies SF, Sarosi GA: Acute cavitary histoplasmosis, *Chest* 73:103–105, 1978.

111. Davis SD, Henschke CI, Chamides BK, et al.: Intrathoracic kaposi sarcoma in AIDS patients: radiographic-pathologic correlation, *Radiology* 163:495–500, 1987.

112. Davis SD, Yankelevitz MD, Wand A, et al.: Juxtaphrenic peak in upper and middle lobe volume loss: assessment with CT, *Radiology* 198(1):143–149, 1996.

113. DeBeer RA, Garcia RL, Alexander SC: Endobronchial metastasis from cancer of the breast, *Chest* 73:94–96, 1978.

114. DeLorenzo LJ, Huang CT, Maguire GP, et al.: Roentgenographic patterns of pneumocystis carinii pneumonia in 104 patients with AIDS, *Chest* 91:323–327, 1987.

115. Dennis LN, Rogers LF: Superior mediastinal widening from spine fractures mimicking aortic rupture on chest radiographs, *AJR Am J Roentgenol* 152:27–30, 1989.

116. Desser TS, Stark P: Pictorial essay: solitary fibrous tumor of the pleura, *J Thorac Imaging* 13:27–35, 1998.

117. Dietrich PA, Johnson RD, Fairbank JT, et al.: The chest radiograph in Legionnaires' disease, *Radiology* 127:577–582, 1978.

118. Dodd III GD, Boyle JJ: Excavating pulmonary metastases, *AJR Am J Roentgenol* 85:277–293, 1961.

119. Dodd III GD, Ledesma-Medina JL, Baron RL, et al.: Posttransplant lymphoproliferative disorder: intrathoracic manifestations, *Radiology* 184:65–69, 1992.

120. Donlan Jr CJ, Reid JW: Endobronchial Hodgkin's disease, *JAMA* 239:1061–1062, 1978.

121. Doppman JL, Skarulis MC, Chen CC, et al.: Parathyroid adenomas in the aorticopulmonary window, *Radiology* 201:456–462, 1996.

122. Doyle TC, Lawler GA: CT features of rounded atelectasis of the lung, *AJR Am J Roentgenol* 143:225–228, 1984.

123. Dyke PC, Mulkey DA: Maturation of ganglioneuroblastoma to ganglioneuroma, *Cancer* 20:1343–1349, 1967.

124. Dynes MC, White EM, Fry WA, et al.: Imaging manifestations of pleural tumors, *Radiographics* 12:1191–1201, 1992.

125. Earls JP, Cerva Jr D, Berman E, et al.: Inhalational Anthrax after bioterrorism exposure: spectrum of imaging findings in two surviving patients, *Radiology* 222:305–312, 2001.

126. Edinburgh KJ, Jasmer RM, Huang L, et al.: Multiple pulmonary nodules in AIDS: usefulness of CT in distinguishing among potential causes, *Radiology* 214:427–432, 2000.

127. Eklof O, Gooding CA: Intrathoracic neuroblastoma, *AJR Am J Roentgenol* 100:202–207, 1967.

128. Elicker BM, Jones KD, Henry TS, et al.: Multidisciplinary approach to hypersensitivity pneumonitis, *J Thorac Imaging* 31:92–103, 2016.

129. Ellis AR, Mayers DL, Martone WJ, et al.: Rapidly expanding pulmonary nodule caused by Pittsburgh pneumonia agent, *JAMA* 245:1558–1559, 1981.

130. Ellis K: The adult respiratory distress syndrome (ARDS), *Comtemp Diag Radiol* 1:1–6, 1978.

131. Ellis K, Wolff M: Mesotheliomas and secondary tumors of the pleura, *Semin Roentgenol* 12:303–311, 1977.

132. Ellis R: Incomplete border sign of extrapleural masses, *JAMA* 237:2748, 1977.

133. Engeler CE, Tashjian JH, Trenkner SW, et al.: Ground-glass opacity of the lung paenchyma: a guide to analysis with high-resolution CT, *AJR Am J Roentgenol* 160:249–251, 1993.

134. Epstein DM, Gefter WB, Miller WT: Lobar bronchioloalveolar cell carcinoma, *AJR Am J Roentgenol* 139:463–468, 1982.

135. Erasmus JJ, Connolly JE, McAdams HP, Roggli VL: Solitary pulmonary nodules: part I: morphologic evaluation for differentiation of benign and malignant lesions, *Radiographics* 20:43–58, 2000.

136. Erasmus JJ, McAdams HP, Connolly JE: Solitary pulmonary nodules: part II: evaluation of the indeterminate nodule, *Radiographics* 20:59–66, 2000.

137. Faer MJ, Burnan RE, Beck CL: Transmural thoracic lipoma: demonstration by computed tomography, *AJR Am J Roentgenol* 130:161–163, 1978.

138. Fagan CJ, Swischuk LE: Dumbbell neuroblastoma or ganglioneuroblastoma of the spinal canal, *AJR Am J Roentgenol* 120:453–460, 1974.

139. Fagan CJ, Swischuk LE: Traumatic lung and paramediastinal pneumatoceles, *Radiology* 120:11–18, 1976.

140. Fairbank JT, Mamourian AC, Dietrich PA, et al.: The chest radiograph in Legionnaires' disease, *Radiology* 147:33–34, 1983.

141. Fairbank JT, Tampas JP, Longstreth G: Superior vena cava obstruction in histoplasmosis, *AJR Am J Roentgenol* 115:488–494, 1972.

142. Fang W, Lacey W, Kumar N: Imaging manifestations of blastomycosis: a pulmonary infection with potential dissemination, *Radiographics* 27:641–655, 2007.

143. Fartoukh M, Humbert M, Carpron F, et al.: Severe pulmonary hypertension in histiocytosis X, *Am J Respir Crit Care Med* 161:216–223, 2000.

144. Feigin DS: Misconceptions regarding the pathogenicity of silicas and silicates, *J Thorac Imaging* 4:68–80, 1989.

145. Feigin DS: Nocardiosis of the lung: chest radiographic findings in 21 cases, *Radiology* 159:9–14, 1986.

146. Feigin DS: Vasculitis in the lung, *J Thorac Imaging* 3:33–48, 1988.

147. Feigin DS, Eggleston JC, Siegelman SS: The multiple roentgen manifestations of sclerosing mediastinitis, *Johns Hopkins Med J* 144:1–8, 1979.

148. Feigin DS, Fenoglio JJ, McAllister HA, et al.: Pericardial cysts: a radiologic-pathologic correlation and review, *Radiology* 125:15–20, 1977.

149. Felker RE, Tonkin ILD: Imaging of pulmonary sequestration, *AJR Am J Roentgenol* 154:241–249, 1990.

150. Felson B: *Chest Roentgenology*, Philadelphia, 1973, WB Saunders.

151. Felson B: The extrapleural space, *Semin Roentgenol* 12:327–333, 1977.

152. Felson B: Lung torsion: radiographic findings in nine cases, *Radiology* 162:631–638, 1987.

153. Ferguson DD, Westcott JL: Lipoma of the diaphragm, *Radiology* 118:527–528, 1976.

154. Fernández Pérez ER, Swigris JJ, Forssén AV, et al.: Identifying an inciting antigen is associated with improved survival in patients with chronic hypersensitivity pneumonitis, *Chest* 144:1644–1651, 2013.

155. Ferris RA, White AF: The round nipple shadow, *Radiology* 121:293–294, 1976.

156. Feuerstein IM, Archer A, Pluda JM, et al.: Thin-walled cavities, cysts, and pneumothorax in Pneumocystis carinii pneumonia: further observations with histopathologic correlation, *Radiology* 174:697–702, 1990.

157. Fink IJ, Kurtz DW, Cazenave L, et al.: Malignant thoracopulmonary small-cell ("Askin") tumor, *AJR Am J Roentgenol* 145:517–520, 1985.

158. Firooznia H, Pudlowski R, Golimbu C, et al.: Diffuse interstitial calcification of the lungs in chronic renal failure mimicking pulmonary edema, *AJR Am J Roengenol* 129:1103–1105, 1977.

159. Fischman RA, Marschall KE, Kislak JW, et al.: Adult respiratory distress syndrome caused by Mycoplasma pneumoniae, *Chest* 74:471–473, 1978.

160. Fisher ER, Godwin JD: Extrapleural fat collections: pseudotumors and other confusing manifestations, *AJR Am J Roentgenol* 161:47–52, 1993.

161. Fisher JK: Skin fold versus pneumothorax, *AJR Am J Roentgenol* 130:791–792, 1978.

162. Fleischner FG: The visible bronchial tree: a roentgen sign in pneumonic and other pulmonary consolidations, *Radiology* 50:184–189, 1948.

163. Fleischner FG, Berenberg AL: Idiopathic pulmonary hemosiderosis, *Radiology* 62:522–526, 1954.

164. Flynn MW, Felson B: The roentgen manifestations of thoracic actinomycosis, *AJR Am J Roentgenol* 110:707–716, 1970.

165. Forrest JV, Shackelford GD, Bramson RT, et al.: Acute mediastinal widening, *AJR Am J Roentgenol* 117:881–885, 1973.

166. Forrest ME, Skerker LB, Nemiroff MJ: Hard metal pneumoconiosis: another cause of diffuse interstitial fibrosis, *Radiology* 128:609–612, 1978.

167. Fortier M, Mayo JR, Swensen SJ, et al.: MR imaging of chest wall lesions, *Radiographics* 14:597–606, 1994.

168. Fortman BJ, Kuszyk BS, Urban BA, Fishman EK: Neurofibromatosis type 1: a diagnostic mimicker at CT, *Radiographics* 21:601–612, 2001.

169. Foster Jr WL, Gimenez EI, Roubidoux MA, et al.: The emphysemas: radiologic-pathologic correlations, *Radiographics* 13:311–328, 1993.

170. Foy HM, Loop J, Clarke ER, et al.: Radiographic study of Mycoplasma pneumoniae pneumonia, *Am Rev Respir Dis* 108:469–474, 1973.

171. Franquet T, Erasmus JJ, Giménez A, et al.: The retrotracheal space: normal anatomic and pathologic appearances, *Radiographics* S231–S246, 2002.

172. Franquet T, Müller NL, Giménez A, et al.: Spectrum of pulmonary aspergillosis: histologic, clinical, and radiologic findings, *Radiographics* 21:825–837, 2001.

173. Franquet T, Müller NL, Lee KS, et al.: Pulmonary candidiasis after hematopoietic stem cell transplantation: thin-section CT findings, *Radiology* 236:332–337, 2005.

174. Fraser RG: The radiologist and obstructive airway disease, *AJR Am J Roentgenol* 120:737–775, 1974.

175. Fraser RS, Müller NL, Colman N, Pare PD: *Fraser and Páre's diagnosis of diseases of the chest*, ed 4, Philadelphia, 1999, WB Saunders.

176. Frazier AA, Franks TJ, Cooke EO, et al.: From the archives of the AFIP: pulmonary alveolar proteinosis, *Radiographics* 28:883–899, 2008.

177. Frazier AA, Rosado-de-Christenson ML, Galvin JR, Fleming MV: Pulmonary angiitis and granulomatosis: radiologic-pathologic correlation, *Radiographics* 18:687–710, 1998.

178. Freundlich IM, McGavran MH: Abnormalities of the thymus, *J Thorac Imaging* 11:58–65, 1996.

179. Friedman AC, Fiel SB, Fisher MS, et al.: Asbestos-related pleural disease and asbestosis: a comparison of CT and chest radiology, *AJR Am J Roentgenol* 150:269–275, 1988.

180. Fulcher AS, Proto AV, Jolles H: Cystic teratoma of the mediastinum: demonstration of fat/fluid level, *Amer J Roentgenol* 154:259–260, 1990.

181. Gaensler EA, Carrington CB: Peripheral opacities in chronic eosinophilic pneumonia: the photographic negative of pulmonary edema, *AJR Am J Roentgenol* 128:1–13, 1977.

182. Gaensler EA, Carrington CB, Contu RE, et al.: Pathological, physiological, and radiological correlations in the pneumoconioses, *Ann NY Acad Sci* 200:574–607, 1972.

183. Gaerte SC, Meyer CA, Winer-Muram HT, et al.: Fat-containing lesions of the chest, *Radiographics* 22:S61–S78, 2002.

184. Gamsu G, Aberle DR, Lynch D: Computed tomography in the diagnosis of asbestos-related thoracic disease, *J Thorac Imaging* 4:61–67, 1989.
185. Garg K, Lynch DA, Newell JD, et al.: Proliferative and constrictive bronchiolitis: classification and radiologic features, *AJR Am J Roentgenol* 162:803–808, 1994.
186. Gavant ML, Flick P, Menke P, Gold RE: CT aortography of thoracic aortic rupture, *AJR Am J Roentgenol* 166:955–961, 1996.
187. Genereux GP: The Fleischner lecture: computed tomography of diffuse pulmonary disease, *J Thorac Imaging* 4:50–87, 1989.
188. Gierada DS, Glazer HS, Slone RM: Pseudomass due to atelectasis in patients with severe bullous emphysema, *AJR Am J Roentgenol* 168:85–92, 1997.
189. Giménez A, Franquet T, Erasmus JJ, et al.: Thoracic complications of esophageal disorders, *Radiographics* S247–S258, 2002.
190. Giménez A, Franquet T, Prats R, et al.: Unusual primary lung tumors: a radiologic-pathologic overview, *Radiographics* 22:601–619, 2002.
191. Gladish GW, Sabloff BM, Munden RF, et al.: Primary thoracic sarcomas, *Radiographics* 22:621–637, 2002.
192. Glazer HS, Anderson DJ, Sagel SS: Bronchial impaction in lobar collapse: CT demonstration and pathologic correlation, *AJR Am J Roentgenol* 153:485–488, 1989.
193. Glazer HS, Duncan-Meyer J, Aronberg DJ, et al.: Pleural and chest wall invasion in bronchogenic carcinoma: CT evaluation, *Radiology* 157:191–194, 1985.
194. Glazer HS, Siegel MJ, Sagal SS: Low-attenuation mediastinal masses on CT, *AJR Am J Roentgenol* 152:1173–1177, 1989.
195. Glazer HS, Wick MR, Anderson DJ, et al.: CT of fatty thoracic masses, *AJR Am J Roentgenol* 159:1181–1187, 1992.
196. Godwin JD, Ravin CE, Roggli VL: Fatal Pneumocystis pneumonia, cryptococcosis, and Kaposi sarcoma in a homosexual man, *AJR Am J Roentgenol* 138:580–581, 1982.
197. Good CA, Wilson TW: The solitary circumscribed pulmonary nodule, *JAMA* 166:210–215, 1958.
198. Goodman PC: Pulmonary tuberculosis in patients with acquired immunodeficiency syndrome, *J Thorac Imaging* 5:38–45, 1990.
199. Goodwin Jr RA, Snell Jr JR: The enlarging histoplasmoma, *Am Rev Respir Dis* 100:1–12, 1969.
200. Gordonson J, Birnbaum W, Jacobson G, et al.: Pulmonary cryptococcosis, *Radiology* 112:557–561, 1974.
201. Gotway MB, Marder SR, Hanks DK, et al.: Thoracic complications of illicit drug use: an organ system approach, *Radiographics* S119–S135, 2002.
202. Gray JE, Taylor KW, Hobbs BB: Detection accuracy in chest radiography, *AJR Am J Roentgenol* 131:247–253, 1978.
203. Greenberg SD, Frager D, Suster B, et al.: Active pulmonary tuberculosis in patients with AIDS: spectrum of radiographic findings (including a normal appearance), *Radiology* 193:115–119, 1994.
204. Greene R: Lung alterations in thoracic trauma, *J Thorac Imaging* 2:1–11, 1987.
205. Greganti MA, Flowers Jr WM: Acute pulmonary edema after the intravenous administration of contrast media, *Radiology* 132:583–585, 1979.
206. Gronner AT, Ominsky SH: Plain film radiography of the chest: findings that simulate pulmonary disease, *AJR Am J Roentgenol* 163:1343–1348, 1994.
207. Groskin SA, Panicek DM, Ewing DK, et al.: Bacterial lung abscess: a review of the radiographic and clinical features of 50 cases, *J Thorac Imaging* 6(3):62–67, 1991.
208. Grossman CB, Bragg DG, Armstrong D: Roentgen manifestations of pulmonary nocardiosis, *Radiology* 96:325–330, 1970.
209. Gruden JF, Huang L, Webb WR: AIDS-related Kaposi sarcoma of the lung: radiographic findings and staging system with bronchoscopic correlation, *Radiology* 195:545–552, 1995.
210. Guest Jr JL, Anderson JN: Osteomyelitis involving adjacent ribs, *JAMA* 239:133, 1978.
211. Gurney JW: Missed lung cancer at CT: imaging findings in nine patients, *Radiology* 199:117–122, 1996.

212. Gurney JW, Bates FT: Pulmonary cystic disease: comparison of Pneumocystis carinii pneumatoceles and bullous emphysema due to intravenous drug abuse, *Radiology* 173:27–31, 1989.

213. Gurney JW, Goodman LR: Pulmonary edema localized in the right upper lobe accompanying mitral regurgitation, *Radiology* 171:397–399, 1989.

214. Gurney JW, Schroeder BA: Upper lobe lung disease: physiologic correlates, *Radiology* 167:359–366, 1988.

215. Hadlock FP, Park SK, Awe RJ, et al.: Unusual radiographic findings in adult pulmonary tuberculosis, *AJR Am J Roentgenol* 134:1015–1018, 1980.

216. Halvorsen RA, Duncan JD, Merten DF: Pulmonary blastomycosis: radiologic manifestations, *Radiology* 150:1–5, 1984.

217. Hamman L, Rich A: Acute diffuse interstitial fibrosis of the lungs, *Johns Hopkins Med J* 74:177–212, 1944.

218. Hampton AO, Castleman B: Correlation of postmortem chest teleroentgenograms with autopsy findings: with special reference to pulmonary embolism and infarction, *AJR Am J Roentgenol* 43:305–326, 1940.

219. Han SS, Wills JS, Allen OS: Pulmonary blastoma: case report and literature review, *AJR Am J Roentgenol* 127:1048–1049, 1976.

220. Hanna JW, Reed JC, Choplin RH: Pleural infections: a clinical-radiologic review, *J Thorac Imaging* 6(3):68–79, 1991.

221. Hansell DM, Bankier AA, MacMahon H, et al.: Fleischner Society: glossary of terms for thoracic imaging, *Radiology* 246(3):697–722, 2008.

222. Haque AK: Pathology of carcinoma of lung: an update on current concepts, *J Thorac Imaging* 7(1):9–20, 1991.

223. Haramati LB, Jenny-Avital ER: Approach to the diagnosis of pulmonary disease in patients infected with the human immunodeficiency virus, *J Thorac Imaging* 13:247–260, 1998.

224. Haramati LB, Schulman LL, Austin JHM: Lung nodules and masses after cardiac transplantation, *Radiology* 188:491–497, 1993.

225. Harisinghani MG, McLoud TC, Shepard JAO, et al.: Tuberculosis from head to toe, *Radiographics* 20:449–470, 2000.

226. Harris VJ, Brown R: Pneumatoceles as a complication of chemical pneumonia after hydrocarbon ingestion, *AJR Am J Roentgenol* 125:531–537, 1975.

227. Hartman TE, Jensen E, Tazelaar HD, et al.: CT findings of granulomatous pneumonitis secondary to mycobacterium avium-intracellulare inhalation: hot tub lung, *AJR Am J Roentgenol* 191:1032–1039, 2008.

228. Hartman TE, Müller NL, Primack SL, et al.: Metastatic pulmonary calcification in patients with hypercalcemia: findings on chest radiographs and CT scans, *AJR Am J Roentgenol* 162:799–802, 1994.

229. Hatcher Jr CR, Sehdeva J, Waters III WC, et al.: Primary pulmonary cryptococcosis, *J Thorac Cardiovasc Surg* 61:39–49, 1971.

230. Hayashi K, Aziz A, Ashizawa K, et al.: Radiographic and CT appearances of the major fissures, *Radiographics* 21:861–874, 2001.

231. Heater K, Revzani L, Rubin JM: CT evaluation of empyema in the postpneumonectomy space, *AJR Am J Roentgenol* 145:39–40, 1985.

232. Heelan RJ, Hehinger BJ, Melamed MR, et al.: Non–small-cell lung cancer: results of the New York screening program, *Radiology* 151:289–293, 1984.

233. Heithoff KB, Sane SM, Williams HJ, et al.: Bronchopulmonary foregut malformations, *AJR Am J Roentgenol* 126:46–55, 1976.

234. Heitzman ER: Bronchogenic carcinoma: radiologic-pathologic correlations, *Semin Roentgenol* 12:165–174, 1977.

235. Heitzman ER: *The lung: radiologic-pathologic correlations*, ed 2, St. Louis, 1984, Mosby.

236. Heitzman ER: Lymphadenopathy related to anticonvulsant therapy: roentgen findings simulating lymphoma, *Radiology* 89:311–312, 1967.

237. Heitzman ER: *The Mediastinum: Radiologic Correlations with Anatomy and Pathology*, ed 2, Berlin, 1988, Springer-Verlag.

238. Heitzman ER, Markarian B, Berger I, et al.: The secondary pulmonary lobule: a practical concept for interpretation of chest radiographs, *Radiology* 93:513–519, 1969.

239. Heller RM, Janower ML, Weber AL: The radiological manifestations of malignant pleural mesothelioma, *AJR Am J Roentgenol* 108:53–59, 1970.

240. Henry DA, Kiser PE, Scheer CE, et al.: Multiple imaging evaluation of sarcoidosis, *Radiographics* 6:75–95, 1986.

241. Henry TS, Little BP, Veeraraghavan S, et al.: The spectrum of interstitial lung disease in connective tissue disease, *J Thorac Imaging* 31:65–77, 2016.

242. Henschke CI, McCauley DI, Yankelevitz DF, et al.: Early lung cancer action project: overall design and findings from baseline screening, *Lancet* 354:99–105, 1999.

243. Henschke CI, Yankelevitz DF, Naidich DP, et al.: CT screening for lung cancer: suspiciousness of nodules according to size on baseline scans, *Radiology* 231:164–168, 2004.

244. Heo J, Choi YW, Jeon SC, et al.: Pulmonary tuberculosis: another disease showing clusters of small nodules, *AJR Am J Roentgenol* 184:639–642, 2005.

245. Hillerdal G, Nou E: Large infiltrate with air bronchogram in a symptomless woman, *Chest* 82:481–482, 1982.

246. Himmelfarb E, Wells S, Rabinowitz JG: The radiologic spectrum of cardiopulmonary amyloidosis, *Chest* 72:327–332, 1977.

247. Hirakata K, Nakata H, Haratake J: Appearance of pulmonary metastases on high-resolution CT scans: comparison with histopathologic findings from autopsy specimens, *AJR Am J Roentgenol* 161:37–43, 1993.

248. Hoagland RJ: The clinical manifestations of infectious mononucleosis: a report of two hundred cases, *Am J Med Sci* 240:21–29, 1960.

249. Holbert JM, Costello P, Li W, et al.: CT features of pulmonary alveolar proteinosis, *AJR Am J Roentgenol* 176:1287–1294, 2001.

250. Holt S, Ryan WF, Epstein EJ: Severe mycoplasma pneumonia, *Thorax* 32:112–115, 1977.

251. Homer MJ, Wechsler RJ, Carter BL: Mediastinal lipomatosis: CT confirmation of a normal variant, *Radiology* 128:657–661, 1978.

252. Houk VN, Moser KR: Pulmonary cryptococcosis, *Ann Intern Med* 63:583–596, 1965.

253. Hourihane JB, Owens AP: A pitfall in the diagnosis of lobar collapse, *Clin Radiol* 40:468–470, 1989.

254. Hultgren HN, Marticorena EA: High altitude pulmonary edema, *Chest* 74:372–376, 1978.

255. Hung Jr KK, Enquist RW, Bowel TE: Multiple pulmonary nodules with central cavitation, *Chest* 69:529–530, 1976.

256. Hutchinson WB, Friedenberg MJ: Intrathoracic mesothelioma, *AJR Am J Roentgenol* 80:937–945, 1963.

257. Ichikado K, Johkoh T, Ikezoe J, et al.: Acute interstitial pneumonia: high-resolution CT findings correlated with pathology, *AJR Am J Roentgenol* 168:333–338, 1997.

258. Ikezoe J, Godwin JD, Hunt KJ, et al.: Pulmonary lymphangitic carcinomatosis: chronicity of radiographic findings in long-term survivors, *AJR Am J Roentgenol* 165:49–52, 1995.

259. Ikezoe J, Johkoh T, Kohno N, et al.: High-resolution CT findings of lung disease in patients with polymyositis and dermatomyositis, *J Thorac Imaging* 11:250–259, 1996.

260. Im JG, Kong Y, Shin YM, et al.: Pulmonary paragonimiasis: clinical and experimental studies, *Radiographics* 13:575–586, 1993.

261. Im JG, Song KS, Kang HS, et al.: Mediastinal tuberculous lymphadenitis: CT manifestations, *Radiology* 164:115–119, 1987.

262. Im JG, Whang HY, Kim WS, et al.: Pleuropulmonary paragonimiasis: radiologic findings in 71 patients, *AJR Am J Roentgenol* 159:39–43, 1992.

263. Iochum S, Ludig T, Walter F, et al.: Imaging of diaphragmatic injury: a diagnostic challenge? *Radiographics* S103–S118, 2002. 22 Spec No.

264. Israel RH: Mycosis fungoides with rapidly progressive pulmonary infiltration, *Radiology* 125:10, 1977.

265. Itzchak Y, Rosenthal T, Adar R, et al.: Dissecting aneurysm of thoracic aorta: reappraisal of radiologic diagnosis, *AJR Am J Roentgenol* 125:559–570, 1975.

266. Jacoby CG, Mindell HJ: Lobar consolidation in pulmonary embolism, *Radiology* 118:287–290, 1976.

267. Jagannath AS, Sos TA, Lockhart SH, et al.: Aortic dissection: a statistical analysis of the usefulness of plain chest radiographic findings, *AJR Am J Roentgenol* 147:1123–1126, 1986.

268. Jang HJ, Lee KS, Kwon OJ, et al.: Bronchioloalveolar carcinoma: focal area of ground-glass attenuation at thin-section CT as an early sign, *Radiology* 199:485–488, 1996.

269. Janower ML, Blennerhassett JB: Lymphangitic spread of metastatic cancer to the lung, *Radiology* 101:267–273, 1971.

270. Jariwalla AG, Al-Nasiri NK: Splenosis pleurae, *Thorax* 34:123–124, 1979.

271. Jaskolka J, Wu L, Chan RP, et al.: Imaging hereditary hemorrhagic telangiectasia, *AJR Am J Roentgenol* 183:307–314, 2004.

272. Jasmer RM, McCowin MJ, Webb WR: Miliary lung disease after intravesical bacillus Calmette-Guerin immunotherapy, *Radiology* 201:43–44, 1996.

273. Jay SJ, Johanson Jr WG, Pierce AK: The radiographic resolution of Streptococcus pneumoniae pneumonia, *N Engl J Med* 293:798–801, 1975.

274. Jeong YJ, Kim K-L, Seo IJ, et al.: Eosinophilic lung diseases: a clinical, radiologic, and pathologic overview, *Radiographics* 27:617–639, 2007.

275. Jeung MY, Gasser B, Gangi A, et al.: Bronchial carcinoid tumors of the thorax: spectrum of radiologic findings, *Radiographics* 22:351–365, 2002.

276. Jeung MY, Gasser B, Gangi A, et al.: Imaging of cystic masses of the mediastinum, *Radiographics* 22:S79–S93, 2002.

277. Joffe N: The adult respiratory distress syndrome, *AJR Am J Roentgenol* 122:719–732, 1974.

278. Joffe N: Roentgenologic findings in post-shock and postoperative pulmonary insufficiency, *Radiology* 94:369–375, 1970.

279. Johkoh T, Ikezoe J, Tomiyama N, et al.: CT findings in lymphangitic carcinomatosis of the lung: correlation with histologic findings and pulmonary function tests, *AJR Am J Roentgenol* 15:1217–1222, 1992.

280. Johnson GL, Askin FB, Fishman EK: Thoracic involvement from osteosarcoma: typical and atypical CT manifestations, *AJR Am J Roentgenol* 168:347–349, 1997.

281. Jones RN, McLoud T, Rockoff SD: The radiographic pleural abnormalities in asbestos exposure: relationship to physiologic abnormalities, *J Thorac Imaging* 3:57–66, 1988.

282. Kadir S, Kalisher L, Schiller AL: Extramedullary hematopoiesis in Paget's disease of bone, *AJR Am J Roentgenol* 129:493–495, 1977.

283. Kalifa LG, Schimmel DH, Gamsu G: Multiple chronic benign pulmonary nodules, *Radiology* 121:275–279, 1976.

284. Kang EY, Grenier P, Laurent F, Müller NL: Interlobular septal thickening: patterns at high-resolution computed tomography, *J Thorac Imaging* 11:260–264, 1996.

285. Kangarloo H, Beachley MC, Ghahremani GG: The radiographic spectrum of pulmonary complications in burn victims, *AJR Am J Roentgenol* 128:441–445, 1977.

286. Kantor HG: The many radiologic facies of pneumococcal pneumonia, *AJR Am J Roentgenol* 137:1213–1220, 1981.

287. Kattan KR, Wiot JF: Cardiac rotation in left lower lobe collapse, *Radiology* 118:275–276, 1976.

288. Katz S, Stanton J, McCormick G: Miliary calcification of the lungs after treated miliary tuberculosis, *N Engl J Med* 253:135–137, 1955.

289. Kazerooni E: High-resolution CT of the lungs, *AJR Am J Roentgenol* 177:501–519, 2001.

290. Kelsey CA, Moseley RD, Brogdon BG, et al.: Effect of size and position on chest lesion detection, *AJR Am J Roentgenol* 129:205–208, 1977.

291. Ketai LH, Godwin JD: A new view of pulmonary edema and acute respiratory distress syndrome, *J Thorac Imaging* 13:147–171, 1998.

292. Khouri NF, Eggleston JD, Siegelman SS: Angioimmunoblastic lymphadenopathy: a cause for mediastinal nodal enlargement, *AJR Am J Roentgenol* 130:1186–1188, 1978.

293. Khoury MB, Godwin JD, Ravin CE, et al.: Thoracic cryptococcosis: immunologic competence and radiologic appearance, *AJR Am J Roentgenol* 141:893–896, 1984.

294. Kim EA, Johkoh T, Lee KS, et al.: Quantification of ground-glass opacity on high-resolution CT of small peripheral adenocarcinoma of the lung: pathologic and prognostic implications, *AJR Am J Roentgenol* 177:1417–1422, 2001.

295. Kim EA, Lee KS, Primack SL, et al.: Viral pneumonias in adults: radiologic and pathologic findings, *Radiographics* S137–S149, 2002. 22 Spec No.

296. Kim EA, Lee SL, Johkoh T, et al.: Interstitial lung diseases associated with collagen vascular diseases: radiologic and histologic findings, *Radiographics* S151–S165, 2002. 22 Spec No.

297. Kim FM, Fennessy JJ: Pleural thickening caused by leukemic infiltration: CT findings, *AJR Am J Roentgenol* 162:293–294, 1994.

298. Kim HY, Song KS, Goo JM, et al.: Thoracic sequelae and complications of tuberculosis, *Radiographics* 21:839–860, 2001.

299. Kim KI, Kim CW, Lee MK, et al.: Imaging of occupational lung disease, *Radiographics* 21:1371–1391, 2001.

300. Kim TS, Han J, Koh W, et al.: Thoracic actinomycosis: CT features with histopathologic correlation, *AJR Am J Roentgenol* 186:225–231, 2006.

301. Kim YK, Kim H, Lee KS, et al.: Airway leiomyoma: imaging findings and histopathologic comparisons in 13 patients, *Am J Roentengol* 189:393–399, 2007.

302. Kirchner SG, Heller RM, Smith CW: Pancreatic pseudocyst of the mediastinum, *Radiology* 123:37–42, 1977.

303. Klein DL, Gamsu G, Gant TD: Intrathoracic desmoid tumor of the chest wall, *AJR Am J Roentgenol* 129:524–525, 1977.

304. Klein JS, Warnock M, Webb WR, et al.: Cavitating and noncavitating granulomas in AIDS patients with pneumocystis pneumonitis, *AJR Am J Roentgenol* 152:753–754, 1989.

305. Kligerman SJ, Groshong S, Brown KK, et al.: Nonspecific interstitial pneumonia: radiologic, clinical, and pathologic considerations, *Radiographics* 29:73–87, 2009.

306. Kountz PD, Molina PL, Sagel SS: Fibrosing mediastinitis in the posterior thorax, *AJR Am J Roentgenol* 153:489–490, 1989.

307. Koyama M, Johkoh Y, Honda O, et al.: Pulmonary involvement in primary Sjögren's syndrome: spectrum of pulmonary abnormalities and computed tomography findings in 60 patients, *J Thorac Imaging* 16:290–296, 2001.

308. Koyama T, Ueda H, Kaori T, et al.: Radiologic manifestations of sarcoidosis in various organs, *Radiographics* 24:87–104, 2004.

309. Kozuka T, Johkoh T, Honda O, et al.: Pulmonary involvement in mixed connective tissue disease, *J Thorac Imaging* 16:94–98, 2001.

310. Kradin RL, Spirn PW, Mark EJ: Intrapulmonary lymph nodes, *Chest* 87(5): 662–667, 1985.

311. Kroboth FJ, Yu VL, Reddy SC, et al.: Clinicoradiographic correlation with the extent of legionnaire disease, *AJR Am J Roentgenol* 141:263–268, 1983.

312. Kruse BT, Vadeboncoeur TF: Methicillin-resistant staphylococcus aureus sepsis presenting with septic pulmonary emboli, *J Emer Med* 37(4):383–385, 2009.

313. Kuhlman JE, Bouchardy L, Fishman EK, et al.: CT and MR imaging evaluation of chest wall disorders, *Radiographics* 14:571–595, 1994.

314. Kuhlman JE, Fishman EK, Hruban RH, et al.: Diseases of the chest in AIDS: CT diagnosis, *Radiographics* 9:827–857, 1989.

315. Kuhlman JE, Fishman EK, Ko-Pen W, et al.: Esophageal duplication cyst: CT and transesophageal needle aspiration, *AJR Am J Roentgenol* 145:531–532, 1985.

316. Kuhlman JE, Knowles MC, Fishman EK, et al.: Premature bullous pulmonary damage in AIDS: CT diagnosis, *Radiology* 173:23–26, 1989.

317. Kuhlman JE, Reyes BL, Hruban RH, et al.: Abnormal air-filled spaces in the lung, *Radiographics* 13:47–75, 1993.

318. Kuhlman JE, Singha NK: Complex disease of the pleural space: radiographic and CT evaluation, *Radiographics* 17:63–79, 1997.

319. Kulwiec EL, Lynch DA, Aguayo SM, et al.: Imaging of pulmonary histiocytosis X, *Radiographics* 12:515–526, 1992.

320. Kundel HL: Predictive value and threshold detectability of lung tumors, *Radiology* 139:25–29, 1981.

321. Lacomis JM, Costello P, Vilchez R, Kusne S: The radiology of pulmonary crypto-coccosis in a tertiary medical center, *J Thorac Imaging* 16:139–148, 2001.

322. Lai EKY, Deir H, Lamere EA, et al.: Severe acute respiratory syndrome: quantitative assessment from chest radiographs with clinical and prognostic correlation, *AJR Am J Roentgenol* 184:255–263, 2005.

323. Landay MJ: Anterior clear space: how clear? How often? How come? *Radiology* 192:165–169, 1994.

324. Landay MJ, Christensen EE, Bynum LJ, et al.: Anaerobic pleural and pulmonary infections, *AJR Am J Roentgenol* 134:233–240, 1980.

325. Latour A, Shulman HS: Thoracic manifestations of renal cell carcinoma, *Radiology* 121:43–48, 1976.

326. Lau KK, Philips G, McKenzie A: Pseudotumoral paraesophageal varices, *Gastrointest Radiol* 17:193–194, 1992.

327. Lautin EM, Rosenblatt M, Friedman AC, et al.: Calcification in non-Hodgkin lymphoma occuring before therapy: identification on plain films and CT, *AJR Am J Roentgenol* 155:739–740, 1990.

328. Lee KS, Kim Y, Primack SL: Imaging of pulmonary lymphomas, *AJR Am J Roentgenol* 168:339–345, 1997.

329. Lee KS, Kullnig P, Hartman TE, et al.: Cryptogenic organizing pneumonia: CT findings in 43 patients, *AJR Am J Roentgenol* 162:543–546, 1994.

330. Lee KS, Logan PM, Primack SL, et al.: Combined lobar atelectasis of the right lung: imaging findings, *AJR Am J Roentgenol* 163:43–47, 1994.

331. Lee KS, Song KS, Lim TH, et al.: Adult-onset pulmonary tuberculosis: findings on chest radiographs and CT scans, *AJR Am J Roentgenol* 160:753–758, 1993.

332. Lee VW, Fuller JD, O'Brien MJ, et al.: Pulmonary Kaposi sarcoma in patients with AIDS: scintigraphic diagnosis with sequential thallium and gallium scanning, *Radiology* 180:409–412, 1991.

333. Lees RF, Harrison RB, Williamson BRJ, et al.: Radiographic findings in Rocky Mountain spotted fever, *Radiology* 129:17–20, 1978.

334. Lemire P, Trepanier A, Hubert G: Bronchocele and blocked bronchiectasis, *AJR Am J Roentgenol* 110:687–693, 1970.

335. Lenique F, Brauner MW, Grenier P, et al.: CT assessment of bronchi in sarcoidosis: endoscopic and pathologic correlations, *Radiology* 194:419–423, 1995.

336. LeRoux BT: Supraphrenic herniation of perinephric fat, *Thorax* 20:376–381, 1965.

337. Lewis ER, Caskey CI, Fishman EK: Lymphoma of the lung: CT findings in 31 patients, *AJR Am J Roentgenol* 156:711–714, 1991.

338. Lewis JE, Sheptin C: Mycoplasma pneumonia associated with abscess of the lung, *Calif Med* 117:69–72, 1972.

339. Li C, Miller WT, Jiang J: Pulmonary edema due to ingestion of organophosphate insecticide, *AJR Am J Roentgenol* 152:265–266, 1989.

340. Libshitz HI, Atkinson GW, Israel HL: Pleural thickening as a manifestation of aspergillus superinfection, *AJR Am J Roentgenol* 120:883–886, 1974.

341. Libshitz HI, Baber CC, Hammond CB: The pulmonary metastases of choriocarcinoma, *Obstet Gynecol* 49:412–416, 1977.

342. Libshitz HI, Pannu HK, Elting LS, Cooksley CD: Tuberculosis in cancer patients: an update, *J Thorac Imaging* 12:41–46, 1997.

343. Liebow AA: Pulmonary angitis and granulomatosis, *Am Rev Respir Dis* 108:1–18, 1973.

344. Liebow AA, Carrington CB: Hypersensitivity reactions involving the lung. In *Transactions and studies of the College of Physicians of Philadelphia 34.* Fourth Series; 1966-1967; pp 47–70.

345. Liebow AA, Carrington CB, Friedman PJ: Lymphomatoid granulomatosis, *Hum Pathol* 3:457–532, 1972.

346. Lindell RM, Hartman TE, Nadrous HF, et al.: Pulmonary cryptococcosis: CT findings in immunocompetent patients, *Radiology* 236:326–337, 2005.

347. Link KM, Samuels LJ, Reed JC, et al.: Magnetic resonance imaging of the mediastinum, *J Thorac Imaging* 8(1):34–53, 1993.

348. Liu YC, Tomashefski Jr JF, Tomford JW, et al.: Necrotizing Pneumocystis carinii vasculitis associated with lung necrosis and cavitation in a patient with acquired immunodeficiency syndrome, *Arch Pathol Lab Med* 113:494–497, 1989.

349. Longuet R, Phelan J, Tanous H, et al.: Criteria of the silhouette sign, *Radiology* 122:581–585, 1977.

350. Lowenthal B, Shiau MC, Garcia R: Metastatic melanoma: an unusual diagnosis for a large anterior mediastinal mass, *Radiographics* 24:1714–1718, 2004.

351. Lundius B: Intrathoracic kidney, *AJR Am J Roentgenol* 125:678–681, 1975.

352. Ly JQ, Sanders TG: Hemangioma of the chest wall, *Radiology* 229:726–729, 2003.

353. Lynch DA, Newell JD, Logan PM, et al.: Can CT distinguish hypersensitivity pneumonitis from idiopathic pulmonary fibrosis, *AJR Am J Roentgenol* 165:807–811, 1995.

354. MacDonald SLS, Rubens MB, Hansell DM, et al.: Nonspecific interstitial pneumonia and usual interstitial pneumonia: comparative appearances at and diagnostic accuracy of thin-section CT, *Radiology* 221:600–605, 2001.

355. Madan R, Matalon S, Vivero M: Spectrum of smoking-related lung diseases, *J Thorac Imaging* 31:78–91, 2016.

356. Madewell JE, Daroca PJ, Reed JC: RPC1 from the AFIP2, *Radiology* 117:555–559, 1975.

357. Madewell JE, Stocker JT, Korsower JM: Cystic adenomatoid malformation of the lung, *AJR Am J Roentgenol* 124:436–448, 1975.

358. Maher GC, Berger HW: Massive pleural effusion: malignant and nonmalignant causes in 46 patients, *Am Rev Respir Dis* 105:458–460, 1972.

359. Maile CW, Rodan BA, Godwin JD, et al.: Calcification in pulmonary metastases, *Br J Radiol* 55:108–113, 1982.

360. Mallens WMC, Nijhuis-Heddes JM, Bakker W: Calcified lymph node metastases in bronchioloalveolar carcinoma, *Radiology* 161:103–104, 1986.

361. Marglin SI, Mortimer J, Castellino RA: Radiologic investigation of thoracic metastases from unknown primary sites, *J Thorac Imaging* 38–43, 1987.

362. Marglin SI, Soulen RL, Blank N, et al.: Mycosis fungoides, *Radiology* 130:35–37, 1979.

363. Marinelli DL, Albelda SM, Williams TM, et al.: Nontuberculous mycobacterial infection in AIDS: clinical, pathologic and radiographic features, *Radiology* 160:77–82, 1986.

364. Martin MD, Chung JH, Kanne JP: Idiopathic pulmonary fibrosis, *J Thorac Imaging* 31:127–139, 2016.

365. Martin III W, Choplin RH, Shertzer ME: The chest radiograph in Rocky Mountain spotted fever, *AJR Am J Roentgenol* 139:889–893, 1982.

366. Martinez S, McAdams HP, Batchu CS: The many faces of pulmonary nontuberculous mycobacterial infection, *AJR Am J Roentgenol* 189:177–186, 2007.

367. Masur H, Ognibene FP, Yarchoan R, et al.: CD4 counts as predictors of opportunistic pneumonias in human immunodeficiency virus (HIV) infection, *Ann Intern Med* 111:223–231, 1989.

368. Matthay RA, Schwarz MI, Ellis Jr JH, et al.: Pulmonary artery hypertension in chronic obstructive pulmonary disease: determination by chest radiography, *Invest Radiol* 16:95–100, 1981.

369. Mays EE: Rheumatoid pleuritis: observations in eight cases and suggestions for making the diagnosis in patients without the "typical findings", *Dis Chest* 53:202–214, 1968.

370. McAdams HP, Rosado-de-Christenson ML, Fishback NF, et al.: Castleman disease of the thorax: radiologic features with clinical and histopathologic correlation, *Radiology* 209:221–228, 1998.

371. McAdams HP, Rosado-de-Christenson ML, Lesar M, et al.: Thoracic mycoses from endemic fungi: radiologic-pathologic correlation, *Radiographics* 15:255–270, 1995.

372. McAdams HP, Rosado-de-Christenson ML, Templeton PA, et al.: Thoracic mycoses from opportunistic fungi: radiologic-pathologic correlation, *Radiographics* 15:271–286, 1995.

373. McGahan JP, Graves DS, Palmer PES, et al.: Classic and contemporary imaging of coccidioidomycosis, *AJR Am J Roentgenol* 136:393–404, 1981.

374. McGuinness G, Scholes JV, Jagirdar JS, et al.: Unusual lymphoproliferative disorders in nine adults with HIV or AIDS: CT and pathologic findings, *Radiology* 197:59–65, 1995.

375. McHugh K, Blaquiere RM: CT features of rounded atelectasis, *AJR Am J Roentgenol* 153:257–260, 1989.

376. McLoud TC: Asbestos-related diseases: the role of imaging techniques. In Abrams HL, editor: *Postgraduate radiology*, 9. Littleton, MA: PSG Publishing, 1989 pp 65–74.

377. McLoud TC, Epler GR, Colby TV, et al.: Bronchiolitis obliterans, *Radiology* 159:1–8, 1986.

378. McLoud TC, Isler RJ, Novelline RA, et al.: Review: the apical cap, *AJR Am J Roentgenol* 137:299–306, 1981.

379. McLoud TC, Kalisher L, Stark P, et al.: Intrathoracic lymph node metastases from extrathoracic neoplasms, *AJR Am J Roentgenol* 131:403–407, 1978.

380. Meighan JW: Pulmonary cryptococcosis mimicking carcinoma of the lung, *Radiology* 103:61–62, 1972.

381. Menon B, Aggarwal B, Iqbal A: Mounier-Kuhn syndrome: report of 8 cases of tracheobronchomegaly with associated complications, *South Med J* 101:83–87, 2008.

382. Mermelstein RH, Freireich AW: Varicella pneumonia, *Ann Intern Med* 55:456–463, 1961.

383. Meszaros WT, Guzzo F, Schorsch H: Neurofibromatosis, *AJR Am J Roentgenol* 98:557–569, 1966.

384. Meyer JE: Thoracic effects of therapeutic irradiation for breast carcinoma, *AJR Am J Roentgenol* 130:877–885, 1978.

385. Millar JK: The chest film findings in "Q" fever—a series of 35 cases, *Clin Radiol* 29:371–375, 1978.

386. Miller MH, Rosado-de-Christenson ML, McAdams HP, et al.: Thoracic sarcoidosis: radiologic-pathologic correlation, *Radiographics* 15(2):421–437, 1995.

387. Miller WT, Aronchick JM, Epstein DM, et al.: The troublesome nipple shadow, *AJR Am J Roentgenol* 145:521–523, 1985.

388. Miller WT, MacGregor RR: Tuberculosis: frequency of unusual radiographic findings, *AJR Am J Roentgenol* 130:867–875, 1978.

389. Miller Jr WT: Spectrum of pulmonary nontuberculous mycobacterial infection, *Radiology* 191:343–350, 1994.

390. Milne ENC, Pistolesi M, Miniati M, et al.: The radiologic distinction of cardiogenic and noncardiogenic edema, *AJR Am J Roentgenol* 144:879–894, 1985.

391. Milos M, Aberle DR, Parkinson BT, et al.: Maternal pulmonary edema complicating beta-adrenergic therapy of preterm labor, *AJR Am J Roentgenol* 151:917–918, 1988.

392. Mintzer RA, Neiman HL, Reeder MM: Mucoid impaction of a bronchus, *JAMA* 240:1397–1398, 1978.

393. Morgan DE, Nath H, Sanders C, et al.: Mediastinal actinomycosis, *AJR Am J Roentgenol* 155:735–737, 1990.

394. Morgan H, Ellis K: Superior mediastinal masses: secondary to tuberculous lymphadenitis in the adult, *AJR Am J Roentgenol* 120:893–897, 1974.

395. Moser Jr ES, Proto AV: Lung torsion: case report and literature review, *Radiology* 162:639–643, 1987.

396. Moser KM: Pulmonary embolism, *Am Rev Respir Dis* 115:829–852, 1977.

397. Mountain CF: Revisions in the international system for staging lung cancer, *Chest* 111:1710–1717, 1997.

398. Mueller-Mang C, Grosse C, Schmid K, et al.: What every radiologist should know about idiopathic interstitial pneumonias, *Radiographics* 27:595–615, 2007.

399. Muhm JR, Brown LR, Crowe JK: Detection of pulmonary nodules by computed tomography, *AJR Am J Roentgenol* 128:267–270, 1977.

400. Muhm JR, Miller WE, Fontana RS, et al.: Lung cancer detected during a screening program using four-month chest radiographs, *Radiology* 148:609–615, 1983.

401. Müller NL, Chiles C, Kullnig P: Pulmonary lymphangiomyomatosis: correlation of CT with radiographic and functional findings, *Radiology* 175:335–339, 1990.

402. Müller NL, Webb WR, Gamsu G: Paratracheal lympnadenopathy: radiographic findings and correlation with CT, *Radiology* 156:761–765, 1985.

403. Müller NL, Webb WR, Gamsu G: Subcarinal lymph node enlargement: radiographic findings and CT correlation, *AJR Am J Roentgenol* 145:15–19, 1985.

404. Murray HW, Masur H, Senterfit LB, et al.: The protean manifestations of mycoplasma pneumoniae infection in adults, *Am J Med* 58:229–242, 1975.

405. Murray HW, Tuazon CU, Kirmani N, et al.: The adult respiratory distress syndrome associated with miliary tuberculosis, *Chest* 73:37–43, 1978.

406. Naidich DP, Garay SM, Leitman BS, et al.: Radiographic manifestations of pulmonary disease in the acquired immunodeficiency syndrome (AIDS), *Semin Roentgenol* 22:14–30, 1987.

407. Nakata H, Kimoto T, Nakayama T, et al.: Diffuse peripheral lung disease: evaluation by high-resolution computed tomography, *Radiology* 157:181–185, 1985.

408. Narinder SP, Taebong C, Konen E, et al.: Prognostic significance of the radiographic pattern of disease patients with severe acute respiratory syndrome, *AJR Am J Roentgenol* 182:493–498, 2004.

409. Narla LD, Newman B, Spottswood SS, et al.: Inflammatory pseudotumor, *Radiographics* 23:719–729, 2003.

410. Neiman HL, Wolson AH, Berenson JE: Pulmonary and pleural manifestations of Waldenstrom's macroglobulinemia, *Radiology* 107:301–302, 1973.

411. Nguyen ET, Kanne JP, Hoang LM, et al.: Community-acquired methicillin resistant staphylococcus aureus pneumonia: radiographic and computed tomography findings, *J Thorac Imaging* 23:13–19, 2008.

412. Nicolau S, Al-Nakshabandi NA, Müller NL: SARS: imaging of severe acute respiratory syndrome, *AJR Am J Roentgenol* 180:1247–1249, 2003.

413. Nishino M, Ashiku SK, Kocher ON, et al.: The thymus: a comprehensive review, *Radiographics* 26:335–348, 2006.

414. Numan F, Islak C, Berkmen T, et al.: Behcet disease: pulmonary arterial involvement in 15 cases, *Radiology* 192:465–468, 1994.

415. O'Connell RS, McLoud TC, Wilkins EW: Superior sulcus tumor: radiographic diagnosis and workup, *AJR Am J Roentgenol* 140:25–30, 1983.

416. Ogakwu M, Nwokolo C: Radiological findings in pulmonary paragonimiasis as seen in Nigeria: a review based on one hundred cases, *Br J Radiol* 46:699–705, 1973.

417. Oldham SAA, Castillo M, Jacobson FL, et al.: HIV-associated lymphocytic interstitial pneumonia: radiologic manifestations and pathologic correlation, *Radiology* 170:83–87, 1989.

418. Ominsky SH, Kricun ME: Roentgenology of sinus of Valsalva aneurysms, *AJR Am J Roentgenol* 125:571–581, 1975.

419. Ontell FK, Moore EH, Shepard JAO, Shelton DK: The costal cartilages in health and disease, *Radiographics* 17:571–577, 1997.

420. Ooi GC, Khong PL, Müller NL, et al.: Severe acute respiratory syndrome: temporal lung changes at thin-section CT in 30 patients, *Radiology* 230:836–844, 2004.

421. Ostendorf P, Birzle H, Vogel W, et al.: Pulmonary radiographic abnormalities in shock, *Radiology* 115:257–263, 1975.

422. Oswalt CE, Gates GA, Holmstrom FMG: Pulmonary edema as a complication of acute airway obstruction, *JAMA* 238:1833–1835, 1977.

423. Pagani JJ, Libshitz HI: Opportunistic fungal pneumonias in cancer patients, *AJR Am J Roentgenol* 137:1033–1039, 1981.

424. Pallisa E, Sanz P, Roman A, et al.: Lymphangioleiomyomatosis: pulmonary and abdominal findings with pathologic correlation, *Radiographics* S185–S198, 2002.

425. Park KJ, Chung JY, Chun MS, Suh JH: Radiation-induced lung disease and the impact of radiation methods on imaging features, *Radiographics* 20:83–98, 2000.

426. Parra O, Ruiz J, Ojanguren I, et al.: Amiodarone toxicity: recurrence of interstitial pneumonitis after withdrawal of the drug, *Eur Respir J* 2:905–907, 1989.

427. Paul NS, Chung T, Konen E, et al.: Prognostic significance of the radiographic pattern of disease in patients with severe acute respiratory syndrome, *AJR Am J Roentgenol* 182:493–498, 2004.

428. Pearlberg JL, Haggar AM, Saravolatz L: Hemophilus influenzae pneumonia in the adult, *Radiology* 151:23–26, 1984.

429. Pendergrass EP: An evaluation of some of the radiologic patterns of small opacities in coal worker's pneumoconioses, *AJR Am J Roentgenol* 115:457–461, 1972.

430. Pickford HA, Swensen SJ, Utz JP: Thoracic cross-sectional imaging of amyloidosis, *AJR Am J Roentgenol* 168:351–355, 1997.

431. Pinckney L, Parker BR: Primary coccidioidomycosis in children presenting with massive pleural effusion, *AJR Am J Roentgenol* 130:247–249, 1978.

432. Pinsker KL: Solitary pulmonary nodule in sarcoidosis, *JAMA* 240:1379–1380, 1978.

433. Plavsic BM, Robinson AE, Freundlich IM, et al.: Melanoma metastatic to the bronchus: radiologic features in two patients, *J Thorac Imaging* 9(2):67–70, 1994.

434. Podoll LN, Winkler SS: Busulfan lung, *AJR Am J Roentgenol* 120:151–156, 1974.

435. Polat P, Kantarci M, Alper F, et al.: Hydatid disease from head to toe, *Radiographics* 23:475–494, 2003.

436. Pope Jr TL, Armstrong P, Thompson R, et al.: Pittsburgh pneumonia agent: chest film manifestations, *AJR Am J Roentgenol* 138:237–241, 1982.

437. Potchen EJ, Bisesi MA: When is it malpractice to miss lung cancer on chest radiographs? *Radiology* 175:29–32, 1990.

438. Press GA, Glazer HS, Wassermann TH, et al.: Thoracic wall involvement by Hodgkin disease and non-Hodgkin lymphoma: CT evaluation, *Radiology* 158:195–198, 1985.

439. Price Jr JE, Rigler LG: Widening of the mediastinum resulting from fat accumulation, *Radiology* 96:497–500, 1970.

440. Primack SL, Hartman TE, Hansell DM, et al.: End-stage lung disease: CT findings in 61 patients, *Radiology* 189:681–686, 1993.

441. Primack SL, Miller RR, Müller NL: Diffuse pulmonary hemorrhage: clinical, pathologic, and imaging features, *AJR Am J Roentgenol* 164:295–300, 1995.

442. Prince JS, Duhamel DR, Levin DL, et al.: Nonneoplastic lesions of the tracheobronchial wall: radiologic findings with bronchoscopic correlation, *Radiographics* S215–S230, 2002.

443. Proto AV, Corcoran HL, Ball Jr JB: The left paratracheal reflection, *Radiology* 171:625–628, 1989.

444. Proto AV, Lane EJ: Air in the esophagus: a frequent radiographic finding, *Am J Roentgenol* 129:433–440, 1977.

445. Proto AV, Moser Jr ES: Upper lobe volume loss: divergent and parallel patterns of vascular reorientation, *Radiographics* 7:875–887, 1987.

446. Putman CE, Loke J, Matthay RA, et al.: Radiographic manifestations of acute smoke inhalation, *AJR Am J Roentgenol* 129:865–870, 1977.

447. Putman CE, Minagi H, Blaisdell FW: The roentgen appearance of disseminated intravascular coagulation (DIC), *Radiology* 109:13–18, 1973.

448. Putman CE, Tummillo AM, Myerson DA, et al.: Drowning: another plunge, *AJR Am J Roentgenol* 125:543–548, 1975.

449. Quint LE, Park CH, Iannettoni MD: Solitary pulmonary nodules in patients with extrapulmonary neoplasms, *Radiology* 217:257–261, 2000.

450. Rabinowitz JG, Busch J, Buttram WR: Pulmonary manifestations of blastomycosis, *Radiology* 120:25–32, 1976.

451. Raider L: Calcification in chickenpox pneumonia, *Chest* 60:504–507, 1971.

452. Rami-Porta R, Crowley JJ, Goldstraw P: The revised TNM staging system for lung cancer, *Ann Thorac Cardiovasc Surg* 15:4–9, 2009.

453. Ravenel JG, Gordon LL, Block MI, et al.: Primary posterior mediastinal seminoma, *AJR Am J Roentgenol* 183:1835–1837, 2004.

454. Ravin CE: Pulmonary vascularity: radiographic considerations, *J Thorac Imaging* 3:1–13, 1988.

455. Ravin CE, Smith GW, Ahern MJ, et al.: Cytomegaloviral infection presenting as a solitary pulmonary nodule, *Chest* 71:220–222, 1977.

456. Raymond GS, Miller RM, Müller NL, Logan PM: Congenital thoracic lesions that mimic neoplastic disease on chest radiographs of adults, *AJR Am J Roentgenol* 168:763–769, 1997.

457. Reed JC: Pathologic correlations of the air-bronchogram: a reliable sign in chest radiology, *CRC Crit Rev Diagn Imaging* 10:235–255, 1977.

458. Reed JC, Choplin RH: Pulmonary and pleural complications of pneumonias, *Contemp Diagn Radiol* 12:1–5, 1989.

459. Reed JC, Hallet KK, Feigin DS: Neural tumors of the thorax: subject review from the AFIP, *Radiology* 126:9–17, 1978.

460. Reed JC, Madewell JE: The air bronchogram in interstitial disease of the lungs, *Radiology* 116:1–9, 1975.

461. Reed JC, McLelland R, Nelson P: Legionnaires' disease, *AJR Am J Roentgenol* 131:892–894, 1978.

462. Reed JC, Reeder MM: Honeycomb lung (interstitial fibrosis), *JAMA* 231:646–647, 1975.

463. Reed JC, Sobonya RE: Morphologic analysis of foregut cysts in the thorax, *AJR Am J Roentgenol* 120:851–860, 1974.

464. Reed JC, Sobonya RE: RPC from the AFIP, *Radiology* 117:315–319, 1975.

465. Reeder MM: Gamut: causes of pleural fluid, *Semin Roentgenol* 12:255, 1977.

466. Reeder MM: Gamut: pleural-based lesion arising from the lung, pleura, or chest wall, *Semin Roentgenol* 12:261–262, 1977.

467. Reeder MM, Bradley Jr WG: *Reeder and Felson's gamuts in radiology*, ed 3, New York, 1993, Springer-Verlag.

468. Reeder MM, Hochholzer L: RPC of the month from the AFIP, *Radiology* 92:1106–1111, 1969.

469. Reeder MM, Reed JC: Solitary pulmonary nodule (<4 cm in diameter), *JAMA* 231:1080–1082, 1975.

470. Reinke RT, Coel MN, Higgins CB: Calcified nonsyphilitic aneurysms of the sinuses of Valsalva, *AJR Am J Roentgenol* 122:783–787, 1974.

471. Renner RR, Markarian B, Pernice NJ, et al.: The apical cap, *Radiology* 110:569–573, 1974.

472. Renner RR, Pernice NJ: The apical cap, *Semin Roentgenol* 12:299–302, 1977.

473. Restrepo CS, Carrillo JA, Martinez S, et al.: Pulmonary complications from co-caine and cocaine-based substances: imaging manifestations, *Radiographics* 27:941–956, 2007.

474. Reynders CS, Whitman GJ, Chew FS: Posttransplant lymphoproliferative disorder of the lung, *AJR Am J Roentgenol* 165:1118, 1995.

475. Rice RP, Loda F: A roentgenographic analysis of respiratory syncytial virus pneumonia in infants, *Radiology* 87:1021–1027, 1966.

476. Rich S, Brundage BH: Primary pulmonary hypertension: current update, *JAMA* 251:2252–2254, 1984.

477. Rigler LG: An overview of cancer of the lung, *Semin Roentgenol* 12:161–164, 1977.

478. Rigler LG: An overview of diseases of the pleura, *Semin Roentgenol* 12:265–268, 1977.

479. Rigler LG: The natural history of untreated lung cancer, *Ann NY Acad Sci* 114:755–766, 1964.

480. Roach HD, Davies GJ, Attanoos R, et al.: Asbestos: when the dust settles—an imaging review of asbestos-related disease, *Radiographics* S167–S184, 2002.

481. Rohlfing BM: The shifting granuloma: an internal marker of atelectasis, *Radiology* 123:283–285, 1977.

482. Rohlfing BM, White EA, Webb WR, et al.: Hilar and mediastinal adenopathy caused by bacterial abscess of the lung, *Radiology* 128:289–293, 1978.

483. Rosado-de-Christenson ML, Abbott GF, McAdams HP, et al.: From the archives of the AFIP: localized fibrous tumors of the pleura, *Radiographics* 23:759–783, 2003.

484. Rosado-de-Christenson ML, Frazier AA, Stocker JT, et al.: Extralobar sequestration: radiologic-pathologic correlation, *Radiographics* 13:425–441, 1993.

485. Rosado-de-Christenson ML, Pugatch RD, Moran CA, et al.: Thymolipoma: analysis of 27 cases, *Radiology* 193:121–126, 1994.

486. Rosado-de-Christenson ML, Templeton PA, Moran CA: Mediastinal germ cell tumors: radiologic and pathologic correlation, *Radiographics* 12:1013–1030, 1992.

487. Rosen SH, Castleman B, Liebow AA: Pulmonary alveolar proteinosis, *N Engl J Med* 258:1123–1142, 1958.

488. Rosenbloom SA, Ravin CE, Putman CE, et al.: Peripheral middle lobe syndrome, *Radiology* 149:17–21, 1983.

489. Rossi SE, Erasmus JJ, McAdams HP, et al.: Pulmonary drug toxicity: radiologic and pathologic manifestations, *Radiographics* 20:1245–1259, 2000.

490. Rossi SE, Erasmus JJ, Volpacchio M, Franquet T, et al.: "Crazy-paving" pattern at thin-section CT of the lungs: radiologic-pathologic overview, *Radiographics* 23:1509–1519, 2003.

491. Rossi SE, Goodman PC, Franquet T: Nonthrombotic pulmonary emboli, *AJR Am J Roentgenol* 174:1499–1508, 2000.

492. Rossi SE, McAdams HP, Rosado-de-Christenson ML, et al.: Fibrosing mediastinitis, *Radiographics* 21:737–757, 2001.

493. Roucos S, Tabet G, Jebara VA, et al.: Thoracic splenosis: case report and literature review, *J Thorac Cardiovasc Surg* 99:361–363, 1990.

494. Rovner AJ, Westcott JL: Pulmonary edema and respiratory insufficiency in acute pancreatitis, *Radiology* 118:513–520, 1976.

495. Rozenshtein A, Hao F, Starc MT, et al.: Radiographic appearance of pulmonary tuberculosis: dogma disproved, *AJR Am J Roentgenol* 204:974–978, 2015.

496. Rubin SA: Radiographic spectrum of pleuropulmonary tularemia, *AJR Am J Roentgenol* 131:277–281, 1978.

497. Rubin SA: Radiology of immunologic diseases of the lung, *J Thorac Imaging* 3:21–39, 1988.

498. Ryerson GG, Lauwassesr ME, Block AJ, et al.: Legionnaires' disease: a sporadic case, *Chest* 73:113–115, 1978.

499. Sagel SS, Forrest JV: Multiple pulmonary nodules in an alcoholic man, *Chest* 66:571–572, 1974.

500. Sahin AA, Cöplü L, Selcuk ZT, et al.: Malignant pleural mesothelioma caused by environmental exposure to asbestos or erionite in rural Turkey: CT findings in 84 patients, *AJR Am J Roentgenol* 161:533–537, 1993.

501. Sahin H, Brown KK, Curran-Everett D, et al.: Chronic hypersensitivity pneumonitis: CT features—comparison with pathologic evidence of fibrosis and survival, *Radiology* 244(2):591–598, 2007.

502. Sakowitz AJ, Sakowitz BH: Disseminated cryptococcosis, *JAMA* 236:2429–2430, 1976.

503. Saltzstein SL, Ackerman LV: Lymphadenopathy induced by anticonvulsant drugs and mimicking clinically and pathologically malignant lymphomas, *Cancer* 12:164–182, 1959.

504. Salyer WR, Salyer DC: Pleural involvement in cryptococcosis, *Chest* 66:139–140, 1974.

505. Samei E, Flynn MJ, Eyler WR: Detection of subtle lung nodules: relative influence of quantum and anatomic noise on chest radiographs, *Radiology* 213:727–734, 1999.

506. Samuel S, Kundel HL, Nodine CF, et al.: Mechanism of satisfaction of search: eye position recordings in the reading of chest radiographs, *Radiology* 194:895–902, 1995.

507. Samuels ML, Howe CD, Dodd Jr GD, et al.: Endobronchial malignant lymphoma, *AJR Am J Roentgenol* 85:87–95, 1961.

508. Sandhu JS, Goodman PC: Pulmonary cysts associated with Pneumocystis carinii pneumonia in patients with AIDS, *Radiology* 173:33–35, 1989.

509. Santana L, Givica A, Camacho C: Best cases from the AFIP: thymoma, *Radiographics* 22:S95–S102, 2002.

510. Sargent EN, Barnes RA, Schwinn CP: Multiple pulmonary fibroleiomyomatous hamartomas, *AJR Am J Roentgenol* 110:694–700, 1970.

511. Sargent EN, Gordonson J, Jacobson G, et al.: Bilateral pleural thickening: a manifestation of asbestosis dust exposure, *AJR Am J Roentgenol* 131:579–585, 1978.

512. Sargent EN, Jacobson G, Gordonson JS: Pleural plaques: a signpost of asbestos dust inhalation, *Semin Roentgenol* 12:287–297, 1977.

513. Sargent EN, Jacobson G, Wilkinson EE: Diaphragmatic pleural calcification following short occupational exposure to asbestos, *AJR Am J Roentgenol* 115:473–478, 1972.

514. Sargent EN, Wilson R, Gordonson J, et al.: Granular cell myoblastoma of the trachea, *AJR Am J Roentgenol* 114:89–92, 1972.

515. Saurborn DP, Fishman JE, Boiselle PM: The imaging spectrum of pulmonary tuberculosis in AIDS, *J Thorac Imaging* 17:28–33, 2002.

516. Savic B, Birtel FJ, Tholen W, et al.: Lung sequestration: report of seven cases and review of 540 published cases, *Thorax* 34:96–101, 1979.

517. Savoca CJ, Austin JHM, Goldberg HI: The right paratracheal stripe, *Radiology* 122:295–301, 1977.

518. Saxon RR, Klein JS, Bar MH, et al.: Pathogenesis of pulmonary edema during interleukin-2 therapy: correlation of chest radiographic and clinical findings in 54 patients, *AJR Am J Roentgenol* 156:281–285, 1991.

519. Schachter EN, Kreisman H, Putman C: Diagnostic problems in suppurative lung disease, *Arch Intern Med* 136:167–171, 1976.

520. Schmitt WGH, Hübener KH, Rücker HC: Pleural calcification with persistent effusion, *Radiology* 149:633–638, 1983.

521. Schwartz EE, Holsclaw DS: Pulmonary involvement in adults with cystic fibrosis, *AJR Am J Roentgenol* 122:708–718, 1974.

522. Schwartz EE, Teplick JG, Onesti G, et al.: Pulmonary hemorrhage in renal disease: goodpasture's syndrome and other causes, *Radiology* 122:39–46, 1977.

523. Schwarz MI: Pulmonary and cardiac manifestations of polymyositis-dermatomyositis, *J Thorac Imaging* 7(2):46–54, 1992.

524. Scott Jr WW, Kuhlman JE: Focal pulmonary lesions in patients with AIDS: percutaneous transthoracic needle biopsy, *Radiology* 189:419–421, 1991.

525. Seltzer SE, Balikian JP, Birnholz JC, et al.: Giant hyperplastic parathyroid gland in the mediastinum—partially cystic and calcified, *Radiology* 127:43–44, 1978.

526. Seo JB, Im JG, Goo JM, et al.: Atypical pulmonary metastases: spectrum of radiologic findings, *Radiographics* 21:403–417, 2001.

527. Seo JB, Song K-S, Lee JS, et al.: Broncholithiasis: review of the causes with radiologic-pathologic correlation, *Radiographics* S199–S213, 2002.

528. Septimus EJ, Awe RJ, Greenberg SD, et al.: Acute tuberculous pneumonia, *Chest* 71:774–776, 1977.

529. Shackelford GD, Sacks EJ, Mullins JD, et al.: Pulmonary venoocclusive disease: case report and review of the literature, *AJR Am J Roentgenol* 128:643–648, 1977.

530. Shaffer Jr HA: Multiple leiomyomas of the esophagus, *Radiology* 118:29–34, 1976.

531. Shah RM, Kaji AV, Ostrum BJ, Friedman AC: Interpretation of chest radiographs in AIDS patients: usefulness of CD4 lymphocyte counts, *Radiographics* 17:47–58, 1997.

532. Shannon TM, Gale ME: Noncardiac manifestations of rheumatoid arthritis in the thorax, *J Thorac Imaging* 7(2):19–29, 1992.

533. Sharma A, Fidias P, Hayman LA, et al.: Patterns of lymphadenopthy in thoracic malignancies, *Radiographics* 24:419–434, 2004.

534. Sheflin JR, Campbell JA, Thompson GP: Pulmonary blastomycosis: findings on chest radiographs in 63 patients, *AJR Am J Roentgenol* 154:1177–1180, 1990.

535. Shin MS, Bradley JL: Chest wall lesions mimicking intrapulmonary pathological conditions, *JAMA* 239:535–536, 1978.

536. Shopfner CE: Aeration disturbances secondary to pulmonary infection, *AJR Am J Roentgenol* 120:261–273, 1974.

537. Sicuranza BJ, Tisdall LH: Amniotic fluid embolism, *NY State J Med* 75:1517–1519, 1975.

538. Sider L, Gabriel H, Curry DR, et al.: Pattern recognition of the pulmonary manifestations of AIDS on CT scans, *Radiographics* 13:771–784, 1993.

539. Sider L, Weiss AJ, Smith MD, et al.: Varied appearance of AIDS-related lymphoma in the chest, *Radiology* 171:629–632, 1989.

540. Siegler DIM: Lung abscess associated with Mycoplasma pneumoniae infection, *Br J Dis Chest* 67:123–127, 1973.

541. Silver TM, Farber SJ, Bole GG, et al.: Radiological features of mixed connective tissue disease and scleroderma-systemic lupus erythematosus overlap, *Radiology* 120:269–275, 1976.

542. Sinner WN, Sandstedt B: Small-cell carcinoma of the lung, *Radiology* 121:269–274, 1976.

543. Sirajuddin A, Raparia K, Lewis VA, et al.: Primary pulmonary lymphoid lesions: radiologic and pathologic findings, *Radiographics* 36:53–70, 2016.

544. Sites VR, Poland JD: Mediastinal lymphadenopathy in bubonic plague, *AJR Am J Roentgenol* 116:567–570, 1976.

545. Sivit CJ, Schwartz AM, Rockoff SD: Kaposi's sarcoma of the lung in AIDS: radiologic-pathologic analysis, *AJR Am J Roentgenol* 148:25–28, 1987.

546. Smith RC, Mann H, Greenspan RH, et al.: Radiographic differentiation between different etiologies of pulmonary edema, *Invest Radiol* 22:859–863, 1987.

547. Smith SD, Cho CT, Brahmacupta N, et al.: Pulmonary involvement with cytomegalovirus infections in children, *Arch Dis Child* 52:441–446, 1977.

548. Smith TR, Khoury PT: Aneurysm of the proximal thoracic aorta simulating neoplasm: the role of CT and angiography, *AJR Am J Roentgenol* 144:909–910, 1985.

549. Sone S, Higashihara T, Kotake T, et al.: Pulmonary manifestations in acute carbon monoxide poisoning, *AJR Am J Roentgenol* 120:865–871, 1974.

550. Sones Jr PJ, Torres WE, Colvin RS, et al.: Effectiveness of CT in evaluating intrathoracic masses, *AJR Am J Roentgenol* 139:469–475, 1982.

551. Sostman HD, Putnam CE, Gamsu G: Review: diagnosis of chemotherapy lung, *AJR Am J Roentgenol* 136:33–40, 1981.

552. Souza CA, Finley R, Müller NL: Birt-Hogg-Dube syndrome: a rare cause of pulmonary cysts, *AJR Am J Roentgenol* 185:1237–1239, 2005.

553. Souza CA, Müller NL, Flint J, et al.: Idiopathic pulmonary fibrosis: spectrum of high-resolution CT findings, *AJR Am J Roentgenol* 185:1531–1539, 2005.

554. St. Clair EW, Rice JR, Synderman R: Pneumonitis complicating low-dose methotrexate therapy in rheumatoid arthritis, *Arch Intern Med* 145:2035–2038, 1985.

555. Stansell JD: Fungal disease in HIV-infected persons: cryptococcosis, histoplasmosis, and coccidioidomycosis, *J Thorac Imaging* 6(4):28–35, 1991.

556. Staples CA, Gamsu G, Ray CS, et al.: High resolution computed tomography and lung function in asbestos-exposed workers with normal chest radiographs, *Am Rev Respir Dis* 139:1502–1508, 1989.

557. Stark DD, Federle MP, Goodman PC, et al.: Differentiating lung abscess and empyema: radiography and computed tomography, *AJR Am J Roentgenol* 141:163–167, 1983.

558. Stark P, Thordarson S, McKinney M: Manifestations of esophageal disease on plain chest radiographs, *AJR Am J Roentgenol* 155:729–734, 1990.

559. Stein DS, Korvick JA, Vermund SH: CD4+ lymphocyte cell enumeration for prediction of clinical course of human immunodeficiency virus disease: a review, *J Infect Dis* 165:352–363, 1992.

560. Stein MG, Mayo J, Müller N, et al.: Pulmonary lymphangitic spread of carcinoma: appearance on CT scans, *Radiology* 162:371–375, 1987.

561. Stelling CB, Woodring JH, Rehm SR: Miliary pulmonary blastomycosis, *Radiology* 150:7–13, 1984.

562. Stephan WC, Parks RD, Tempest B: Acute hypersensitivity pneumonitis associated with carbamazepine therapy, *Chest* 74:463–464, 1978.

563. Stern RG, Gamsu G, Golden JA, et al.: Intrathoracic adenopathy: differential features of AIDS and diffuse lymphadenopathy syndrome, *AJR Am J Roentgenol* 142:689–692, 1984.

564. Stokes D, Sigler A, Khouri NF, et al.: Unilateral hyperlucent lung (Swyer-James syndrome) after severe Mycoplasma pneumoniae infection, *Am Rev Respir Dis* 117:145–152, 1978.

565. Stolz JL, Arger PH, Benson JM: Mushroom worker's lung disease, *Radiology* 119:61–63, 1976.

566. Streiter ML, Schneider HJ, Proto AV: Steroid-induced thoracic lipomatosis: paraspinal involvement, *AJR Am J Roentgenol* 139:679–681, 1982.

567. Strollo DC, Rosado-de-Christenson ML: Tumors of the thymus, *J Thorac Imaging* 14:152–171, 1999.

568. Sugimoto H, Ohsawa T: Unilateral hyperlucent thorax on plain chest radiographs after neck dissection: importance of atrophy of the trapezius muscle, *AJR Am J Roentgenol* 163:1079–1082, 1994.

569. Sumikawa H, Johkoh T, Ichikado K, et al.: Usual interstitial pneumonia and chronic idiopathic interstitial pneumonia: analysis of CT appearance in 92 patients, *Radiology* 241:258–266, 2006.

570. Summer WR, Dwyer P, Hales ED, et al.: Hypersensitivity pneumonitis, *Johns Hopkins Med J* 146:80–87, 1980.

571. Sundaram B, Gross BH, Martinez FJ, et al.: Accuracy of high-resolution CT in the diagnosis of diffuse lung disease: effect of predominance and distribution of findings, *AJR Am J Roentgenol* 191:1032–1039, 2008.

572. Swensen SJ, Brown LR, Colby TV, et al.: Lung nodule enhancement at CT: prospective findings, *Radiology* 201:447–455, 1996.

573. Swensen SJ, Jett JR, Hartman TE, et al.: CT screening for lung cancer: five year prospective experience, *Radiology* 235:259–265, 2005.

574. Talner LB, Gmelich JT, Liebow AA, et al.: The syndrome of bronchial mucocele and regional hyperinflation of the lung, *AJR Am J Roentgenol* 110:675–686, 1970.

575. Tan RT, Kuzo RS: High-resolution CT findings of mucinous bronchioloalveolar carcinoma: a case of pseudopulmonary alveolar proteinosis, *AJR Am J Roentgenol* 168:99–100, 1997.

576. Tanaka N, Kim JS, Newell JD, et al.: Rheumatoid arthritis-related lung diseases: CT findings, *Radiology* 232:81–91, 2004.

577. Tang ER, Schreiner AM, Pua BB: Advances in lung adenocarcinoma classification: a summary of the new internal multidisciplinary classification system (IASLC/ATS/ERS), *J Thorac Dis* 6(S5):S489–S501, 2014.

578. Taryle DA, Potts DE, Sahn SA: The incidence and clinical correlates of parapneumonic effusions in pneumococcal pneumonia, *Chest* 74:170–173, 1978.

579. Tateishi U, Gladish GW, Kusumoto M, et al.: Chest wall tumors: radiologic findings and pathologic correlation. Part 1. Benign tumors, *Radiographics* 23:1477–1490, 2003.

580. Tateishi U, Gladish GW, Kusumoto M, et al.: Chest wall tumors: radiologic findings and pathologic correlation. Part 2. Malignant tumors, *Radiographics* 23:1491–1508, 2003.

581. Teixidor HS, Bachman AL: Multiple amyloid tumors of the lung, *AJR Am J Roentgenol* 111:525–529, 1971.

582. Templeton AW: Malignant mediastinal teratoma with bone metastases, *Radiology* 76:245–247, 1961.

583. Teplick JG, Nedwich A, Haskin ME: Roentgenographic features of thymolipoma, *AJR Am J Roentgenol* 117:873–877, 1973.

584. Teplick JG, Teplick SK, Haskin ME: Granular cell myoblastoma of the lung, *AJR Am J Roentgenol* 125:890–894, 1975.

585. Theros EG: RPC of the month from the AFIP, *Radiology* 92:1557–1561, 1969.

586. Theros EG: RPC of the month from the AFIP, *Radiology* 93:677–681, 1969.

587. Theros E: Varying manifestations of peripheral pulmonary neoplasms: a radiologic-pathologic correlative study, *AJR Am J Roentgenol* 128:893–914, 1977.

588. Theros EG, Feigin DS: Pleural tumors and pulmonary tumors: differential diagnosis, *Semin Roentgenol* 12:239–247, 1977.

589. Theros EG, Reeder MM, Eckert JF: An exercise in radiologic-pathologic correlation, *Radiology* 90:784–791, 1968.

590. Thiessen R, Seely JM, Matzinger FRK, et al.: Necrotizing granuloma of the lung: imaging characteristics and imaging-guided diagnosis, *AJR Am J Roentgenol* 189:1397–1401, 2007.

591. Thompson BH, Stanford W, Galvin JR, et al.: Varied radiologic appearances of pulmonary aspergillosis, *Radiographics* 15:1273–1284, 1995.

592. Thompson PL, Mackay IR: Fibrosing alveolitis and polymyositis, *Thorax* 25:504–507, 1970.

593. Thurlbeck WM, Müller NL: Emphysema: definition, imaging and quantification, *AJR Am J Roentgenol* 163:1017–1025, 1994.

594. Thurlbeck WM, Simon G: Radiographic appearance of the chest in emphysema, *AJR Am J Roentgenol* 130:429–440, 1978.

595. Timmons RG, Siegel JS, Metheny Jr RS: Fatal pulmonary hemorrhage complicating infectious mononucleosis, *Pa Med* 74:65–67, 1971.

596. Tocino IM, Miller MH, Fairfax WR: Distribution of pneumothorax in the supine and semirecumbent critically ill adult, *AJR Am J Roentgenol* 144:901–905, 1985.

597. Travis WD: Pathology of lung cancer, *Clinics in Chest Medicine* 32:669–692, 2011.

598. Travis WD, Travis LB, Devesa SS: Lung cancer, *Cancer* 75(Suppl 1):191–202, 1995.

599. Triebwasser JH, Harris RE, Bryant RE, et al.: Varicella pneumonia in adults, *Medicine* 46:409–423, 1967.

600. Truong MT, Sabloff BS, Gladish GW, et al.: Invasive thymoma, *AJR Am J Roentgenol* 181:1504, 2003.

601. Tuddenham WJ: Glossary of terms for thoracic radiology: recommendations of the nomenclature of the Fleishner society, *AJR Am J Roentgenol* 143:509–517, 1984.

602. Tunaci M, Özkorkmaz B, Tunaci, et al.: CT findings of pulmonary artery aneurysms during treatment for Behcet's disease, *AJR Am J Roentgenol* 172:729–733, 1999.

603. Unger JM, Schuchmann GG, Grossman JE, et al.: Tears of the trachea and main bronchi caused by blunt trauma: radiologic findings, *AJR Am J Roentgenol* 153:1175–1180, 1989.

604. Urban BA, Fishman EK, Goldman SM, et al.: CT evaluation of amyloidosis: spectrum of disease, *Radiographics* 13:1295–1308, 1993.

605. Vanley GT, Huberman R, Lufkin RB: Atypical Pneumocystis carinii pneumonia in homosexual men with unusual immunodeficiency, *AJR Am J Roentgenol* 138:1037–1041, 1982.

606. Wadsworth DT, Siegel MJ, Day DL: Wegener's granulomatosis in children: chest radiographic manifestations, *AJR Am J Roentgenol* 163:901–904, 1994.

607. Wagenvoort CA, Wagenvoort N: Primary pulmonary hypertension: a pathologic study of the lung vessels in 156 clinically diagnosed cases, *Circulation* 42:1163–1184, 1970.

608. Wagner AL, Szabunio M, Hazlett KS, Wagner SG: Radiologic manifestations of round pneumonia in adults, *AJR Am J Roentgenol* 170:723–726, 1998.

609. Wagner RB, Crawford WO, Schmipf PP: Classification of parenchymal injuries of the lung, *Radiology* 167:77–82, 1988.

610. Wallace LS, Robinson AE: Unusual radiological manifestations of acquired pulmonary cysts in children, *JAMA* 248:85–87, 1982.

611. Walter JF, Rottenberg RW, Cannon WB, et al.: Giant mediastinal lymph node hyperplasia (Castleman's disease): angiographic and clinical features, *AJR Am J Roentgenol* 130:447–450, 1978.

612. Washington L, Miller Jr WT: Mycobacterial infection in immunocompromised patients, *J Thorac Imaging* 13:271–281, 1998.

613. Webb WR: Radiologic evaluation of the solitary pulmonary nodule, *AJR Am J Roentgenol* 154:701–708, 1990.

614. Webb WR: Thin-section CT of the secondary pulmonary lobule: anatomy and the image: the 2004 Fleischner lecture, *Radiology* 239:322–338, 2006.

615. Webb WR, Gamsu G: Cavitary pulmonary nodules with systemic lupus erythematosus: differential diagnosis, *AJR Am J Roentgenol* 136:27–31, 1981.

616. Webb WR, Gatsonis C, Zerhouna EA, et al.: CT and MR imaging in staging non–small cell bronchogenic carcinoma: report of the Radiologic Diagnostic Oncology Group, *Radiology* 178:705–713, 1991.

617. Webb WR, Müller NL, Naidich DP: Standardized terms for high-resolution computed tomography of the lung: a proposed glossary, *J Thorac Imaging* 8(3):167–175, 1993.

618. Webb WR, Sagel SS: Actinomycosis involving the chest wall: CT findings, *AJR Am J Roentgenol* 139:1007–1009, 1982.

619. Weber WN, Margolin FE, Nielson SL: Pulmonary histiocytosis X, *AJR Am J Roentgenol* 107:280–289, 1969.

620. Weick JK, Kiely JM, Harrison Jr EG, et al.: Pleural effusion in lymphoma, *Cancer* 31:848–853, 1973.

621. Weisbrod GL, Chamberlain D, Herman SJ: Cystic change (pseudocavitation) associated with bronchioloalveolar carcinoma: a report of four patients, *J Thorac Imaging* 10(2):106–111, 1995.

622. Weisbrod GL, Todd TR: Congenital left superior vena cava with absent right superior vena cava: a cause of progressive mediastinal widening, *J Can Assoc Radiol* 36: 155–157, 1985.

623. Weisbrod GL, Towers MJ, Chamberlain DW, et al.: Thin-walled cystic lesions in bronchioalveolar carcinoma, *Radiology* 185:401–405, 1992.

624. Wellner LJ, Putnam CE: Imaging of occult pulmonary metastases: state of the art, *Cancer* 36:48–58, 1986.

625. Westcott JL, Volpe JP: Peripheral bronchopleural fistula: CT evaluation in 20 patients with pneumonia, empyema, or postoperative air leak, *Radiology* 196:175–181, 1995.

626. Wexler HA, Dapena MV: Congenital cystic adenomatoid malformation, *Radiology* 126:737–741, 1978.

627. Whalen JP, Lane Jr EJ: Bronchial rearrangements in pulmonary collapse as seen on the lateral radiograph, *Radiology* 93:285–288, 1969.

628. Whitcomb ME, Schwartz MI: Pleural effusion complicating intensive mediastinal radiation therapy, *Am Rev Respir Dis* 103:100–107, 1971.

629. White CS, Haramati LB, Elder KH, et al.: Carcinoma of the lung in HIV-positive patients: findings on chest radiographs and CT scans, *AJR Am J Roentgenol* 164: 593–597, 1995.

630. White CS, Romney BM, Mason AC, et al.: Primary carcinoma of the lung overlooked at CT: analysis of findings in 14 patients, *Radiology* 199:109–115, 1996.

631. Whitten CR, Khan S, Munneke GJ, et al.: A diagnostic approach to mediastinal abnormalities, *Radiographics* 27:657–671, 2007.

632. Wiedemann HP, Matthay RA: Pulmonary manifestations of systemic lupus erythematosus, *J Thorac Imaging* 7(2):1–18, 1992.

633. Wieder S, Rabinowitz JG: Fibrous mediastinitis: a late manifestation of mediastinal histoplasmosis, *Radiology* 125:305–312, 1977.

634. Wieder S, White III TJ, Salazar J: Pulmonary artery occlusion due to histoplasmosis, *AJR Am J Roentgenol* 138:243–251, 1982.

635. Wilen SB, Rabinowitz JG, Ulreich S, et al.: Pleural involvement in sarcoidosis, *Am J Med* 57:200–209, 1974.

636. Williams JL, Moller GA: Solitary mass in the lungs of coal miners, *AJR Am J Roentgenol* 117:765–770, 1973.

637. Williams JR, Wilcox WC: Pulmonary embolism, *AJR Am J Roentgenol* 89:333–342, 1963.

638. Williams NS, Lewis CT: Bronchopleural fistula: a review of 86 cases, *Br J Surg* 63:520–522, 1976.

639. Wilson ES: Pleuropulmonary amebiasis, *AJR Am J Roentgenol* 111:518–524, 1971.

640. Wimbish KJ, Agha FP, Brady TM: Bilateral pulmonary sequestration: computed tomographic appearance, *AJR Am J Roentgenol* 140:689–690, 1983.

641. Winer-Muram HT, Rubin SA: Thoracic complications of tuberculosis, *J Thorac Imaging* 5:46–63, 1990.

642. Winterbauer RH, Belic N, Moores KD: A clinical interpretation of bilateral hilar adenopathy, *Ann Intern Med* 78:65–71, 1973.

643. Winterbauer RH, Riggins RCK, Griesman FA, et al.: Pleuropulmonary manifestations of Waldenstrom's macroglobulinemia, *Chest* 66:368–375, 1974.

644. Wiot JF, Spitz HB: Atypical pulmonary tuberculosis, *Radiol Clin North Am* 11:191–196, 1973.

645. Wolson AH: Pulmonary findings in Gaucher's disease, *AJR Am J Roentgenol* 123:712–715, 1975.

646. Wolson AH, Rohwedder JJ: Upper lobe fibrosis in ankylosing spondylitis, *AJR Am J Roentgenol* 124:466–471, 1975.

647. Wong JSL, Weisbrod GL, Chamberlain D, et al.: Bronchioloalveolar carcinoma and the air bronchogram sign: a new pathologic explanation, *J Thorac Imaging* 9(3):141–144, 1994.

648. Wood BJ, DeFranco B, Ripple M, et al.: Inhalational anthrax: radiologic and pathologic findings in two cases, *AJR Am J Roentgenol* 181:1071–1078, 2003.

649. Wood BP, Anderson VM, Mauk JE, et al.: Pulmonary lymphatic air: locating "pulmonary interstitial emphysema" of the premature infant, *AJR Am J Roentgenol* 138:809–814, 1982.

650. Woodring JH: Determining the cause of pulmonary atelectasis: a comparison of plain radiography and CT, *AJR Am J Roentgenol* 150:757–763, 1988.

651. Woodring JH: Pitfalls in the radiologic diagnosis of lung cancer, *AJR Am J Roentgenol* 154:1165–1175, 1990.

652. Woodring JH, Fried AM, Chuang VP: Solitary cavities of the lung: diagnostic implications of cavity wall thickness, *AJR Am J Roentgenol* 135:1269–1271, 1980.

653. Woodring JH, Halfhill II H, Reed JC: Pulmonary strongyloidiasis: clinical and imaging features, *AJR Am J Roentgenol* 162:537–542, 1994.

654. Woodring JH, Howard TA, Kanga JF: Congenital pulmonary venolobar syndrome revisited, *Radiographics* 14:349–369, 1994.

655. Woodring JH, King JG: Determination of normal transverse mediastinal width and mediastinal-width to chest-width (M/C) ratio in control subjects: implications for subjects with aortic or brachiocephalic arterial injury, *J Trauma* 29:1268–1272, 1989.

656. Woodring JH, Reed JC: Radiographic manifestations of lobar atelectasis, *J Thorac Imaging* 11:109–114, 1996.

657. Woodring JH, Reed JC: Types and mechanisms of pulmonary atelectasis, *J Thorac Imaging* 11:92–108, 1996.

658. Woodring JH, Rhodes III RA: Posterosuperior mediastinal widening in aortic coarctation, *AJR Am J Roentgenol* 144:23–25, 1985.

659. Woolley K, Stark P: Pulmonary parenchymal manifestations of mitral valve disease, *Radiographics* 19:965–972, 1999.

660. Worsley DF, Alavi A, Aronchick JM, et al.: Chest radiographic findings in patients with acute pulmonary embolism: observations from the PIOPED study, *Radiology* 189:133–136, 1993.

661. Young LW, Smith DI, Glasgow LA: Pneumonia of atypical measles, *AJR Am J Roentgenol* 110:439–448, 1970.

662. Zagoria RJ, Choplin RH, Karstaedt N: Pulmonary gangrene as a complication of mucormycosis, *AJR Am J Roentgenol* 114:1195–1196, 1985.

663. Zapol WM, Trelstad RL, Coffey JW, et al.: Pulmonary fibrosis in severe acute respiratory failure, *Am Rev Respir Dis* 119:547–554, 1979.

664. Zelefksy MN, Lutzker LG: The target sign: a new radiologic sign of septic pulmonary emboli, *AJR Am J Roentgenol* 129:453–455, 1977.

665. Zerhouni EA, Stitik FP, Siegelman SS, et al.: CT of the pulmonary nodule: a cooperative study, *Radiology* 160:319–327, 1986. 826.

666. Ziskind MM, George RB, Weill H: Acute localized and diffuse alveolar pneumonias, *Semin Roentgenol* 2:49–60, 1967.

667. Ziter Jr FMH, Westcott JL: Supine subpulmonary pneumothorax, *AJR Am J Roentgenol* 137:699–701, 1981.

668. Zwiebel BR, Austin JHM, Grimes MM: Bronchial carcinoid tumors: assessment with CT of location and intratumoral calcification in 31 patients, *Radiology* 179:483–486, 1991.

669. Zwirewich CV, Vedal S, Miller RR, et al.: Solitary pulmonary nodule: high-resolution CT and radiologic-pathologic correlation, *Radiology* 179:469–476, 1991.

670. Zylak CJ, Eyler WR, Spizarny DL, et al.: Developmental lung anomalies in the adult: radiologic-pathologic correlation, *Radiographics* 22:S25–S43, 2002.

671. Zyroff J, Slovis TL, Nagler J: Pulmonary edema induced by oral methadone, *Radiology* 112:567–568, 1974.

INDEX

Page numbers followed by *f* indicate figure, by *t* table, and by *b* box.